The Role of New Technologies in Medical Microbiological Research and Diagnosis

Edited By

John P. Hays and W.B. van Leeuwen

Department of Medical Microbiology and Infectious Diseases
Erasmus University Medical Centre (Erasmus MC)
Rotterdam
The Netherlands

eBooks End User License Agreement

CONTENTS

CHAPTERS

FOREWORD

The field of medical microbiology, and particularly bacteriology, has evolved rather slowly over the last century, with the widely accepted "gold standard" method for microbial detection/identification having remained (since the golden days of Koch and Pasteur!) the selective isolation of microorganisms on suitable growth medium. Selective isolation is then followed by identification to species level, using biochemical or serological testing, and the determination of antimicrobial susceptibility profiles.

However, over the last decade, major developments in automation and in the rapid diagnosis of clinical disease, have led to great improvements in the methods available for the early detection, isolation, characterisation, and quantification of microorganisms (and their products), within clinical samples. Further, the development of these "cutting-edge" technologies has brought about major advances in the fields of genomics, proteomics, transcriptomics and metabolomics, generating major impacts in many fields of scientific research and diagnosis, including microbiology. Among these, rapid developments has been a trend towards the improvement of high-throughput testing possibilities and the miniaturization of components. Further, the accelerated development of accompanying apparatus, and affordable hardware and software, now means that these new technologies have the potential to provide added value (and to a certain extent even replace) the more traditional techniques that have previously been used in microbiological research and diagnostic laboratories. The adoption of these new techniques will generate; i) savings in "time-to-diagnosis", ii) provide a more accurate picture of the disease process itself, and iii) subsequently lead to improvements in both treatment regimens and costs for clinicians, microbiologists, hospital managers, and ultimately patients.

The aim of this e-Book is to introduce the reader to some of the key technologies that are likely to impact the field of medical microbiology within the next few years. The e-Book is edited by Dr. J.P. Hays, with editing support provided by Dr. W.B. van Leeuwen, both have the experience in the development and evaluation of new technologies in the field of microbiological research and diagnosis.

The e-Book will be of interest to microbiologists, infectious disease doctors, laboratory workers, and hospital managers, as well as (current or future) manufacturers of new technologies that have potential application in the field of microbiological research and diagnosis.

Thierry Naas,
Patrice Nordmann,
University of South Paris Medical School
France

PREFACE

In this e-Book 'primer' the editors have attempted to provide the reader with an overview of some of the most important 'new technologies' that are currently being developed, evaluated and validated for use in medical microbiological diagnosis and research laboratories throughout the world. Though the definition of 'new' is open to interpretation, and several of these 'new technologies' have already found a niche within (medical) microbiological research and diagnostic laboratories, the true potential of these technologies have yet to be realised, and it may yet be some time before any of the new technologies described in this e-book become firmly established within the majority of global microbiological research and diagnostic laboratories.

The choice of new technologies possessing the potential to replace (or at least augment) traditional "gold standard" culture and serological methods in microbiological research and diagnostic laboratories is surprisingly large, with most of these new technologies having been developed into commercially viable options within the previous 10 years. Bearing this in mind, the authors have attempted to include in this e-book primer, a broad range of chapters describing innovative new technologies that are being/have been developed within several different fields of scientific research. These fields include nano-culture, nucleic acid amplification and detection (genomics), protein-based detection (proteomics), growth and metabolism (metabolomics), and immunological/serological markers. Further, the authors of each chapter have included descriptions of how their technology is being/may be used in both theory and practice within medical microbiological diagnosis and research, including relevant lists of references.

In Chapter 1, Ingham and Schneeberger discuss a new technology that take the traditional approach to microbiological research and diagnosis (with its emphasis on the selective culture to obtain pure microbial colonies) a step further. They describe the advantages associated with new nanoporous materials (especially porous aluminium oxide or PAO), and their use in the development of highly subdivided microbial culture chips, with up to a million separate, miniaturized growth areas.

Chapters 2 and 3 describe new technologies associated with proteins and proteomics and their use in medical microbiological diagnostics. In Chapter 2, Hwang *et al.*, describe recent advances in peptide-based probes and biosensor technology, including methods associated with mass perturbance, electrical perturbance, and optical methods. Special emphasis is placed on the possible impact of peptide-based biosensors in pandemic disease surveillance. Martin Welker in Chapter 3 explains the technique of Matrix Assisted Laser Desorption/Ionization Time-of-Flight Mass Spectrometry (MALDI-TOF MS) and its potential application in rapidly identifying microorganisms and cellular components, including the advantages and disadvantages of this new technology in microbial identification and taxonomy.

The field of metabolomics and metabolomic-related technology is described in Chapters 4 and 5, Guazzaroni *et al.*, provide a general overview of the techniques, problems and prospects encountered in the analysis of small metabolite compounds. One of their objectives is to provide the reader with information on how (meta-) metabolomic fingerprinting studies can be used to assess microbial community and microbe-host interactions. In a similar manner, Bruins *et al.*, provide a brief overview of the problems and recent technological developments associated with the development of 'electronic nose' technology, with particular emphasis on their own company's technology. Their embryonic electronic nose technology monitors the production of volatile metabolic molecules during bacterial growth.

The use of nanoparticles in medical microbiological research and diagnosis is described in Chapter 6, where Ikonomopoulis *et al.*, explain the possible uses of nanoparticles (conjugated to oligonucleotide, antibodies and peptides) in identifying the genetic or immunogenic footprint of pathogens. Manmohan *et al.* in Chapter 7, describe the potential use of a novel DNA nucleic acid amplification system (Loop Mediated Isothermal Amplification or LAMP) as a tool that offers rapid, accurate, and cost-effective diagnosis for infectious diseases. This technology has already been developed into several commercial kits, but the full potential of this technology has yet to be realised.

In chapter 8, Nuutila describes recent research investigating the use of flow cytometric quantitative analysis in the detection of new specific and sensitive phagocytic cell surface markers. He shows how these findings may be incorporated into novel algorithms in order to rapidly determine the presence/absence of bacterial or viral infections in hospitalised patients. In Chapter 9, Verkaik *et al.,* provide a brief description of the Luminex bead-based flow cytometry technique, which allows the simultaneous quantification of multiple antibodies antigens (or oligonucleotide) in a single sample. They include an example of how this technology is being used to determine the importance of IgG immunoglobulin levels in *Staphylococcus aureus* colonisation.

Finally, the editors predict that advances in at least some of the 'new technologies' described in this e-Book 'primer', will eventually be developed into successful 'point-of-care' or 'near-patient' testing technologies, not least due to concomitant advances currently being made in 'accessory' technological fields such as microfluidics, microengineering, photonics, increased signal detection sensitivity, and the miniaturization of essential components. The development and application of point-of-care/near-patient testing in the context of medical microbiological diagnosis (and to a lesser extent medical microbiological research), will provide immediate benefits both for the patient and the attending physician, allowing more rapid and better informed diagnoses and treatment schemes to be made. The net effect will be; i) to provide a better health service for patients, ii) to better understand disease epidemiology and the infection process, iii) to help reduce health-care costs, and iv) to limit the development and spread of infectious disease and antimicrobial resistance.

One thing is certain, research into 'new technologies' in medical microbiological research and diagnosis is continuing, financed by all types of business, including large industrial concerns, small / medium enterprises and university campuses, all of whom are working to push back the boundaries of our current scientific knowledge and technological innovation. This means that the 'next generation of new technologies' in the field of medical microbiological research and diagnosis promise to generate even greater benefits for physicians, patients and society as a whole .

John P. Hays and W. B. van Leeuwen

Department of Medical Microbiology and Infectious Diseases
Erasmus University Medical Centre (Erasmus MC)
The Netherlands

List of Contributors

van Belkum, A.	-	Erasmus Medical Center Rotterdam, Department of Medical Microbiology and Infectious Diseases, 's -Gravendijkwal 230, 3015 CE Rotterdam, The Netherlands.
Bos, A.	-	C-it BV, Marspoortstraat 2, 7201 JB Zutphen, The Netherlands.
Bruins, M.	-	C-it BV, Marspoortstraat 2, 7201 JB Zutphen, The Netherlands.
Emmanouil, L.	-	Faculty of Animal Science, Laboratory of Anatomy-Physiology, Agricultural University of Athens, 75, Iera Odos st., 11855Athens, Greece.
Fernández-Arrojo, L.	-	Department of Applied Biocatalysis, Institute of Catalysis, CSIC, Marie Curie 2, 28049 Madrid, Spain.
Ferrer, M.	-	Department of Applied Biocatalysis, Institute of Catalysis, CSIC, Marie Curie 2, 28049 Madrid, Spain.
Gazouli, M.	-	Laboratory of Biology, School of Medicine, University of Athens, 11527, Athens, Greece.
Guazzaroni, M.-E.	-	Department of Applied Biocatalysis, Institute of Catalysis, CSIC, Marie Curie 2, 28049 Madrid, Spain.
Hwang, G.M.	-	The MITRE Corporation, 7515 Colshire Drive, McLean, VA, 22102, United States.
Ikonomopoulos, J.	-	Faculty of Animal Science, Laboratory of Anatomy-Physiology, Agricultural University of Athens, 75, Iera Odos st., 11855Athens, Greece.
Ingham, C.	-	MicroDish BV, Hazenakker 18, 3994EJ, Houten, The Netherlands.
Korves, T.M.	-	The MITRE Corporation, 202 Burlington Road, Bedford, MA, 01730, United States.
Lakshmana Rao, P.V. Establishment,	-	Division of Virology, Defence Research & Development Gwalior – 474002, M.P, India.
López-Cortés, N.	-	Department of Applied Biocatalysis, Institute of Catalysis, CSIC, Marie Curie 2, 28049 Madrid, Spain.
Nuutila, J.	-	University of Turku, Department of Biochemistry, Vatselankatu 2 20014 Turku, Finland.
Parida, M. Establishment,	-	Division of Virology, Defence Research & Development Gwalior – 474002, M.P, India.
Renda, P.F.	-	The MITRE Corporation, 202 Burlington Road, Bedford, MA, 01730, United States.
Schneeberger, P.M.	-	Department of Medical Microbiology and Infection Control, Jeroen Bosch Hospital,'s-Hertogenbosh, The Netherlands.

Sharma, S. Establishment,	-	Division of Virology, Defence Research & Development Gwalior – 474002, M.P, India.
Shukla, I. Establishment,	-	Division of Virology, Defence Research & Development Gwalior – 474002, M.P, India.
Suh, S-J	-	Auburn University, Department of Biological Science, 101 Life Sciences Building, Auburn, AL, 36849, United States.
Tachtsidis, I.	-	Department of Medical Physics and Bioengineering, Malet Place Engineering Building, University College London, Gower st., WC1E 6BT, London, United Kingdom.
Verkaik, N. J.	-	Erasmus Medical Center Rotterdam, Department of Medical Microbiology and Infectious Diseases, 's -Gravendijkwal 230, 3015 CE Rotterdam, The Netherlands.
de Vogel, C.P.	-	Erasmus Medical Center Rotterdam, Department of Medical Microbiology and Infectious Diseases, 's -Gravendijkwal 230, 3015 CE Rotterdam, The Netherlands.
van Wamel, W.J.B.	-	Erasmus Medical Center Rotterdam, Department of Medical Microbiology and Infectious Diseases, 's -Gravendijkwal 230, 3015 CE Rotterdam, The Netherlands.
Welker, M.	-	BioMérieux – R&D Microbiology, 3 route de Port Michaud, La Balme les Grottes, 38390, France.

CHAPTER 1

Can We Improve on the Petri Dish with Porous Culture Supports?

Colin Ingham* and Peter M. Schneeberger

MicroDish BV, Hazenakker 18, 3994EJ, Houten, The Netherlands and the Department of Medical Microbiology and Infection Control, Jeroen Bosch Hospital, 's-Hertogenbosh, The Netherlands

Abstract: Microbial culture is exemplified by the Petri dish, a tool that (one century after its invention) still remains one of the "gold standards" for microbiological analysis. However, current trends towards automation, massively paralleled assays, and miniaturization (as well as the observation that we still cannot culture most microorganisms), suggest that new ideas in microbial culture are required. In the Petri dish, nutrient containing agar is typically used as the matrix on which microorganisms are cultured. However, new materials such as nanofibres and nanoporous materials may be better choices as supporting matrixes. Further, emerging techniques in microengineering and the fabrication of low cost materials are helping to create new porous disposables that are of sufficiently low cost that they may be used in the routine microbiology laboratory. These disposables are in turn allowing the development of novel miniature culture methods to take place, methods such as microchemostats, cages for growing microorganisms, and "habitats on a chip". One particularly useful porous ceramic is Porous Aluminium Oxide (PAO), which can be utilized to generate highly subdivided culture chips that possess up to one million separate, miniaturized, growth areas. Indeed, this material has applications in microbiological diagnostics, microbiological research and industrial microbiology. In this chapter, the applications, advantages, and limitations of porous matrixes and accompanying culture chips will be examined. It is expected that these advances will yield significant improvements in microbial culture when compared to the classical Petri dish.

Keywords: Nanoculture, Petri Dish, Nanoporous Aluminium Oxide (PAO), Chemostat, Membrane Enrichment, Microdish Culture Chip (MDCC), High Throughput.

1. THE PETRI DISH

Much of modern microbiology is founded upon simple but powerful concepts that derive from the ability to grow pure strains of microorganisms in a controlled fashion. Before the development of axenic (microbiologically pure) culture in defined media, microbiology was not a coherent science. Microscopists such as Hooke and van Leeuwenhoek knew that there existed a complex and fascinating world on the micron-scale, but could perform very few actual experiments using their findings [1]. It was not until the development of microbial culture methods using "Petri" dish technology, (Petri being one of Robert Koch's students) that the role of microorganisms in disease could be experimentally verified [2]. It was the growth of microorganisms in a Petri dish filled with a nutrient gel matrix (most commonly agar), that allowed the segregation and manipulation of microorganisms into colony forming units (Robert Koch's description of a microbial community). This process of microbial culture was then refined *via* the use of selective agents, specific nutrients and indicators that allowed the characteristics of unusual colony phenotypes (including shape, smell, and colour) to be determined. This resulted in advances in the identification of particular bacterial species, eventually facilitating strain identification and microbial genetics [3]. The functionality of agar culture was further increased *via* the use of simple additional tools, such as metabolic indicator dyes and a velvet pad which was used to reproducibly replicate colonies (printing them by a simple stamping action) [4].

So far so good. Billions of Petri dishes are used each year, having become the workhorses of basic and applied microbiology. Indeed, the use of microbial culture is still the "gold standard" method for the

*Address correspondence to Colin Ingham:** MicroDish BV, Hazenakker 18, 3994EJ, Houten, The Netherlands; E-mail: colin.ingham@wur.nl

detection of many microorganisms, with developments in agar-based microbial culture having been primarily limited to a switch from glass to disposable plastic Petri dishes, as well as the subdivision of single plate culture into multiwell plate formats. However, the persistence of this technology is an indication of the value of such a simple tool. The advent of modern microbiological analysis techniques now means that the basic limitations of Petri dish-based culture are becoming increasingly apparent, particularly with respect to microbiological diagnosis and research. One of the major limitations associated with conventional agar protocols is that the Petri-dish culture process per se is difficult to automate with respect to high-throughput applications, there being particular problems related to the automation of specimen preparation, inoculation, incubation, and result interpretation. Moreover, though separate solutions for each of these issues exist, the result of integrating these systems into a functional robotic platform generates a system that is too large and/or inflexible for most microbiology laboratories [5]. Further, automated systems tend to be relatively expensive, limiting their application to centralized laboratories that perform a limited range of repetitive assays, meaning that small microbiology laboratories tend to be unable to automate at all. Finally, other limitations of conventional culture are: 1) agar-based microbiology creates a great deal of infectious waste, yet growth on agar usually involves the detection or assaying of visible colonies, a process that may be regarded as overkill in many situations, 2) agar may be an undesirable contaminant, or even inhibitory, in some downstream assay processes, 3) metabolic studies of bacteria have benefited greatly from continuous culture in a chemostat, but this is a situation effectively impossible to achieve on (or in) agar, 4) biofilms required for research purposes may be optimally formed on solid supports rather than on a gel, and 5) the vast majority of microorganisms have never been cultured in a Petri dish, and some may never be cultured due to their exacting growth requirements. All of these issues raise the question as to whether, in the long term, it is desirable to perform microbial culture in the laboratory at all. If yes, then the Petri dish is probably not the best format! If not, then what is the solution?

The aim of this chapter is to address the issues mentioned above by specifically discussing the advantages of porous supports in microbial culture, and how these supports have been engineered and/or modified to create useful culture formats with great potential for the future of microbiological diagnosis and research. Particularly relevant to the discussion are the recent advances made in materials and fabrication technology, advances that fall within the broad areas of microengineering, Lab-On-A-Chip (LOC) and nanotechnology [6-8]. The most promising of these advances involves the fabrication and application of "culture chips" based around an interesting ceramic, namely Porous Aluminium Oxide (PAO) [9].

2. NANOPOROUS AND NANOFIBROUS MATERIALS

By definition, porous materials contain "open space" as well as "solid matter", with most of these materials possessing a porosity (ratio of the volume of open space to solid) of 0.2 to 0.95 [10]. Further, porous materials may be divided into 2 main types. "Open porous materials" possess pores connected to the exterior, whilst "closed porous materials" possess pores that are internal. Additionally, "penetrating pores", such as those in a membrane filter, go completely through a material, and pores with many twists and turns have a high tortuosity. For the microbiologist, the most interesting materials are usually open porous materials that possess penetrating pores.

The classification of pore sizes themselves can be rather confusing. In the IUPAC scheme a microporous material has a pore size less than 2 nm, a mesoporous material from 2 to 50 nm and a macroporous material has pores above 50 nm [10]. A rather more intuitive definition of a nanoporous material is a material containing a pore size from 1 to 100 nm with a porosity >0.4. The term microporous will be used in this chapter to describe porous materials with larger pore sizes, including most conventional (polycarbonate) sterilizing filters. Standard microscale filters, such as those used to sterilize liquids, are relevant but will not be described in detail as they are familiar to most microbiologists.

Porous materials have a high surface to area ratio, which is particularly relevant for some nanoporous materials. Oxides, metals, alumino-silicates, carbon and certain types of glass can all be nanoporous, and some commonly used materials are also nanoporous, such as the smaller (30 nm) polycarbonate filters. Additionally, a number of materials such as crystalline cellulose are nanofilamentous, with meshes created from layers of such materials being essentially nanoporous (Fig. **1**). Further, the study of nanoporous materials is a large and expanding field, with roles in particle separation, catalysis, energy generation, development as storage sensors, as well as applications as self-assembling materials.

3. BASIC MEMBRANE CULTIVATION SYSTEMS

It is worth briefly describing a few of the more basic systems utilized for the cultivation of microorganisms on microporous surfaces (in general, these are filters used for sterilization purposes), because they illustrate the usefulness of culture techniques in microbiological research and diagnosis, even if they are conceptually very basic. Further, this understanding will provide us with clues to the opportunities presented more sophisticated systems in the future.

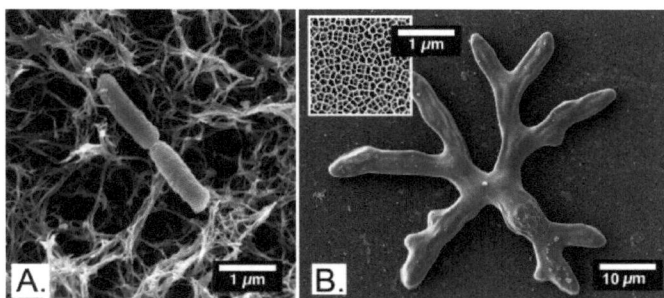

Fig. (1) Examples of culture on nanoporous materials visualized by scanning electron microscopy. **A.** Nanofibrous cellulose used as an inert matrix for microbial growth. A mesophilic bacterium (*Escherichia coli*, cell length c. 2 microns) is shown. The organism was cultured whilst supported by cellulose fibres [8]. N.B. Nanofibrous cellulose is extremely heat-stable and therefore also shows promise in the culture of thermophiles at temperatures where conventional gel-matrices fail. Image shown with permission of S. Deguchi, Japan Agency for Marine-Earth Science and Technology (JAMSTEC). **B.** Growth of *Aspergillus fumigatus* (under stress from a triazole drug) growing on planar Porous Aluminium Oxide (PAO) engineered with pore sizes from 20 to 200 nm. The material is extremely porous and inert. Here the fungal hyphae are growing on the surface with nutrients supplied through the pores. **Inset to Panel B:** Detail of PAO surface structure.

Screening Microbial Libraries on Nylon Membranes. The culture of microorganisms containing DNA libraries on porous membranes is a well established screening method in molecular biology [11]. The advantages of this system include the fact that bacterial colonies can be lysed *in situ* on the membrane (for example by washing and alkaline lysis treatment), the naked DNA being immobilized, which allows for further molecular analysis *e.g.* Southern blotting. In this case, the porous support comprises part of an integrated assay that combines microbial culture with molecular detection techniques.

Culture of Agarose Degrading Bacteria on Membranes. In some situations *Streptomyces coelicolor* and other bacteria are highly destructive to agar plates due to their production of agarase, an enzyme that can digest agarose. Such bacteria may be cultivated on a membrane that has been placed on an agar plate. The purpose of the intervening membrane is to separate the organism from the agar/nutrient matrix, thereby preserving the integrity of the plate and preventing the bacterium from becoming embedded in the agar. This simple method then allows the organism to be recovered for further microbiological analysis.

Counting Microorganisms on a Filter. A common practice in the water industry is to count microorganisms after filtration, *e.g.* for the enumeration of coliforms [12]. Essentially, the filter support acts to concentrate the sample, and provides advantages with respect to manual and automated colony imaging and counting. Filter membranes can also be colored for high contrast imaging or to reduce autofluorescence. Further, microbial staining with fluorogenic or colored dyes is possible, for example to assist in strain identification.

Subdivided Membranes. A logical development to counting microorganisms on a filter is the Hydrophobic Grid Membrane (HPGM), where the filter is subdivided by a grid to create over a thousand culture areas [13]. These large numbers of small compartments facilitate colony counting over a wider range (typically 3 orders of magnitude) than the simple Petri dish (it is generally accepted that <30 colonies on a plate represent too few colonies for accurate statistical analysis, whilst >300 colonies per plate results in confluent growth which prevents accurate counting). Large numbers of countable colonies (typically thousands) may be cultured on HPGMs (dependant on the number of subdivisions present), the grid pattern making it easier to automate colony counting as compared to an unstructured agar surface.

Membrane/Porous Bioreactors. Biofilms can be grown on porous membranes, and planar or hollow fibres *e.g.* polyethersulfone (PES) and polyvinyl difluoride (PVDF). These allow oxygenation through the membrane and hence facilitate a higher oxygen utilization capacity and generally more efficient growth than culture in shaken flasks [14]. Immobilization in porous particles is another common bioreactor system that facilitates higher oxygen utilization. An interesting variant of this form of immobilization is the use of printable latex formulation technologies that contain nanopores. In some applications, microorganisms are designed to function as catalysts or sensors that are embedded within the thin latex coatings [15].

4. MICROBIAL PENETRATION OF PORES - LEARNING FROM THE CONFINEMENT OF MICRO-ORGANISMS AND THE CREATION OF COMPLEX, MICRO-ENGINEERED, HABITATS

The traditional sterilizing filter used in microbiology has pores with a diameter of 220 nm, meaning that most microorganisms cannot pass through, though very small bacteria or even quite large microorganisms with little or no cell wall (*e.g.* L-forms) are exceptions. Howver, pore size considerations are not normally a problem with respect to the creation of porous culture systems, though some applications have exploited pore penetration as a research tool, using adaptations where microorganisms are in some way restricted or confined within the pores. For example, the creation of narrow and very precise apertures in silica, by means of microengineering, has been used to investigate how the geometry of the environment affects microbial morphology and behavior. Using these systems, it is possible to create complex habitats containing discrete growth areas that are connected by communicating pores that allow limited (or no) microbial access, whilst still permitting communication and transfer of metabolites [16]. By creating a large number of such growth areas, a culture format may be achieved that simulates a complex habitat *e.g.* a biofilm or soil, in which many polymicrobial combinations and spatial arrangements are possible. Further, the fact that combinations or geometries of growth areas can be created, allows polymicrobial statistical and modeling approaches to be utilized. Approaches that were previously difficult or impossible to perform. This approach has provided insights into the colonization of constricted situations, cell-cell communication, biofilm formation and morphological adaptation [16, 17]. For example, it has been shown that growth in a pore (or in a confined area) can generate a distorted morphology on a normally rod-shaped bacteria, a morphology that persists through several subsequent cycles of division. Additionally, for motile microorganisms, microengineered pores have been used to create cell concentration systems, where penetration or "traffic flow" is essentially unidirectional [18]. Another interesting research approach has been directed to the study of how fungi generate force. This approach uses physical confinement and shape distortion under stress (created when cells are confined and grown in microwells or pores) to gain insights into the amount of mechanical force a growing cell can exert on its environment. This can be relevant, for example, with respect to soil penetration or the invasion of plants by pathogens [19]. Though currently niche applications, these approaches have resulted in genuine surprises and an increased understanding of the properties of microorganisms. Moreover, conventional culture cannot produce these results.

5. MICROCHEMOSTATS

The chemostat (<u>chem</u>ical environment is <u>stat</u>ic) allows microorganisms to be grown at a physiological steady state. This is pretty much impossible to achieve in a microbial colony on agar, where nutrients are depleted and waste products accumulate as the colony grows. Microchambers have been fabricated that use porous silica or elastomer materials to facilitate nutrient exchange approximating to a chemostat in function. For example, a series of different microfabricated chambers have been created with an accompanying porous membrane (typically polydimethylsiloxane or silicon), that allows extremely rapid exchange of nutrients and waste products due to the small scale of the devices (chamber sizes typically being hundreds of microns across). Such "microchemostats" do allow limited steady state growth [20], though one limitation of, for example, the above mentioned microchemostat array, is that microbial cells cannot be removed and that the steady state does not indefinitely persist (especially once microorganisms have multiplied to such an extent that they completely fill the microchemostat chamber). However, these initial microchemostat experiments are some of the first that have tried to mimic chemostat function in a manner that could eventually lead to high-throughput analysis applications, a process that may be valuable given the technical demands of "macrochemostat" experiments. Another approach (used in the "Tesla" microchemostat), is to use a porous material for the exchange of small molecules and a larger pore, which when coupled to the physical expansion of cells, acts as the dilution factor in removing excess microorganism biomass [21]. This format is a step closer towards the generation of microchemostat technology, though it should be emphasized that to date there is insufficient validation to indicate whether these devices function as true chemostats.

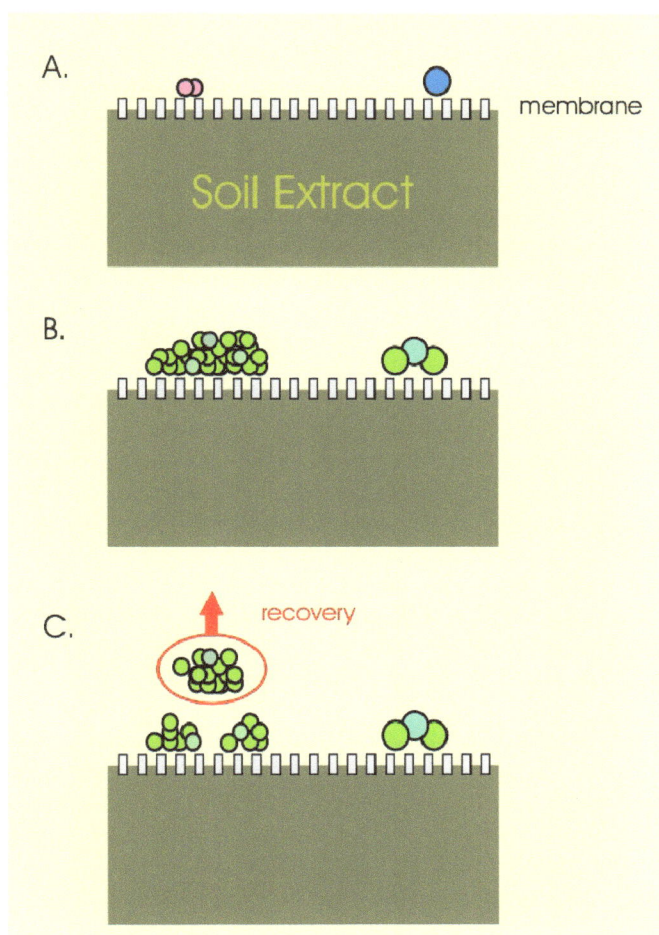

Fig. (2) Simple membrane enrichment system for growth and recovery of previously uncultured soil microorganisms. **A.** Basic set up with a gelled soil extract below a polycarbonate membrane, which is inoculated on the upper surface with microorganisms from the same sample. **B.** After growth the cells are stained to visualize the microcolonies. **C.** Targeted recovery of living cells is possible by laser capture microscopy or using a fine toothpick and a micromanipulator.

6. SIMPLE MEMBRANE ENRICHMENT SYSTEMS

One of the most basic uses of a porous culture system is to allow microorganisms to grow whilst in communication with a complex or natural source of nutrients (Fig. **2**). This rather simple idea has only recently gained favor, with a number of culturing systems now having demonstrated significant improvements in growing previously unculturable microorganisms. In this respect, the nutrient source used is identical to the natural nutrient source utilized by the previously unculturable organism. Further, if the porous support acts as a sterilizing filter, then the nutrient source does not need to be sterile. This property allows the preservation of unstable nutrient molecules that are required for growth (but may be degraded during autoclave sterilization), and facilites polymicrobial co-culture. Finally, the membrane itself may be imaged using optical devices, allowing the identification of microorganisms that only grow to the size of a microcolony and do not generate a visible colony (*e.g.* due to slow growth, limitation by unusual nutrients, lack of stimulation by other organisms or factors etc) [22, 23].

7. POROUS CAGES AS CULTURE SYSTEMS

If it is productive to grow microorganisms in porous enrichment systems, then a logical extension of this idea would be to enclose the growing cells in a "porous cage". This offers the interesting prospect of actually embedding the culture system in appropriate environments. One extraordinarily simple but effective version of this technique is a diffusion chamber bounded by two membranes that function as microbial barriers (Fig. **3A** to **3C**). The chamber may be filled with agar (but not nutrients, as these can diffuse into the system from outside the cage) and then inoculated with an environmental sample [23].

When such a chamber is placed within an (artificial) environment that simulates a natural environment *e.g.* sediment in an aquarium, the result may be an enrichment of previously unculturable microorganisms, with the majority of growing microbes being viewed as microcolonies on the surface of the agar. However, in most cases, further cultivation of microcolonies in pure culture proves difficult, though co-culture of the previously "unculturable" microorganisms may be accomplished using a special "diffusion chamber". An interesting variation on the diffusion chamber system uses asymmetric membranes (Fig. **3D** to **3F**). Essentially, the diffusion chamber comprises an upper membrane that cannot be penetrated by microorganisms, whilst a lower membrane has a pore size that enriches for microbes by selectively permitting size-dependant growth into the chamber. In one such system, it was discovered that if the pore size was decreased to 0.2 μm, then filamentous bacteria (particularly actinomycetes) could be isolated, as they possessed an advantage in being small enough to penetrate the chamber. In contrast, fungi were too large to penetrate [24]. In this case, precision microengineering of pore size successfully excluded fungi, (fungi frequently overgrow and contaminate actinomycetes in environmental screening experiments). This is a promising technique, given that actinomycetes are major antibiotic producers, and that new isolations of useful antibiotic producers are declining. Further, if membranes can be fabricated that are selectively porous (based on additional physical/chemical properties *e.g.* surface charge or hydrophobicity or surface molecules), then refinement of the selective entrapment technique could yield even more interesting culture results.

The diffusion chambers described above are sealed by hand under aseptic conditions. An interesting development however is self-closing chambers, particularly those that can be deployed in challenging environments (*e.g.* the deep sea and the human gastointestinal tract). These devices comprise flat boxes whose sides are all porous cages that self-assemble when the right mechanical stimulation is provided [25]. Further, the boxes can be sorted into artificial communities and are amenable to manipulation by magnetic fields. These properties offer the potential for the creation of artificially structured communities of cells (Fig. **3G** to **J**). Though this technology is still in its infancy, and current cages possess pore sizes that are too large to exclude all but the largest of microorganisms, the technology is amenable to any future microengineering advances that can generate pore sizes that exclude smaller microbial cells.

An alternative format for generating porous microbial cages is the hollow porous fibre, whose geometry provides an exceptionally high surface area for contact with the environment [26]. A hollow-fibre PVDF membrane (0.1 μm mean pore size) forms the basis of this cultivation system (Fig. **3K**). In tests, the system provides a significant enhancement in microbial culture, having been used to culture microorganisms from 3 difficult environmental samples, including tidal flats and 2 forms of activated sludge. Additionally, the total volume of the system can be increased (by extending the length of the hollow porous tubing), allowing larger volumes of microorganisms to be cultured compared to microcolony-based methods.

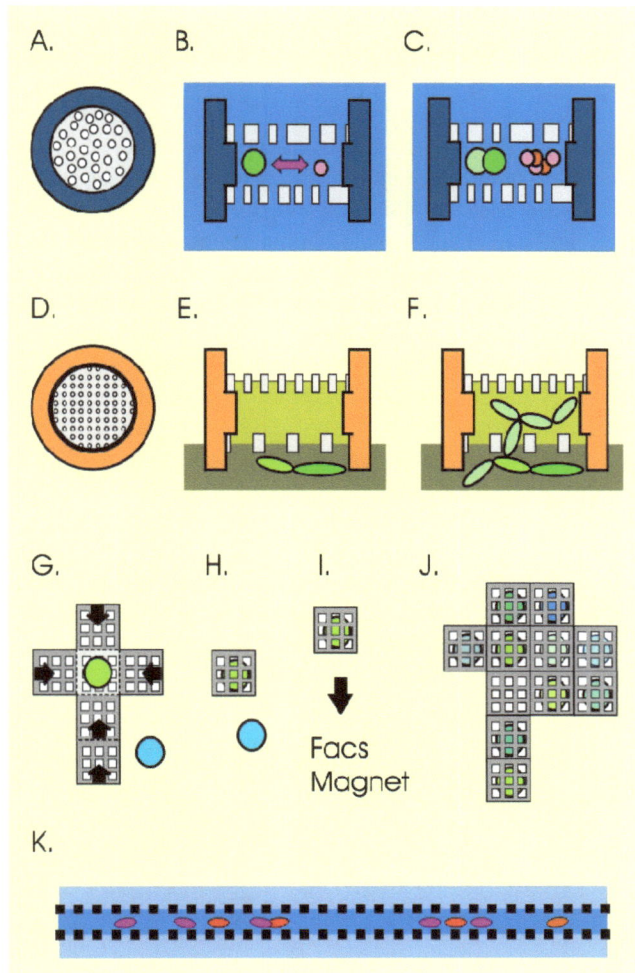

Fig. (3) Cages for Microorganisms – mechanical trapping using porous supports. **Panels A-C** A simple culture chamber constructed from washers and two circles of porous membrane. The chamber can be deployed back into the natural environment [23]. **A.** View from above (c. 1 cm across). **B.** View from the side with two species of microorganisms trapped in the sealed chamber. **C.** If the two species stimulate each other then growth will occur. **Panels D-F.** Chamber with asymmetric membranes, the lower of which can only be penetrated by filamentous microorganisms (*e.g.* actinomycetes or filamentous fungi). dependant on the membrane pore size [24]. **D.** View from above. **E** View from the side; the upper membrane is completely impenetrable to microorganisms, the lower membrane is selectively permeable. **F.** View from the side showing mycelial penetration and entrapment. **Panels G-I.** Cages hundreds of microns across fabricated from metal [25]. **G.** Flat, unfolded cage with nine square holes per side (view from above). Dashed lines indicate flexible hinges. The device traps particles when it is closed. **H.** Organism (green cell trapped, blue cell not) now trapped within a cubical cage but with access to the external medium. **I.** Cages can be moved and sorted; for example the cage can be moved in a magnetic field or a fluorescence activated cell sorter (FACS) could be used. **J.** Cages can also be assembled like building bricks into 2D arrays or stacked into 3D structures to create artificially structured communities. **K.** Flexible, porous microtube allowing the cultivation of large numbers of microorganisms with access to the surrounding medium (lighter blue) [26].

8. NANOPOROUS ALUMINIUM OXIDE CULTURE CHIPS

In this section of the chapter, we will concentrate on "culture chips", with one particular line of development being described in detail, namely culture methods based upon nanoporous aluminium oxide (PAO). As a material, nanoporous aluminium oxide has found applications: 1) as a filter that is resistant to organic solvents, 2) as a scaffold for nanotechnology fabrication (including nanowires), and 3) as a support for microarrays. Within the field of microbiology, the material has been found to be a good imaging support for counting microorganisms from water samples, particularly when combined with fluorogenic dyes [27, 28]. Here the combination of filtration with low background allows accurate microbial counting. Finally, the material has also been proven to be a good support for eubacteria, eukaryotes and even thermophilic archaea [9, 29].

Culture Chip Construction. In order to progress from the base material to a culture chip, the surface material has first to be subdivided with barriers or walls, in order to create distinct growth areas. Initially, polymer deposition methods were used for this purpose, effectively printing a latex barrier [29]. Such printing techniques are robust and can create growth compartments hundreds of microns across, though the construction of smaller compartments are possible by laminating the PAO with a separate material and then selectively removing this material to leave culture compartments surrounded by walls. Further, a mask can be used to direct oxygen plasma to burn away the laminate in the culture areas, whilst preserving the grid of laminate that forms the walls. This protocol works because the laminate is more labile than the PAO. In fact, the precision of this technique is amazing, as it is possible to create an array of 7 x 7 μm culture areas with 10 μm high intervening walls, meaning that on an 8 x 36 mm strip of PAO, a million growth compartments can be fabricated – the most highly subdivided disposable product for microbial growth ever created [9]. Finally, this process allows the creation of flexible formats, with larger microwells comprising several different geometries *e.g.* circles, also being possible (Fig. **4**).

Porous culture chips (MDCC or MicroDish Culture Chips) have several advantages over non-porous microwell plates. Firstly the medium can be readily exchanged from beneath the culture chip. Secondly, desiccation is not an issue despite the small volume of the wells (a major disadvantage of handling small liquid volumes involves the rapid desiccation of the sample).

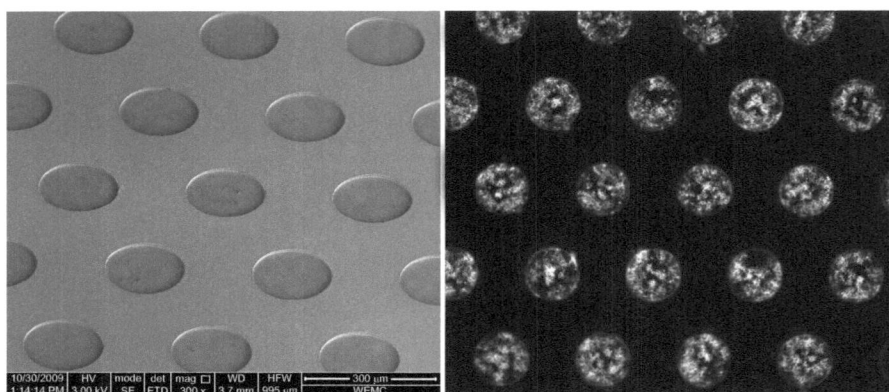

Fig. (4) Example of part of a culture chip containing thousands of circular culture wells. Left. View from above by SEM (at 45° angle) of round culture areas under 200 μm in diameter with PAO (nanoPorous Aluminium Oxide) at the base and 10 μm high walls. Right. View from above of bacteria growing in wells (as panel A). Bacteria are stained with the fluorogenic dye Syto 9 (c. 100 bacteria/well shaded white) and imaged by fluorescence microscopy.

Microbial Colony Counting. Subdivided surfaces, such as the HPGM mentioned earlier, provide advantages over the commonly used Petri dish when counting Colony-Forming Units (CFU). The dynamic range for counting CFU is larger in subdivided surfaces than in the Petri Dish, which can only effectively count from between 30 to 300 CFU per plate, necessitating the traditional use of a 1/10 dilution series in order to provide the 30–300 CFU required per Petri dish. Highly subdivided surfaces are more robust in this respect, reducing dilution steps before inoculation. Additionally, the grid-like pattern of microcolonies that form is more predictable, facilitating automated image analysis (Fig. **5**). The same advantages apply to micropetri dishes, which provide a 4-fold dynamic range for commonly cultured microorganisms [9]. Further, there exists a speed advantage in using subdivided surfaces, as these generate results approximately 5 times faster compared to Petri dish colony counting, particularly important with respect to slower growing microorganisms. Indeed, using sub-divided surface techniques for basic colony counting and sterility testing probably generates the greatest advantage in processes where the culture of slow growing microorganisms has a disproportionately serious impact, such as sterility testing in high value manufacturing processes and contaminant detection in industrial fermentations.

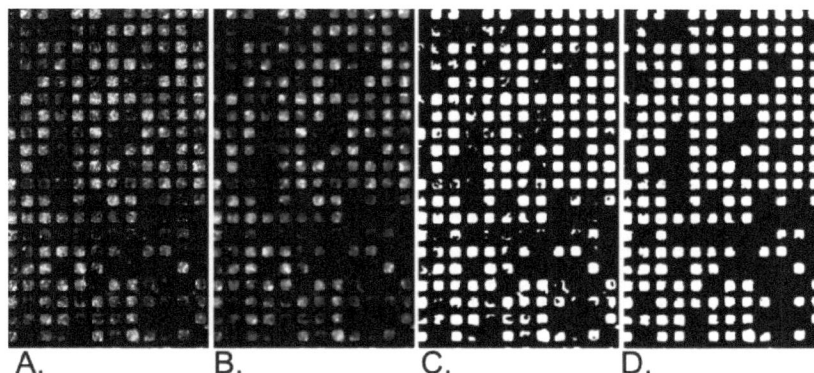

Fig. (5) Example of image processing during a viable count on the MDCC40.10. **A.** Raw image of *Candida albicans* cultured for 5 h (small portion of chip with 40 x 40 μm compartments with 10 μm high walls, hence MDCC40.10, with > 200 growth compartments out of 60,000 shown). **B.** First step in image processing: a median filter is applied using ImageJ software [30]. **C.** Binary threshold tranformation converts microcolonies to white outlines. **D.** Scoring of growth (168 CFU in field of view).

Culturing the Recalcitrant. MDCC can be used to culture microorganisms that are not normally cultivable, a technique also available using some of the porous cage methods previously mentioned. Indeed, some of the common advantages relating to porous systems also apply to MDCC systems as well. These include the fact that: a) many organisms grow as microcolonies, and MDCC systems can be used alongside various imaging techniques to visualize these microcolonies; b) complex and natural substrates can be used (without sterilization if growth media nutrients are destroyed by autoclaving) so that organisms on the chip can be cultured in a near-natural environment and in close communication with other organisms in the medium beneath, for example culture chips have been used to screen for phosphate-metabolizing, previously unculturable, bacteria from the river Rhine using actual Rhine river water as the culture medium [9]; c) MDCC chips may possess many subdivisions, allowing the segregation of samples, and thereby including protecting samples from "spreading" or "swarming" organisms that can move across unsegregated porous surfaces and overgrow undivided culture plates; and d) the miniaturized nature of MDCC suits the use of samples that are limited in volume, such as surgical material or samples from other microscale niches.

High Throughput Screening (HTS). MDCC compartmentalization allows hundreds of thousands of strains to be screened provided that appropriate automation exists and that the target phenotype is identifiable at the microcolony level. One example of HTS is provided above in Fig. **5**, where a fluorogenic dye that is sensitive to phosphate metabolism was used to target microcolonies from the environment [9]. The recovery of "hits" (separate microcolonies) is facilitated by use of a micromanipulator, which can generally be used to obtain hundreds of cells for further culture and validation. Additionally, the chips do not easily dry out and the environment experienced by the cultured microcolonies can be easily changed, which are distinct advantages in some high-throughput screening protocols. Currently, HTS are mainly used for industrial strain improvement in the overproduction of low molecular weight metabolites and in the identification of microorganisms expressing novel lytic enzymes.

Rapid Diagnostics. Susceptibility testing is a major issue in microbial diagnostics. Although molecular techniques exist for some antimicrobials *e.g.* rifampicin, testing is still primarily phenotypic, *i.e.* growth based. In part, this is because of the number and diversity of mutations and genes that may generate an antimicrobial resistance phenotype, a diversity that makes it challenging to cover all possibilities using, for example, a nucleic acid amplification technique. The continued spread of antimicrobial resistance throughout microbial species and around the world remains a challenge, including antimicrobial resistance in species for which species identification used to be considered a relatively accurate guide for antibiotic treatment *e.g. Aspergillus fumigatus* [31]. Additionally, in the clinical setting, the speed and accuracy of antimicrobial testing is an issue, with the accurate determination of breakpoints often being highly subjective. In this context, microcolony imaging on PAO culture platforms can help speed-up this process, with susceptibility testing of *Mycobacterium tuberculosis* being possible within 3 days, compared to the approximately 10 days required by standard culture bottles *e.g.* BacT Alert, and 2 weeks or more required using agar dilution methods [32]. Additionally, more traditional antimicrobial resistance assays may be transferred to culture chips in an approach that leads to greater quantification. An example of this is shown in Fig. **6**, which compares the E-test with microcolony imaging on unstructured PAO and an MDCC with 20 x 20 µm compartments. In this example, in both traditional and MDCC cases, the E-strip is used to create a gradient of Voriconazole, for direct *Candida albicans* testing either on agar, under PAO, or under the culture chip. The zone of clearing on agar after 36 hours allows reading of the Minimal Inhibitory Concentration (MIC), though it should be noted that this is not a sharp endpoint. Culture on PAO for 12 hours demonstrates the effect of the antimicrobial drug more quickly, but is harder to quantify. Culture on culture chips allows quantification in the same time period, whilst facilitating automated image processing.

Environmental Monitoring. Environmental quality (water, air, soil, human habitation) may also be monitored using culture methods that extend beyond the traditional use of water-quality testing filters. For example, for "re-growth" assays (used to determine water pipe contamination), it may take several weeks to predict contaminating nutrients and microorganisms using a biofilm / ATPase activity assay [33]. Such culture-based assays may be improved by automation and more rapid culture chip-based approaches, possibly *via* the placement of culture chips within pipelines and in combination with low cost imaging apparatus.

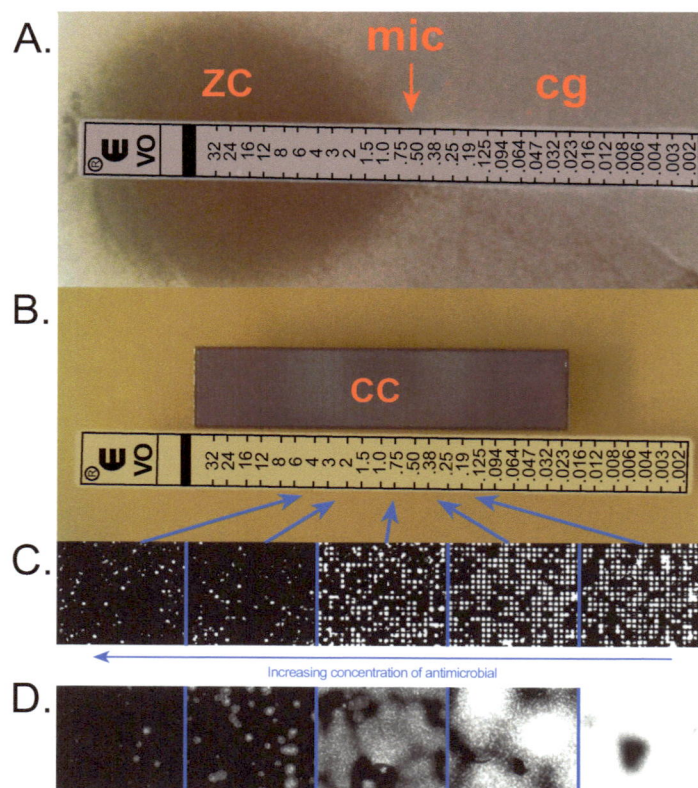

Fig. (6) Example of susceptibility testing on the MDCC20.10. **A.** E-strip on an agar plate spread with *C. albicans* and incubated for 36 h. Diffusion of the antimicrobial (Voriconazole, VOR) in a gradient from the E-strip creates a zone of clearing (zc) which is in contrast to confluent growth (cg). The MIC (µg/ml) can be read from the E-strip, where the zone of clearing intersects the strip, though determining a precise MIC can be difficult. **B.** An E-strip can also be used to create a gradient of VOR under a culture chip (shown) or an unstructured strip of PAO (not shown). In these cases the *C. albicans* is spread on top of the chip and incubated for 9 h. **C.** After staining the effect of VOR can be assessed by counting compartments (20 microns wide, 10 micron high walls, hence the designation MDCC20.10) with significant growth. Arrows show which concentrations (µg/ml) each region of the chip is dosed with. **D.** The effect can also be seen on PAO without barriers walls but it is hard to quantify.

Limitations. Miniaturization brings with it problems as well as benefits. Though an MDCC may be utilized as a "sterile filter", it cannot be used to capture microorganisms from large volumes (hundreds of ml) of liquids, particularly if these liquids are viscous or highly particulate. This limitation produces an upper limit on culture sensitivity. Containment may also be an issue, as overgrowth will ultimately occur if incubation is prolonged, though this problem may be minimized by the correct choice of chip. Additionally, a reader or detection method is required (this can be a microscope), though microcolony visualization may require the use of fluorogenic dye staining techniques. A more convenient protocol would eliminate this step, using instead non-intrusive detection methods such as polarized light microscopy or infrared spectroscopy wherever possible. With respect to High Throughput Screening (HTS), limitations include the fact that a high degree of robotics/automation is required, including an automated "XY table" recognition device that allows a micromanipulator to return to exactly the same position for microcolony recovery. Further, for many applications, improved detection reagents (*e.g.* fluorogenic dyes) are desirable in order to increase sensitivity or facilitate lower cost imaging. Though indiscriminate dye techniques are useful for MDCC applications (for example for equally detecting all microorganisms in enumeration and sterility assays), the development of highly specific dyes for strain identification, metabolic process detection, phenotyping characterization and HTS strain improvement is desirable. Ultimately, this means that fluorogenic dyes are currently most useful when: i) they possess a high dynamic range, ii) become fluorescent when the desired phenotype is apparent, and iii) are resistant to photobleaching. Though not yet perfected, there is an encouraging trend in recent years towards expanding the types of reagents suitable for nanoculture protocols, particularly in the field of functionalized nanoparticles such as pH sensitive quantum dots or silica nanoparticles.

9. FUTURE DEVELOPMENTS AND PROSPECTS

Broadly, the future for nanoporous materials looks good, especially within specific defined applications. However, to capture a wider market, both materials and fabrication techniques must become cheaper, and it remains to be seen to what degree porous culture chips are able to replace the areas of diagnostic and research microbiology that are traditionally reliant on the Petri dish. Based on the microbial culture applications already mentioned in this chapter, the authors foresee an emphasis towards the development of simple automation methods as an attractive developmental path for nanoculture technology. In this respect, automated culture formats that reduce the need for sample manipulation *e.g.* plating-out dilution series of microorganisms, and increase the ease of data capture and interpretation, are likely candidates for automation. The use of MDCC technology is one format that may facilitate this change.

The current growth in imaging technologies available also provides new opportunities for the use of nanoculture in microbiological diagnosis and research. One pleasing trend lies in the reduction of costs, with LED imaging systems becoming cheaper, but at the same time more versatile [34]. For example, low cost LED systems are found in USB microscopes that are capable of visualizing microcolonies on the MDCC [35]. Additionally, LED imaging systems are being adapted to new applications, for example acting as polarized light sources [36].

In terms of fluorescence, cheaper and more versatile reagents may help extend the use of culture chips, including the detection of TB using intrinsic fluorescence [37].

With respect to detection systems, functionalized nanoparticles (quantum dots and variants) are in theory capable of acting as sensors that can be integrated into MDCCs. Whilst currently at an early stage, this is an exciting technology that offers to expand the range of assays available, and at the same time may facilitate the use of low cost miniaturized detection platforms. In terms of more sophisticated detection systems, methods such as MALDI-TOF mass spectrometry and Raman spectroscopy are emerging in diagnostics laboratories, primarily for strain identification [38]. These may also combine well with culture chips in the future.

Current advances in Microelectro-Mechanical Systems (MEMS) offers the ability to embed a culture chip (and even a disposable lens or imaging system) in a culture/detection device [39, 40]. Indeed, there may be a number of interesting possibilities here. Using MEMS and porous cages (Fig. **3**), it may be possible to devise a miniaturized capture method that is more easily deployed for microorganism culture from difficult situations, for example within the deep sea or the human body. The latter statement is especially important as it suggests that for some applications the best place to grow microorganisms is simply not in the laboratory but *in situ* or even *in vivo*. In fact, the laboratory is an artificial setting, requiring dedicated specimen and microbial transport systems, with consequent delays in diagnosis and treatment, as well as the added risks associated with the transport of biohazardous material. In the future, miniaturized, disposable culture devices that do not need skilled personnel or additional technical facilities may be developed for use *in situ*, in the natural environment or at a point of care location (such as a small peripheral health clinic). However, this line of thought is almost the opposite of the current design philosophy that is associated with the development of automated nanoculture platforms. The current philosophy relying instead on integrated culture and detection platforms based on a single disposable chip, rather than separate high-throughput specimen processing and handling, culture, and image detection platforms. Though it is still a long term vision, it will be interesting to see whether individual disposable chips or high-throughput nanoculture technologies become the most popular culture methods of the future. Certainly, miniaturized methods involving porous supports and a variety of detection technologies are likely to be contributing factors in the development of new culture methods for microbial diagnostics, screening and research in the future.

ACKNOWLEDGEMENTS

The authors would like to acknowledge the JBZ hospital for supporting the development of MDCC for microbial diagnostics.

REFERENCES

[1]   Sutcliffe I, Silver S. *Antonie van Leeuwenhoek* for the era of online academic publishing. Anton Leeuw 2007; 91: 97-98.

[2]   Carter KC. (1987) Essays of Robert Koch. Portsmouth, USA: Greenwood Press, 1987.

[3]   Brock TD. Milestones in Microbiology 1546-1940. Washington, DC, USA: ASM Press, 1999; ch. 1-2, pp. 8-9.

[4]   Lederberg JC, Lederberg EM. Replica plating and indirect selection of bacterial mutants. J Bacteriol 1952; 63: 399-406.

[5]   Kiestra Lab Automation Home Page: http://www.kiestra.nl/ Accessed November 2009.

[6]   Xiong X, Lidstrom ME, Parviz BA. Microorganisms for MEMs. J Microelectromech Syst 2007; 16: 429-44.

[7]   Ingham CJ, van Hylckama Vlieg JET. MEMS and the microbe. Lab Chip 2008; 8: 1604-16.

[8]   Tsudome M, Deguchi S, Tsujii K, Ito S, Horikoshi K. Versatile solidified nanofibrous cellulose-containing media for growth of extremophiles. Appl Environ Microbiol 2009; 75: 4616-4619.

[9]   Ingham CJ, Sprenkels A, Bomer JG, *et al.* The micro-Petri dish, a million-well growth chip for the culture and high-throughput screening of microorganisms. Proc Natl Acad Sci USA 2007; 46: 18217-22.

[10]   Lu GQ, Zhao XS. 1: Nanoporous materials – an overview. In: Nanoporous Materials: Science and Engineering. Lu GQ, Zhao XS, Eds. London: Imperial College Press, London, 2005.

[11]   Kincaid RL, Nightingale MS. A rapid non-radioactive procedure for plaque hybridization using biotinylated probes prepared by random primed labeling. Biotechniques 1988; 6: 42-9.

[12]   Li F, Wichmann K, Otterpohl R. Review of the technological approaches for grey water treatment and reuses. Sci Total Environ 2009; 407: 3439-49.

[13]   Sharpe AN, Michaud GL. Hydrophobic grid-membrane filters: new approach to microbiological enumeration. Appl Microbiol 1974; 28: 223-5.

[14]   Li T, Liu J, Bai R. Membrane aerated biofilm reactors: a brief current review. Recent Pat Biotechnol 2008; 2: 88-93.

[15]   Flickinger MC, Schottel JL, Bond DR, Aksan A, Scriven LE. Painting and printing living bacteria: engineering nanoporous biocatalytic coatings to preserve microbial viability and intensify reactivity. Biotechnol Prog 2007; 23: 2-17.

[16]   Keymer JE, Galajda P, Muldoon C, Park S, Austin RH. Bacterial metapopulations in nanofabricated landscapes. Proc Natl Acad Sci USA 2006; 103: 17290-5.

[17] Mannik J, Driessen R, Galajda P, *et al.* Bacterial growth and motility in sub-micron constrictions. Proc Natl Acad Sci USA 2009; 106: 14861-66.

[18] Galajda P, Keymer J, Chaikin P, Austin R. A wall of funnels concentrates swimming bacteria. J Bacteriol 2007; 189: 8704-7.

[19] Minc N, Boudaoud A, Chang F. Mechanical forces of fission yeast growth. Current Biol 2009; 19: 1096-1101.

[20] Cookson S, Ostroff N, Pang WL, *et al.* Monitoring dynamics of single-cell gene expression over multiple cell cycles. Mol Syst Biol 2005; 1: 2005.0024.

[21] Balagadde FK, You L, Hansen CL, *et al.* Long-term monitoring of bacteria undergoing programmed population control in a microchemostat. Science 2005; 309: 137–140.

[22] Ferrari BC, Winsley T, Gillings M, Binnerup S. Cultivating previously uncultured soil bacteria using a soil substrate membrane system. Nat Protocol 2008; 3: 1261-9.

[23] Kaeberlein T, Lewis K, Epstein SR. Isolating "uncultivable" microorganisms in pure culture in a simulated natural environment. Science 2002; 296: 1127-1129.

[24] Gavrish E, Bollmann A, Epstein S, Lewis K. A trap for *in situ* cultivation of filamentous actinobacteria. J Microbiol Methods 2008; 72: 257–262

[25] Leong TG, Randall, CL Benson, BR Zarafshar, AM Gracias, DH. Self-loading lithographically structured microcontainers: 3D patterned, mobile microwells. Lab Chip 2008; 8: 1621-4.

[26] Aoi Y, Kinoshita T, Hata T, Ohta H, Obokata H, Tsuneda S. Hollow-fiber membrane chamber as a device for *in situ* environmental cultivation. Appl Environ Microbiol 2009; 75: 3826–33.

[27] Jones SE, Ditner SA, Freeman C, Whitaker CJ, Lock MA. Comparison of a new inorganic membrane filter (Anopore) with a track-etched polycarbonate membrane filter (Nuclepore) for direct counting of bacteria. Appl Environ Microbiol 1989; 55: 529-30.

[28] McKenzie CH, Helleur R, Deibel D. Use of inorganic membrane filters (Anopore) for epifluorescence and scanning electron microscopy of nanoplankton and picoplankton. Appl Environ Microbiol 1992; 58: 773-776.

[29] Ingham CJ, van den Ende M, Pijnenburg D, Wever PC, Schneeberger PM. Growth and multiplexed analysis of microorganisms on a subdivided, highly porous, inorganic chip manufactured from anopore. Appl Environ Microbiol 2005; 71: 978-81.

[30] ImageJ: Image processing and analysis in Java. http://rsbweb.nih.gov/ij/ (accessed November 2009).

[31] Verweij, PE, Mellado E, Melchers WJ. Multiple-triazole-resistant aspergillosis, N Engl J Med 2007; 356, 1481–83.

[32] Ingham CJ, Ben Ayad A, Nolsen K, Mulder, B. Growth and drug sensitivity testing of Mycobacterium tuberculosis complex on a novel porous ceramic. Int J Tuberc Lung Dis 2008; 12: 645-50.

[33] Juhna T, Birzniece D, Larsson S, Zulenkovs D, Sharipo A, Azevedo F. Menard-Szczebara F, Castagnet S, Feliers C, Keevil CW. Detection of Escherichia coli in Biofilms from pipe samples and coupons in drinking water distribution networks. Appl Environ Microbiol 2007; 73:7456-64.

[34] Canadian Electronics: Trends in LED design. http://www.electronicsincanada.com/index.php/Trends-in-LED-Design.html (accessed November 2009).

[35] QX5 USB Microscope. http://store.digiblue.com/QX5_Computer_Microscope_for_PC_p/db12011.htm (accessed November 2009).

[36] Morejon IJ, Zhai JL, Haizhang P, Robert J. Polarized light emitting diode (LED) color illumination system and method for providing same US Patent 7325957, 2008.

[37] Hung NV, Sy DN, Anthony RM, Cobelens FG, van Soolingen D. Fluorescence microscopy for tuberculosis diagnosis. Lancet Infect Dis 2007; 7: 238-9.

[38] Willemse-Erix DF, Scholtes-Timmerman MJ, Jachtenberg JW, *et al.* Optical fingerprinting in bacterial epidemiology: Raman spectroscopy as a real-time typing method. J Clin Microbiol 2009; 47: 652-9.

[39] Wolfe DB, Qin D, Whitesides GM. Rapid prototyping of microstructures by soft lithography for biotechnology. Methods Mol Biol 2010; 583: 81-107.

[40] Tsai FS, Cho SH, Lo YH, Vasko B, Vasko J. Miniaturized universal imaging device using fluidic lens. Opt Lett 2008; 1: 291-3.

CHAPTER 2

Peptide-Based Probes and Biosensor Technology in Medical Microbiological Diagnosis and Research

G.M. Hwang[1*], T.M. Korves[2], P.F. Renda[2] and S.-J. Suh[3]

[1]The MITRE Corporation, 7515 Colshire Drive, McLean, VA, 22102, United States; [2]The MITRE Corporation, 202 Burlington Road, Bedford, MA, 01730, United States and [3]Auburn University, Department of Biological Science, 101 Life Sciences Building, Auburn, AL, 36849, United States

Abstract: Biosensors utilizing peptide and protein probes offer the potential to provide rapid, highly sensitive, specific, and economical infectious disease diagnostics. In this respect, the following chapter describes recent advances in peptide-based biosensor technologies, including mass perturbance, electrical perturbance, and optical methods. Further, the applicability of these biosensors in the diagnosis of microbial infections in both laboratory and field settings is described. The chapter also discusses current, competing technologies to peptide-based biosensors, as well as point-of-care testing (with an emphasis on the comparison of influenza diagnostics). In addition, the chapter illustrates; 1) the positive impact that rapid diagnosis from biosensors could have on pandemic disease surveillance, 2) describes the different types of peptide-based probes (including antibodies and oligopeptides), and 3) presents an internationally approved clinical method for determining limits of detection for biosensors. The chapter concludes with predictions on the limitations of peptide-based biosensors, and the promising technological advances that will allow full potential of biosensor applications to be achieved within the field of medical microbiological diagnosis.

Keywords: Petide-Based Probes, Biosensors, ELISA, Flow Cytometry, Luminex, Phage Display, Mass Perturbance Biosensors, Electrical Perturbance Biosensors, Optical Biosensors, Limit Of Detection.

1. INTRODUCTION

Pathogenic microorganisms have affected civilisations throughout history, and many new disease-causing organisms have been discovered in recent decades. Examples include: rotavirus [1], Ebola virus [2], *Legionella pneumophila* [3], toxin-producing *Staphylococcus aureus* [4], SARS [5], pathogenic *E. coli* strains [6], *Borrelia burgdorferi* [7], HIV [8], *Helicobacter pylori* [9], *Vibrio cholera* [10], Hantaviruses that cause pulmonary syndrome [11], Nipah [12], Hendra [13], South American Arenaviruses that cause hemorrhagic fever (Junin, Machupo, Guanarito, Sabia, Chapare, Tacribe, Amapari) [14-16], and novel strains of influenza [17,18]. Moreover, new disease-causing organisms, that have yet to be catalogued as human pathogens, are still likely to be found in nature. Further, some pathogens can rapidly evolve, posing serious challenges to those tasked with preventing the outbreak and spread of infectious diseases. Finally, in recent years, an extra dimension to microbial disease epidemiology and pathogenesis has been the use of bioterrorism. For example, the anthrax attacks that occurred in the United States after 9/11 highlighted the potential dangers posed by the intentional use of biological threat agents against civilian and/or military targets (in fact, "bioterrorists" have tried since ancient times to deliberately spread diseases, but with varying degrees of success) [19- 21].

This e-Book chapter will address the utility of peptide-based probes and biosensors for detecting known pathogens in medical microbiological research and diagnosis, and is divided into the following sections:

1. The importance of developing highly sensitive, specific, fast and economical medical microbial biosensors for bio-threat preparedness and pandemic disease surveillance.

2. Currently available gold-standard technologies.

Address correspondence to G.M. Hwang: The MITRE Corporation, 7515 Colshire Drive, McLean, VA, 22102, United States. Email to: gmhwang@mitre.org

3. Types of peptide probes - antibodies, antibody fragments, bacteriophages that express peptides, and short strands of amino acids.

4. Recent advances in peptide-based biosensors for the capture and detection of various infectious agents from human samples, and their applicability to both laboratory-grade and field-deployable instruments.

5. A survey of patient studies that employed commercially available point-of-care tests, with an emphasis on the Influenza A virus.

6. Methods for generating limits of detection for biosensors, based on an internationally approved clinical methods.

7. Predictions about the future appearance of rapid diagnostics and instrumentation in clinical environments.

1.1. The Need for Rapid Medical Microbial Biosensors

Many diseases show symptoms that do not correspond to a single infectious agent. For example, a variety of viral and bacterial pathogens may cause what are commonly called "flu-like" symptoms, *i.e.* fever, muscle aches and pains, fatigue, and headache. As a result, in the absence of (i) disease-specific findings (such as the characteristic rash of a poxvirus), or (ii) a known outbreak of a particular disease in the community, it may be very difficult to make an etiological assessment of an outbreak early enough to effectively treat many infected persons. Indeed, the earlier specific clinical testing is implemented, the sooner the diagnosis, the earlier treatment can begin, and the better the prognosis will be for infected individuals. This timing is critical for disease outbreaks because sick people will typically buy "over-the-counter" medications first, before going to their personal physicians or to a hospital emergency room when the over-the-counter drugs fail to relieve their symptoms. Doctors seeing such patients may initially make a diagnosis of an unknown viral illness, some type of influenza infection (especially if the outbreak occurs during the influenza season), gastroenteritis, or even encephalitis, with blood and urine samples subsequently being sent to a clinical laboratory for testing. However, it is not until physicians, or emergency room staff, have already seen several patients presenting with an identical "flu-like" illness, that they begin to recognize that something out of the ordinary (possibly a disease outbreak) may be occurring and decide to run additional diagnostic testing in order to pinpoint the pathogen responsible [22].

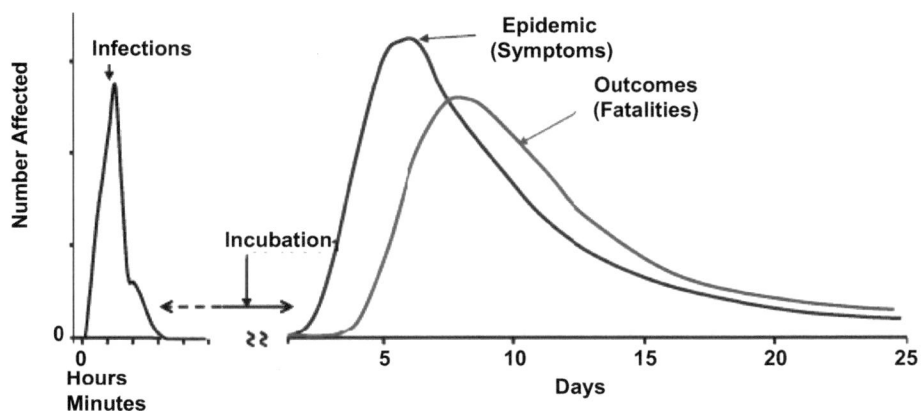

Fig. (1). Typical timeline of a hypothetical disease outbreak. Fig. (1) is adapted and reprinted with permission from Ref. [32].

Fig. **1**. illustrates the timeline of a disease outbreak in which infections occur in the first 12 hours, followed by the onset of symptoms and casualties if all affected individuals remain untreated. From this figure, the benefit of rapid medical microbial diagnosis in outbreaks of potentially fatal diseases is obvious, and the international community is currently implementing a variety of efforts to actually improve early diagnosis [23-28]. For example, several organizations have created databases to monitor emerging outbreaks by collecting data on patient symptoms as they are treated in emergency rooms. Collectively these programs are referred to as "syndromic surveillance", and are aimed at reducing the time it takes for doctors to recognize major infectious disease outbreaks, and to determine whether the outbreaks "natural" in origin. As an example of such a proactive "distributed environmental biosensor system", the United States government has implemented a program involving the deployment of aerosol collectors in 38 locations worldwide, including 30 metropolitan areas in the United States in 2003 [29]. Filters in aerosol collectors are sent daily to local laboratories that are part of the Laboratory Response Network (LRN), with a 10 to 36 hour timeframe between the time that the filter is retrieved from the collector and the time confirmatory test results are produced. This LRN was established in 1999 by the Centers for Disease Control and Prevention and is charged with responding to public health emergencies [22].

Currently, this LRN comprises 150 laboratories distributed in the US, Canada, United Kingdom and Australia [30]. Each LRN lab falls under one of four categories depending on the capabilities within each lab. Typically, level A labs are clinical microbiology laboratories, including hospital and other community clinical laboratories, that can culture and identify pathogens and perform exclusion testing on suspected isolates. If a level A lab cannot rule out a suspected isolate, then the sample is referred to a level B lab. A level B lab typically operates at Biological Safety Level 3 (BSL-3) and can conduct rapid presumptive testing to identify and confirm the presence of the etiological agent. Once a sample is ruled in, it could be sent to a level C lab for strain-typing *e.g. via* nucleic acid testing, and to a level D lab to be further characterized and archived [31].

With respect to fatalities, Fig. **2**. illustrates how rapid diagnosis could substantially reduce fatalities in the event of a disease pandemic, based on predictions provided by Kaufmann *et al.* [33]. Kaufmann postulates that without medical intervention, almost 66% (32,875 out of 50,000) of the people affected would eventually die. The figure shows the percentage of fatalities that would be avoided if antibiotic treatment were initiated on a particular day subsequent to a *Bacillus anthracis* release using an antibiotic efficacy of 95%. Further, while clinical diagnosis on day 5 would prevent 16% of fatalities, successful implementation of more rapid diagnosis on day 3 would save another 44% of the infected population. Overall, Kauffmann's 1997 model suggests that effective, rapid clinical diagnosis could save 16% to 60% more patients than traditional diagnostic methods.

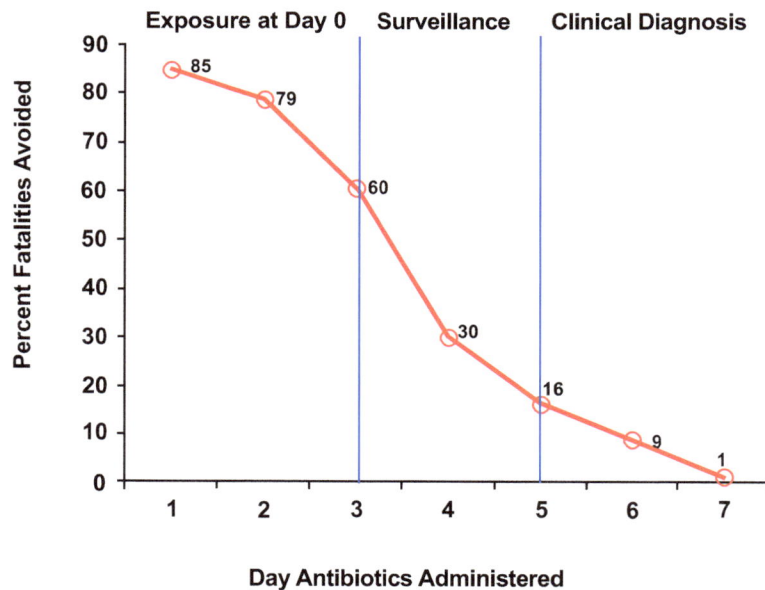

Fig. (2). Percent fatalities avoided as a function of how many days before antibiotics are administered following a pandemic-scale disease. Adapted from Ref. [33]

Instantaneous and accurate information-coupling between biosensor and syndromic surveillance systems *e.g.* [23-28], should enable doctors to rapidly diagnose patients and immediately begin effective antimicrobial therapy. In practice, effective treatment of infected and symptomatic patients, as well as those who have been exposed but do not yet show symptoms, depends on specific anti-microbial or anti-viral therapies. In recent years, many bacteria, including *Staphylococcus aureus* [4] and *Mycobacterium tuberculosis* [34] have become highly resistant to antibiotics and pose a serious problem with respect to finding an effective treatment for infected populations. For most pathogenic bacteria, it may also be necessary to perform antibiotic sensitivity testing in order to determine an effective course of antimicrobial therapy. Unfortunately, this extra step may delay the implementation of an effective treatment for an additional 1-3 days, which could result in an increased risk of people succumbing to infection.

Presently, the traditional approach of culturing and isolating microbial pathogens is still considered the "gold standard" for the positive identification of many infectious disease agents. Unfortunately, isolation and culture techniques may require large quantities of the infectious agent, an understanding of appropriate culture conditions, and up to 10 or more days to complete sample analysis [35]. In recent years, several molecular approaches to identify infectious agents have been developed that will likely replace traditional microbiological methods because these new techniques are more sensitive and yield results in a much shorter time. For example, molecular approaches such as the Polymerase Chain Reaction (PCR) amplification of unique DNA sequences, or sequence analysis of 16S rDNA, are highly accurate and sensitive [36]. Nevertheless, these assays require specialized instruments, highly trained staff, and still may take several hours to perform. Based on these limitations, a new set of techniques are needed that will combine the identification accuracy of current traditional culture techniques (applicable to a wide range of biological samples), with the much higher sensitivity of molecular diagnostic approaches. Further, methods providing a decreased "time-to-diagnosis" and increased cost effectiveness are also necessary in order to detect rapidly propagating infectious diseases, including i) those agents that have not previously been identified, and ii) agents that are resistant to current antimicrobial therapies.

The field of biosensor technology is one that brings together the accuracy of gold-standard (culture-based) approaches with concomitant improvements in the speed and sensitivity of detection. A typical biosensor is composed of a sampler that collects, concentrates, and prepares the biological specimen for identification using a combination of a downstream biodetector/capture device *e.g.* an immunoassay, and a bioidentifier *e.g.* a polymerase chain-reaction amplification step. However, due to the very different operational requirements, environmental and clinical biosensors are likely to employ entirely different front-end sample collection hardware (though peptide-based probes, transducers and other hardware and software could potentially be shared between environmental and clinical applications). A variety of sample collection, concentration, and preparation methods have been described and will not be discussed here [21, 32].

In general, a biosensor platform that detects a specific probe:analyte interaction and generates a measurable signal, needs to be sensitive enough to detect infectious agents at low concentrations and in contaminated (*e.g.* environmental), samples. However, the test should also demonstrate a very low false-positivity rate if it is to become an efficient, field-practical, device.

When considering biosensor design, sensitivity is a term often used interchangeably with the quantity known as the limit of detection (LoD). The LoD is defined as the minimum detectable concentration of an analyte in a Given Sample (see Section 6.0 for details). Biosensor specificity however, is defined as the rate at which analyte-free samples produce correct "true negative" test results. False positivity, on the other hand, are errors in which analyte-free samples produce incorrect "false-positive" test results. Therefore, the sum of the specificity and the rate of false positive results is one. In the clinical setting, sensitivity is measured as the percentage of true positive cases that actually test positive. Similarly, specificity is measured as the percentage of true negative cases that actually test negative (usually in comparison with a 'gold standard'). Although test specificity is a serious concern, due to the fact that responding to false-alarms can be cost prohibitive, biosensor test design should actually be optimized for sensitivity even at the risk of a higher number of false positive results in clinical settings [37,38]. In addition, although specificity is still a challenge in the clinical setting, clinical analysis has the advantage that the range of patient samples measured (*e.g.* blood, sputum, nasopharyngeal aspirate, urine) is easier to characterize compared to the results of uncontrolled in-field environmental sample collection. Therefore, reducing the rate of false negative analyses (missed detections) is the primary challenge for biosensors in the clinical setting. Finally, two statistical terms are typically used to evaluate assays in clinical settings. The positive predictive value (PPV) is a measure of the percentage of positive tests in which the identified disease-causing agent is actually present in the sample. The Negative Predictive Value (NPV) is a measure of the percentage of negative test results in which no identified disease-causing agent is actually present. PPVs and NPVs are values that change with disease prevalence across time and are useful to clinicians in interpreting results and informing their diagnostic decision making.

2. GOLD STANDARDS AND COMPETING TECHNOLOGIES

The isolation and culture of microbial pathogens has remained the "gold standard" testing technology ever since Robert Koch proposed his postulates (comprising 4 criteria for determining the identity of an infectious agent) in the late 19th century. After more than 100 years (and although it is now clear that Koch's postulates do not apply to all infectious agents, for example prions), traditional culturing and identification of microbial organisms is still the most widely used approach for identifying infectious agents, though one notable exception is the use of real-time PCR for the detection of human influenza viruses [37,39]. In fact, culture methods for the detection of viruses, especially influenza viruses, have made several evolutionary advances over the last few decades, including: i) a shell vial culture method that leads to analyte detection within 1-2 days [35], and ii) the development of cryo-preserved cell mixtures capable of replacing conventional tube cell culture and yielding a 52% improvement in the detection of Influenza A and B virus within 1 day of incubation [40,41]. These rapid and sensitive viral culture methods are being adopted in many laboratories [42]. In most cases, however, any sample that produces a negative test result is expected to be examined by traditional culturing methods. That said, the following section will discuss the instruments and approaches that we anticipate will eventually replace conventional 'gold standard' culture methods.

2.1. ELISA - Enzyme-Linked Immunosorbent Assays and Enzyme Immunoassays

Enzyme-Linked Immunosorbent Assay (ELISA), or Enzyme Immunoassay (EIA), is a technique that was simultaneously demonstrated by two research groups in the 1970's, even despite pervasive skepticism, regarding the concept of using large bound enzymes as reporter molecules [43]. The first research group from Stockholm University (Peter Perlmann and Eva Engvall) demonstrated ELISA as a quantitative tool using Immunoglobulin G [44] from rabbit as the antigen (or analyte), sheep-anti-rabbit IgG tethered to microcrystalline cellulose as the immunosorbent material (or probe), and IgG conjugated *via* gluteraldehyde to alkaline phosphatase as the reporter molecule (or label) [45]. Enzyme reactions were stopped and enzyme activity was monitored using an absorbance spectrophototometer and centrifuged samples. The researchers used known concentrations of unlabeled antigens to produce a calibrated dose-response curve based on competitive binding, with unlabeled antigens displacing labeled antigens. Thus the concentration of unlabeled antigens was able to be inferred relative to a sample where no unlabeled antigens were added. The second research group at the Research Laboratories of NV Organon, Oss, The Netherlands (Anton Schuurs and Bauke van Weemen), developed the EIA technique using Human Chorionic Gonadotrophin (HCG) from urine as an antigen, which was conjugated to cellulose as the immunosorbent material. HCG antibodies were used as capture probes, and the Horse Radish Peroxidase (HRP) enzyme as the reporter molecule [46]. HCG-bound HRP was centrifuge-separated and fractions were pooled, then HRP activity was quantified by absorbance measurements. Nearly four decades after the inception of ELISA, it remains broadly used in many assays today. Although the ELISA and EIA assays differ slightly in design, both techniques replaced the need to use the hazardous radioactive isotope iodine-131 with non-hazardous enzymes that served as reporter molecules. In this chapter, rather than describing ELISA in great detail, we highlight its advancement since its initial discovery (Please see Ref. [47] for a more detailed description of ELISA).

Modern day ELISA can be conducted in a variety of formats. Various solid-phase materials employed by ELISA instrument and kit manufacturers include plastic beads, microtiter plates (96 or 384 wells), and plastic strips [48]. Fig. **3**. illustrates several common ELISA approaches. One common approach relies on passive adsorption of antigens onto a solid-phase material, a wash step, the addition of enzyme-linked primary antibodies, a second wash step, which is then followed by the addition of reporter molecules (typically involving color development *e.g.* TMB (3,3',5,5'- tetramethylbenzidine, OPD (*o*-phenylenediamine dihydrochloride), PNPP (*p*-Nitrophenyl Phosphate, Disodium Salt), or ABTS (2,2'-Azinobis [3-ethylbenzothiazoline-6-sulfonic acid]-diammonium salt] – see Fig. **3A**). In situations where primary enzyme-linked antibodies are not available, unlabeled primary antibodies can be added, followed by the addition of secondary enzyme-linked antibodies, before reporter molecules are applied (Fig. **3B**). Instead of relying on passive adsorption of antigens (which is only likely to work well when using high quality samples), an alternative ELISA approach requires that specific antibodies be first bound to a solid phase material, followed by the addition of enzyme-linked antigens, and subsequent color development *via* the addition of reporter molecules (Fig. **3C**). Some protocols call for the addition of secondary enzyme-linked antibodies to complete the "antigen sandwich", followed by the addition of reporter molecules (Fig. **3D**). When designing such antibody sandwich ELISAs, it is critical that the primary and secondary antibodies target different binding sites on the analyte in order to minimize competitive binding. In instances where protocols specify the use of tertiary enzyme-linked antibodies instead of secondary enzyme-linked antibodies (Fig. **3E**), it is critical to note that the tertiary antibodies should be from a different species in order to minimize binding with unoccupied primary antibody sites. Note also, that the overall strategy of relying on secondary or even tertiary enzyme-linked antibodies as reporter molecules is commonly referred to as indirect ELISA (Fig. **3B**), or indirect ELISA sandwich (Fig. **3E**), respectively. The major benefits of ELISA include its affordability, ease of use, acceptance within the research community, and a short "time-to-result", which is typically under 30 minutes. Assay sensitivity however, does vary with the type of antigen and antibody used, and the type of speciemen being tested (see Table **1**).

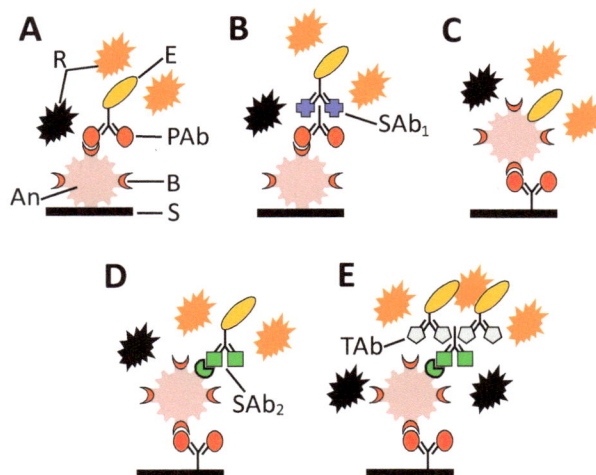

Fig. (3). Schematic illustration of common ELISA approaches **(A)** Direct-labeled antibody, **(B)** Indirect ELISA, **(C)** Direct-labeled Antigen, **(D)** Direct Sandwich ELISA, **(E)** Indirect Sandwich ELISA. Legend: *S* = solid-phase substance, *An* = antigen, *B* = binding site on the antigen, *E* = enzyme-linked, *R* = reporter molecules which are shaded in gray when not in close proximity to the enzyme, *Pab* = primary antibody, *SAb₁* = secondary antibody that binds to an unlabeled primary antibody, *SAb₂* = secondary antibody that binds to an alternate binding site (panel D), *TAb* = tertiary antibody that bind to unlabeled secondary antibody (panel E). See text for additional details. Illustrated by Joe Monaco and Elaine Mullen.

2.2. Flow Cytometry

Flow cytometry is a technique that employs a beam of monochromatic light to illuminate a stream of hydrodynamically focused fluid that carries suspended particles varying in size from 0.2 to 150 μm in diameter. Forward and back-scattered photons emitted from this illuminated fluid can be collected and used to characterize the suspended particles. The first flow cytometer was developed in 1947 by Gucker to detect bacteria in an aerosol using a Ford headlamp as a light source and a Photomultiplier Tube (PMT) to count photons scattered off the bacterial cells [49]. In 1953, flow cytometry was introduced to the scientific community as an analytical technique for cell counting [50]. In 1968, fluorescent flow cytometry was demonstrated by Wolfgang Göhde at the University of Münster in Germany, paving the way for the trademarked Fluorescence Activated Cell Sorter (FACS) developed by Becton Dickinson in 1974. Five decades after the inception of flow cytometry, it continues to expand in application and usage across research laboratories for the detection and identification of proteins *e.g.* cytokines, hormones, and nucleic acids (including gene transcripts). To a lesser extent, FACS is employed in niche research applications for the detection of bacteria and viruses, sometimes from complex samples. A modern example is the versatile unit developed by the Luminex Corporation. Staying true to the concept of flow cytometry, Luminex xMAP® technology utilizes a range of 5.6 micron diameter beads that are colored with precise ratios of red and infrared fluorescent dyes [51]. A total of 100 different bead colors, each with a unique spectral signature, are currently available (Fig. **4**, step 1). The exterior of the bead can be coated with different types of capture probes such as peptide-based probes or nucleic acids (Fig. **4**, step 2).

Table 1: Advantages and Disadvantages of Selected Competing Technologies.

Assay Type	Time-to-Result	Advantages	Disadvantages
Isolation and culturing of microbial pathogens	2-10 days	Affordable (~$2 per test) [73], reliable and sensitive. Many clinically approved tests exist.	Long turn over time. Requires trained personnel. Some organisms are difficult to culture and may require up to 10 days [74].
PCR	1 – 2 hrs	Reliable, sensitive (~20 genomic copies per 0.1 mL), portable, multiplex detection (<120 analytes). Some units do not require highly trained personnel and are intended for field use.	Most primers are designed for known strains, thus novel strains of a disease may result in false negatives. Inhibitors could prevent nucleic acid amplification. Fieldable PCR units are expensive (~$50,000) compared to culture methods. A test for one analyte is <$20.
ELISA	< 1 hour	Rapid and affordable. Plate readers vary in cost, typically <$15,000. Some kits require minimal training. Several clinically approved tests for diseases using peptide-based assays.	Depending on analyte, may not be very sensitive (<100 ng mL^{-1}) or specific (see section 5). Confirmation by an alternative 'gold standard' methodology is often required for negative test results.
Flow Cytometry	< 8 hrs	Reliable and sensitive (antigen dependent: <100 pg mL$^{-1)}$, multiplex detection (< 100 analytes, 20 analytes is a practical limit).	Few clinically approved tests for diseases using peptide-based assays. An instrument costs $50,000 including annual maintenance (< $10,000). A test for one analyte is ~$20 in reagent costs per well (including cost for positive and negative controls). A highly skilled technician is required for some instruments.

The assay is typically conducted in a standard 96-well plate where samples containing analytes of interest are incubated with beads coated with capture probes (Fig. **4**, steps 3 and 4). After mixing (30 minutes on a plate shaker), wells are washed, and a second biotinylated probe is applied (Fig. **4**, step 5). Finally, a reporter molecule (typically streptavidin linked to a phycoerythrin (PE) fluorophore), is added to each well to form an "antigen sandwich" in the presence of the intended analyte (Fig. **4**, steps 6). Some protocols call for the conjugation of the reporter molecule to the secondary probe prior to the addition of the secondary probe into the test well, thereby combining steps 5 and 6 (illustration not shown). Subsequently, the resuspended beads pass through the illumination paths of 2 lasers, one bead at a time (Fig. **4**, step 7).

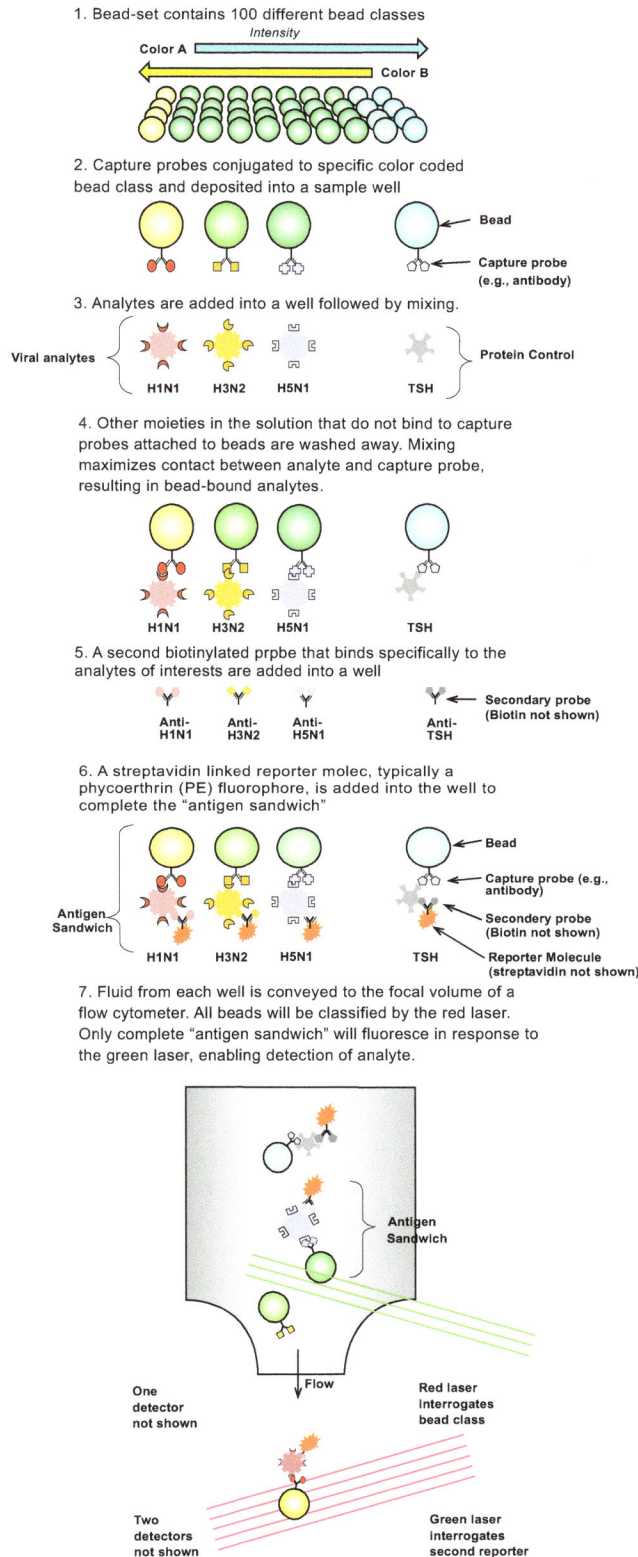

Fig. (4). Schematic of a 100-plex Luminex Liquid array generated from a mix of different red - labeled color A, and infrared dyes - labeled color B (step 1). Beads are first coated with capture probes (step 2), then incubated with analytes (step 3), followed by addition of labeled secondary probes (step 4) and reporter molecules (step 5) to complete the "antigen sandwich" (step 6). The beads are then analyzed by the flow cytometer using 2 distinct lazers (step 7).

Analysis to find the presence of a particular analyte is confirmed by employing two disinct lasers, the first laser (red, 635 nm) is tuned to the absorption band of the dye integral to the bead (which identifies the bead color, >100 classes), while the second laser (green, 532 nm) is tuned to the absorption spectrum of the PE probe. Only beads that form a complete "antigen sandwich" will fluoresce in response to the green laser. By simultaneously monitoring the Mean Fluorescence Intensities (MFI) of the dyes that color the bead, and from the PE probe, many different bead classes and analytes can be detected, all within a single well. The ability to detect many antigens from a single well is referred to as "multiplex" detection and multiplexing is a distinct advantage of the Luminex system as it saves on time, specimen volumes, and reagent costs. Although Luminex offers as many as 100 bead classes, the simultaneous use of 30 different bead classes per well is a practical maximum for peptide-based assays. This limitation is inherent to the use of multiplexed antibodies, as the chances of cross-reactions occurring increase as more antibodies are added. In fact, it may be more resource efficient to separate sets of assays into different wells, as identifying suitable multiplex antibody combinations may require significant effort. Such cross-reactivity is less of a problem when using nucleic acids as capture probes [52]. Finally, the Luminex assay classifies hundreds of beads per second and analyses a well in less than one minute.

Suppliers of Luminex-based assays offer calibration and validation kits intended to ensure that the instrument components (*i.e.* lasers, detectors, optics, fluidics, bead classifier) are functioning within operational tolerance. Errors identified by these calibration kits do not however address variations in Luminex readout caused by batch-to-batch variation in reagents *e.g.* antibody, or analytes *e.g.* influenza viruses. To address issues resulting from inter- and intra-reagent variations, one can employ an internal reference ruler such as a Thyroid Stimulating Hormone standard on each 96-well plate and compare the readings obtained from the internal control to the actual assay results [53].

At present, the Luminex Corporation markets a US-FDA approved test, xTAG™ Respiratory Viral Panel, which is suitable for the detection of a suite of respiratory viruses including influenza A, influenza A subtype H1, influenza A subtype H3, influenza B, respiratory syncytial virus subtype A, respiratory syncytial virus subtype B, parainfluenza 1, parainfluenza 2, and parainfluenza 3 virus, human metapneumovirus, rhinovirus, and adenovirus. Note however that this particular test utilizes DNA as the probe molecule instead of peptide-based probes [54]. Several research groups are working to develop portable flow-cytometry instruments for bedside, point-of-care and medical microbial use. Research to miniaturize the bench scale flow-cytometry unit generally consist of integration of microfluidics, application of dielectrophoresis to aid in fluid movement, and improvements in the optical components which includes the use of microscope objectives, polymer waveguides, or chip-embedded optical fibers [55-57].

2.3. Polymerase Chain Reaction

Real-Time Polymerase Chain Reaction (PCR) is a variant of the nucleic acid amplification technology described by Mullis in the mid-1980s [58]. Real-time PCR amplifies and quantifies the amplification of nucleic acid fragments during the progression of PCR. The relative concentration of the DNA of interest is determined *via* the incorporation of fluorescent dye or by activation of fluorescence attached to a probe specific for the target DNA. Using real-time PCR also allows "melting curve" analysis to be performed, which may be used to differentiate between genetic alleles. Real-time PCR has high sensitivity and specificity, the detection limit typically being 10-100 cells or organisms. Further, some platforms take less than one hour for detection [21]. The major disadvantages of real-time PCR include issues relating to sample preparation (including nucleic acid degradation and contaminants that inhibit PCR) and the ability to detect only the target sequences being searched for, which may not include closely related target sequences containing (single nucleotide) polymorphisms [21]. As examples, 2 real-time PCR platforms that integrate sample preparation with real-time PCR are i) the Gene Xpert (Cepheid; [59]) and ii) the R.A.P.I.D. (Rugged Advanced Pathogen Identification Device; Idaho Tech; [60]) systems. Gene Xpert uses cartridges with reagents for single tests that can be run in under one hour. FDA approved Gene Xpert diagnostic tests include assays for *Clostridium difficile*, Methicillin-resistant *Staphylococcus aureus* (MRSA, sensitivity 95%, specificity 98% [61]), enterovirus, and streptococcal assays; an influenza A virus assay has also recently received emergency use authorization. There is also a 3-agent kit for environmental samples only, which tests for *Bacillus anthracis, Yersinia pestis*, and *Francisella tularensis* [62]. A new automated platform, called Gene Xpert Infinity, is designed to be able to perform more than 2000 diagnostic tests in 24 hours. The R.A.P.I.D. system was developed for military clinical use and designed to be portable and robust for use in rugged environments. It is FDA approved for detecting *Bacillus anthracis, Yersinia pestis*, and *Francisella tularensis*. Other leading platforms that do not integrate sample preparation but provide flexibility in the kinds of real-time PCR reactions that can be run include SmartCycler (Cepheid; [63]), LightCycler (Roche; [64]) and ABI Prism Sequence Detection systems, all of which can be used for the detection of pathogens [65]. Multiplex real-time systems not yet FDA approved include platforms such as the FilmArray (Idaho Tech; [66]).

Table 2: Advantages and Disadvantages of Peptide-Based Probes

Probe Type	Advantages	Disadvantages
Polyclonal antibodies	• Relatively easy to make and widely available commercially • Cheaper than monoclonal and recombinant antibodies • Rapid *in vitro* production • Can be made selective for specific epitopes, and are reproducible • Can determine target epitope	• Sensitive to temperature and other environmental parameters • Reduced specificity due to multiple antibody specificities • Batch to batch variation • Expensive production • Sensitive to temperature and other environmental parameters • Unwanted reactivities can be mediated by Fc portion
Shark and camelid single domain antibodies	• Thermostable and stable to detergents • High solubility • Small size can increase packing density, resulting in greater sensitivity • Can recognize hidden antigenic sites due to small size and loop structure	• More expensive • Not commercially available, few research labs synthesize • Some are difficult to express and produce
Antibody fragments	• Can have very high sensitivity and specificity • Can be engineered for high affinity, stability, and immobilization	• Expensive production • Not as commercially available as other types of antibodies • Some are difficult to express and produce • Stability and aggregation a problem for some fragments
Peptide and landscape phage probes	• Relatively inexpensive production • Thermostable and environmentally stable • Ability to engineer antibodies to specific requirements • No need to engineer for production purposes	• Currently unclear whether specificity and sensitivity are as high as for antibodies • Choosing and screening peptides can be challenging; the number of possible peptides can be very large

Some technologies for infectious disease diagnosis use PCR amplification, but utilize detection methods other than real-time PCR. One such technology is DNA microarrays, reviewed in [67,68]. Another relatively new technology for microbe identification is PCR electrospray-ionization mass spectrometry PCR/ESI-MS [69-71]. This technology uses mass spectrometry to determine molecular weights and base composition of amplified PCR regions, and analyzes this information for pathogen identification.

A platform utilizing PCR/ESI-MS, which is not yet FDA approved, is the Ibis T5000 (Ibis Pharmaceuticals) [72]. A comparison of selected gold standards is included in Table **1**.

3. PEPTIDE-BASED PROBES

In this section and throughout this chapter, antibodies, fragments of antibodies, bacteriophages that express peptides, and short strands of amino acids will all be considered as peptide-based probes. Antibodies and peptides can form a variety of tertiary structures that bind to various molecules with high specificity. Due to these characteristics, peptide-based molecules continue to be utilized as probes in biosensor research for applications where near real-time responses are desired [73,74] The advantages and disadvantages of using these various peptide-based approaches to biosensing will be highlighted throughout this section and are summarised in Table **2** [75]. Lastly, a (non-exhaustive) list of peptide-based probes is provided in Table **3**.

Table 3: Peptide-based Probes for Infectious Microbes and Toxins

Microbe or Toxin	Polyclonal Antibodies in Biosensors	Monoclonal Antibodies in Biosensors	Antibody Fragments	Oligopeptides and Peptide Phage-display
Bacillus anthracis	[127]	[128]	[129-132]	[117, 119]
Brucella species			[133]	
Campylobacter jejuni	[134]			
Chlamydia trachomatis			[135]	
E. coli O157:H7		[84, 136]		
Francisella tularensis	[80, 137]	[137, 138]		
Listeria monocytogenes	[81]	[139]	[109, 140]	
Mycobacterium tuberculosis	[141, 142]	[142]		
Salmonella enterica serovar Typhimurium		[84, 136, 143]		[144, 145]
Vibrio cholerae	[146]	[147]		
Yersinia pestis		[138, 148]		
Plasmodium falciparum			*[149]*[+]	
Ebolavirus	[150]	[150]	[151]	
Epstein Barr virus		[152]		
Hepatitis B virus			[153]	[154, 155]
Hepatitis C virus			[156, 157]	
Herpes simplex virus		[152]	[158]	
Marburg virus			*[97]*[+]	
Norwalk virus		[80]		
Rabies virus			[159, 160]	
SARS	[161]		[162]	
Vaccinia virus			[163]	
Varicella-zoster virus		[152]		
Venezuelan equine encephalitis (VEE) virus			[164]	
Botulinum toxin			*[94-96]*[+]	[165]

Table 3: cont....

Clostridium difficile toxin B			[166]	
Cholera toxin	[167]	[167]	*[168]*[+]	
Diphtherotoxin		[169]		
Ricin	[137, 167]	[80, 137, 167]	*[96, 98, 170]*[+]	
Staphylococcal enterotoxin B	[80, 127, 137, 167]	[167]	*[96]*[+]	[121, 171]

[+]Italicized examples are camelid or shark-derived single domain antibodies.

3.1. Antibodies

Antibodies are an excellent choice for biosensor probes because they possess a high specificity and high affinity for their targets. Antibodies bind to antigens *via* non-covalent bonds with apparent dissociation constants (K_d) ranging from 10^{-7} to 10^{-11} M [76]. This combination of high affinity and high specificity allows antibodies to bind strongly to targets in complex mixtures. In addition, antibodies are well-suited as sensors because they are relatively stable molecules that can be chemically linked to reporter molecules [77, 78].

The earliest antibodies used in microbiological research and diagnosis were polyclonal antibodies, which are antibodies isolated from an animal (usually a rabbit) infected with a target microbe or peptide. Polyclonal antibodies have been used in biosensors to detect avian influenza virus [79], *Francisella tularensis* [80], and *Listeria monocytogenes* [81] (see Table **3** for additional examples). Polyclonal antibodies are composed of a mixture of antibodies with different specificities. This poly-specificity can be a problem for biosensors, as polyclonal antibodies may recognize antigens that are present on closely related, non-pathogenic organisms, leading to false positive pathogen identification. In addition, polyclonal specificity can result in batch-to-batch quality variation [82]. To address these shortcomings, researchers developed monoclonal antibodies, which are produced by hybridomas formed by fusing B lymphocytes with cancer cells.

Monoclonal antibodies can be produced more rapidly and reproducibly than polyclonal antibodies [77, 82], and each monoclonal antibody possesses a single highly-specific binding activity. One example of this high specificity is the fact that certain monoclonal antibodies targeting *Bacillus anthracis* can differentiate between spores and vegetative cells, as well as between the spores of other *Bacillus* species [83]. Monoclonal antibody probes have also been used in biosensors to detect *E. coli* O157:H7, *Salmonella enterica* serovar Typhimurium, *Legionella pneumophila*, and *Yersinia enterocolitica* [84], as well as Norwalk virus [80] (Table **3** provides additional examples). Both monoclonal and polyclonal antibodies are sensitive to high temperature and have a limited shelf life [85]. As a consequence, they may need to be stored under refrigerated conditions, which limits their application outside of the laboratory environment [86, 87]. For improved robustness to environmental conditions, biosensor developers have explored antibodies from sharks and camelids (*e.g.* camels and llamas). Shark and camelid antibodies are composed of only heavy chains with very small antigen-binding domains [86, 88-90]. Shark and camelid antibody fragments that contain only the hypervariable antibody region have been developed as single domain antibodies (sdAbs, see Fig. **5.** for schematic illustration). These single domain antibodies are stable to temperatures as high as 90°C [91, 92], stable to detergents, and highly soluble [90, 91, 93]. In addition, the small size of single domain antibodies (12–15 kDa) increases packing density (which increases test sensitivity), whilst the small size and loop structure enable these antibodies to recognize hidden antigenic sites [93]. Single domain antibodies have been used in the detection of botulinum A neurotoxin [94, 95], cholera toxin, ricin, Staphylococcal Enterotoxin B [96] and Marburg hemorrhagic fever antigens [97] (see Table **3**). Although single domain antibodies are generally thermostable, whether their use can completely eliminate the need for refrigeration over prolonged periods of time of storage remains unclear.

In order to overcome the inherent difficulties of monoclonal and polyclonal antibodies with respect to unpredictable conformational changes upon attachment to surfaces, as well as any unwanted reactivities, biosensor developers have utilized antibody fragments developed through molecular biological techniques [82]. The fragments used include: i) the Fab fragment, consisting of the light chain and the first half of the heavy chain without the Fc part; ii) the Fv fragment, consisting of the V_H and V_L domains; iii) the single-chain Fv (scFv) fragment, which has a polypeptide linker between V_H and V_L domains to increase stability; iv) V_H fragments [82]; and v) V_{HH} fragments, single domain antibodies derived from camelid and shark antibodies (see Fig. **5**).

A major advantage of antibody fragments is that they can be engineered to improve their affinity and stability. Large libraries of antibody fragments can be created by cloning and amplifying cDNA from immunized or naïve animal B cells, with antibody fragment diversity being created through site-directed and random mutagenesis, or *via* the random recombination of antibody fragments [77].

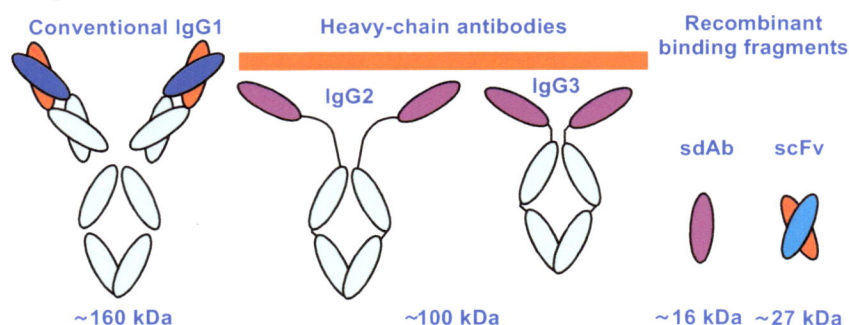

Fig. (5). Schematics showing conventional antibodies, heavy chain antibodies, and their cloned recombinant binding fragments. Variable domains are depicted in red, heavy (VH) and light chains (VL) are shown in blue, and single domain antibodies (sdAb) from the single variable domain are shown in purple. Reprinted with permission from Ref. [98].

The construction and efficient screening of large libraries has been made possible by phage display technology [99-101], and more recently by ribosome display, RNA-peptide fusion display and mRNA display [77]. In phage-display, the DNA coding for specific antibody fragments is fused to a phage protein coat gene, such as bacteriophage pIII gene of filamentous phage (M13 and Fd). Antibody fragments are displayed on the surface of the phage and are linked to the genetic information within the phage. The resultant phage library can contain billions of different antigenic specificities [77]. Phage libraries can be screened for antibody fragments by "biopanning" for a target analyte, and selected antibody fragments may then be recovered by growing the selected phage in pure culture [102, 103]. Antibody fragments selected *via* phage-display technology may possess a higher specificity, sensitivity, and stability than polyclonal and non-recombinant monoclonal antibodies [77, 104-106]. However, scFv and V_H fragments tend to form aggregate bodies [82]. While this is not as problematic for Fab, Fab tend to be less stable than scFv, though the stability of Fab can be improved by using a polypeptide linker between the Fd (fragment difficult) and the light chain to form a single-chain Fab (scFab) [107]. Antibody fragments may also require additional engineering to enhance stability to environmental stresses (*e.g.* [108]). Furthermore, producing antibody fragments in sufficient quantities can be difficult because some antibody fragments are poorly expressed in bacteria [105]. As a technique, phage display has been used to develop antibodies for a number of infectious agents (reviewed in Ref. [77,106] and see Table **3**). In addition, phage-displayed antibody fragments have been used in certain biosensors and may improve detection limits compared to antibody probes [98,109,110].

3.2. Phage-Displayed Oligopeptides, Landscape Phage Probes, and Engineered Affinity Proteins

Protein molecules other than antibodies can also be used to bind and recognize microbes. In particular, short peptides can function as biosensor probes when displayed on the surface of phages. As for antibody fragments, DNA for oligopeptides can be fused to the pIII, pVI, pVIII, or pIX genes of filamentous phage. Fusion to pIII protein, which is the most commonly used protein for phage display, allows the display of approximately five copies of the oligopeptide fragment on the polar ends of phages [103]. Fusion to the pVIII gene results in the display of almost 3000 copies of the oligopeptide per phage, and interactions among these numerous oligopeptide copies form a unique "landscape" on the phage surface. The high copy number of pVIII display results in greater avidity, but only short peptides (up to 12 amino acids) can be used in pVIII display without affecting the function of the pVIII protein [111]. More information on phage displayed peptides can be found in references [103,105,112,113].

Phage-displayed peptides have several advantages compared to antibody probes. First, the production of probes *via* phage display is relatively inexpensive and does not require probe re-engineering (as is the case with antibody fragments) in order to provide sufficient production capacity [103]. Second, peptides displayed on phages may be more thermodynamically stable than monoclonal antibodies [104] and are resistant to environmental stressors such as the presence of proteolytic enzymes and chemicals [111]. However, screening peptide libraries can be technically challenging, and choosing which actual peptides to screen is difficult [114,115]. Currently it is unclear whether phage-displayed antibody peptides have as high a sensitivity and specificity as other antibody types [116]. pIII and pVII phage-displayed oligopeptides have been selected to recognize *Bacillus anthracis* spores [115,117-119], though not with 100% specificity. Phage display of peptides has also been used in sensors to detect *E. coli* [120] and SEB [121]. See Table **3** for additional examples of oligopeptide probes.

In addition to oligopeptides, longer engineered proteins can also be used in biosensors [122-124]. Engineered affinity proteins include alpha-helix structures, such as affibodies, and peptides based on immunity proteins, cytochrome B, ankyrin repeat proteins, and proteins with irregular secondary structures [124,125]. To date, these affinity engineered proteins have been used primarily for the detection of human molecules [123] and rarely for the detection of microbes [126], but they could be used in biosensors in the future.

4. BIOSENSOR PLATFORMS

In this section, various types of biosensor platforms will be discussed with an emphasis on their reported sensitivity, throughput, and time-to-result for each technique (summarized in Table **4**). Sensitivity is the sensor's ability to detect a given quantity of a biological analyte and is expressed in either units of conconcentration *e.g.* organisms mL^{-1}, or surface density *e.g.* ng mm^{-2}. Throughput refers to the number of simultaneous assays that can be executed in a typical situation. Time-to-result is a function of both the size of the fluid volume in the sensor and the mixing techniques required for the analytes to attach to the sensing surface, this time will be reported whenever provided. Specificity is an issue not mentioned in this section as it is largely governed by probe:analyte interactions, interactoins that were described in the previous section. In principle, there are 3 types of biosensor technology platforms, namely; i) mass perturbance biosensors, ii) electrical perturbance biosensors, and iii) optical biosensor platforms. All of the platforms discussed here can be adapted for medical microbiology research and diagnosis.

Table 4: Biosensor Performance Characteristics

Technique	Analyte	Probe Type	Limit of Detection	Throughput	Time-to-result	Ref
Piezoelectric –QCM	*S. enterica* serovar Typhimurium	Landscape phage	100 cells mL^{-1}	1	200 sec	[144]
Piezoelectric –SAW	*Sin Nombre* virus (SNV)	Antibody	7000 particles	4	15 sec	[172]
Piezoelectri – Cantilever	*B. anthracis*	Antibody	300 spores mL^{-1}	1	120 sec	[173]
Piezoelectri – Cantilever	*Cryptosporidium parvum* oocyst	Antibody	1-10 oocyst(s)	1	<30 minutes (min)	[174]
Magnetoelastic	*E. coli* O157:H7	Antibody	100 cells mL^{-1}	4	< 2 hours	[175]
Magnetoelastic	SEB	Antibody	0.5 ng mL^{-1}	4	< 3 hours	[176]
Magnetoelastic	*B. anthracis spores*	Landscape phage	1000 CFU mL^{-1}	10	<15 min	[177]
Amperometric	*E. coli*	Antibody	100 cells mL^{-1}	1	30 min	[178]
Amperometric	*E. coli*	Antibody	100 cells mL^{-1}	1	10 min	[179]

Table 4: cont....

Potentiometric – LAPS	*Y. pestis* *B. globigii*	Antibody	10 cells 15 cells	1	<90 min, inferred	[180]
Potentiometric – LAPS	*B. subtilis*	Antibody	3×10^3 spores mL^{-1}	8	15 min	[118]
Potentiometric – LAPS	VEE	Biotinylated scFv	30 ng mL^{-1}	<4	< 90min	[181]
Impedance - EIS	*S. enterica* serovar Typhimurium	Antibody	10 CFU 100μL^{-1}	1	90 sec	[182]
SPR – prism	SEB Ricin *B. globigii*	Antibody	25 ng mL^{-1} 100 ng mL^{-1} 10^6 spores mL^{-1}	1	~20 min	[183]
SPR – prism	*B. subtilis*	Antibody	9×10^4 CFU mL^{-1}	24	<20 min	[80]
SPR – prism	Ricin	Antibody	200 ng mL^{-1}	1	10 min	[184]
SPR – prism	*E. coli* O157:H7, *S. enterica* serovar Typhimurium, *L. pneumophila, and Y. enterocolitica.*	Antibody	<100 CFU mL^{-1}	4	Not reported	[84]
SPR – prism	*S. aureus*	Lytic phage	10^4 CFU mL^{-1}	1	30 min	[185]
LSPR – Nanochip	Fibronegin	Antibody	100 pg mL^{-1}	300	~30 min	[186]
SPR-nanoarray MMN	Streptavidin	Bovine serum albumin	0.3 nM	4	<30 min	[187]
SPR – nanohole array Imager	Antibody for S-glutathione-S-transferase (GST)	GST	13 nM	25 spots (20,164 spots max)	<10 min	[188]
Optical Interferometry – IRIS	Influenza	Poly-L-lysine	One 100-nm virus under high magnification (mag). 26 pg mm^{-2} per spot of 150 kDa proteins (low mag) or 19 ng mL^{-1}	387	<10 min	[189] [190]

4.1. Mass Perturbance Biosensors

Biosensors that monitor mass-induced perturbations include piezoelectric cantilever arrays, Quartz Crystal Microbalance (QCM) sensors, Surface Acoustic Wave (SAW) devices, and magnetoelastic transducers.

4.1.1. Piezoelectric Sensors

Piezoelectric sensors, commonly referred to as "acoustic wave" or "microbalance" sensors, operate on the principle of efficiently coupling electrical and mechanical energy. In general, piezoelectric biosensors measure changes in the system's natural frequency of vibration, also termed the "resonance frequency". These changes can be caused by an alteration in mass and/or visco-elastic properties at a liquid-solid interface within the system when analyte binding takes place (see Fig. **6**). Further, bulk acoustic wave devices use the entire piezoelectric device for wave propagation, SAW devices operate by confining acoustic energy to a thin surface region on the substrate. In bulk acoustic wave devices, the maximum amplitude of vibration occurs at the top and bottom faces of the crystal, enabling the device to function as a surface detector, typically at frequencies of 10 to 50 MHz. The most common type of bulk acoustic wave device is the QCM sensor, due largely to quartz's tolerance for high temperatures. In SAW devices, acoustic energy confinement is generated and detected using interdigital transducers located on the surface of a piezoelectric crystal (see Fig. **6**). In contrast to bulk wave devices, most SAW devices oscillate at higher resonance frequencies, between 50 MHz and several GHz. The relationship between the change in resonance frequency and mass adsorbed on the SAW device is defined by the Sauerbrey equation:

$$\Delta f = (- 2.3 \times 10^6 \ F^2 \ \Delta m) \ A^{-1}$$

where F is the resonance frequency in MHz, Δm is the mass change in grams, and A is the coated sensing area in cm^2 [191]. It follows that for a given sensing surface area, a SAW device will be more sensitive the higher the frequency of the device. In general, the amount of analyte mass adsorbed by the probe determines the magnitude of change in the oscillator circuit frequency. Interested readers are referred to a comprehensive review of the last 20 years work in this acoustic wave research [192-194]. As an example, to detect *S. enterica* serovar Typhimurium, Olsen *et al.* [144] immobilized a pathogen-specific landscape phage and demonstrated the usefulness of a phage-displayed probe bound to an acoustic wave device. The phage was attached to the transducer *via* physical adsorption and tested against *S. enterica*. The time-to-result was approximately 200 seconds, with a limit of detection of 100 cells mL^{-1}. Similarly, to detect *Sin Nombre* Virus (SNV), Bisoffi *et al.* [172] immobilized monoclonal antibodies to a hand-portable SAW device with a resonance frequency of 325 MHz and demonstrated virus binding from 0.4 mL of sewage samples that were spiked with SNV. The time-to-result was 15 seconds of virus injection with a limit of detection of 7000 SNV particles. In addition, the SAW sensor showed a log-linear dose-response relationship that spanned up to three orders of magnitude in SNV concentrations [particles uL^{-1}]: 1.8×10^1– 1.8×10^4, R^2=0.95. Investigators verified the specificity of their probes by introducing high concentrations of HSV-1 virus (~3.6×10^6 particles uL^{-1}) as a confounding agent, yet observed no false positive effects. Further, the SAW device was able to detect analytes after surface regeneration using organic solvents, ultrasound, and ultraviolet-ozone. Unfortunately, although surface regeneration is a useful feature for real-time environmental testing, it may not be appropriate for clinical applications due to the possibility of residual contamination Fig. **6**.

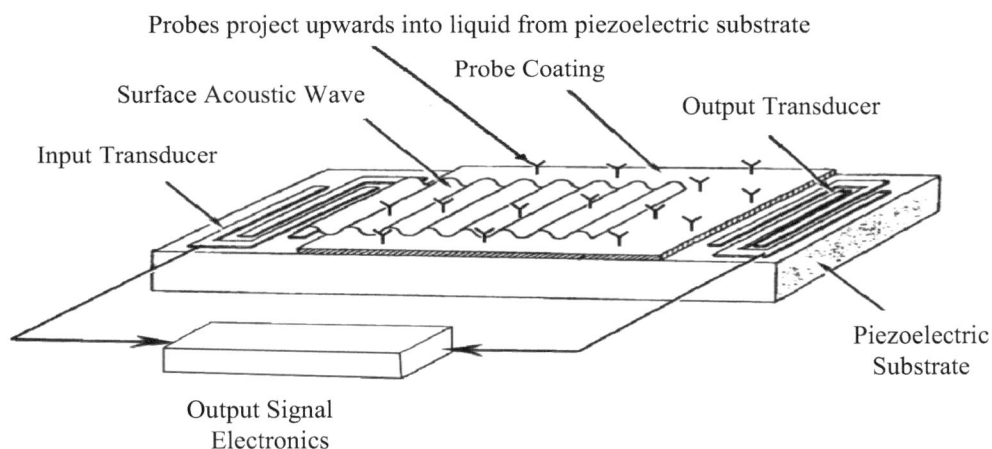

Probes project upwards into liquid from piezoelectric substrate

Probe Coating

Surface Acoustic Wave

Output Transducer

Input Transducer

Output Signal Electronics

Piezoelectric Substrate

Fig. (6). Schematic representation of the principle behind a surface acoustical wave sensor. The transducers are part of an oscillator circuit whose frequency is determined by the speed of the acoustic wave in the quartz substrate. An input transducer generates a SAW that propagates to the output transducer and is fed back through an amplifier. Perturbations at the surface of the piezoelectric crystal induce a detectable change in the resonance frequency of the device and provide information for analysis of the interaction between the probe:analyte. Reprinted with permission from Ref. [75].

The Piezoelectric-Excited Millimeter-Sized Cantilever (PEMC), developed by Campbell and Mutharasan [173], measures changes in resonance frequency caused by an alteration in mass when an analyte binds to the sensing surface. The cantilevers are constructed of a layer of zircon titanite (PZT) bonded to a glass cover slip [195]. To detect *B. anthracis* spores [173], the cantilever surface is cleaned and treated to bond with a *B. anthracis* spore–specific antibody probe. The time-to-result is approximately 120 seconds, with a reported limit of detection of 300 spores mL^{-1}. Campbell and colleagues also analyzed the PEMC sensor for detection of *B. anthracis* spores in a flow cell [196]. Investigators determined that the binding rate between spores and antibodies increased five-fold in the flow cell compared to static conditions. Finally, to detect *Cryptosporidium parvum* oocysts, the cantilever surface was functionalized by adding a specific IgM antibody probe. The time-to-result was under 30 minutes, with a limit of detection of 1-10 oocysts [174].

4.1.2. Magnetoelastic Sensors

Magnetoelastic sensors (Fig. **7**), typically constructed from amorphous ferromagnetic ribbons or wires that efficiently couple magnetic and mechanical energy, measure changes in resonance frequency caused by analyte binding. Magnetoelastic sensors operate on the general principle that when a time-modulated magnetic field is applied to a magnetoelastic material, it exhibits a mechanical vibration with a dominant characteristic resonance frequency. This resonance frequency is dependent on the shape, physical dimensions and mass of the sensor. The binding of the biological analyte to the surface of the sensor causes a drop in the sensor resonance frequency which can be described by the equation in which M is the initial mass of the sensor, Δm is the mass change, and Δf is the change in resonance frequency [175].

$$\Delta f = -f\left(\Delta m \, (2M)^{-1}\right)$$

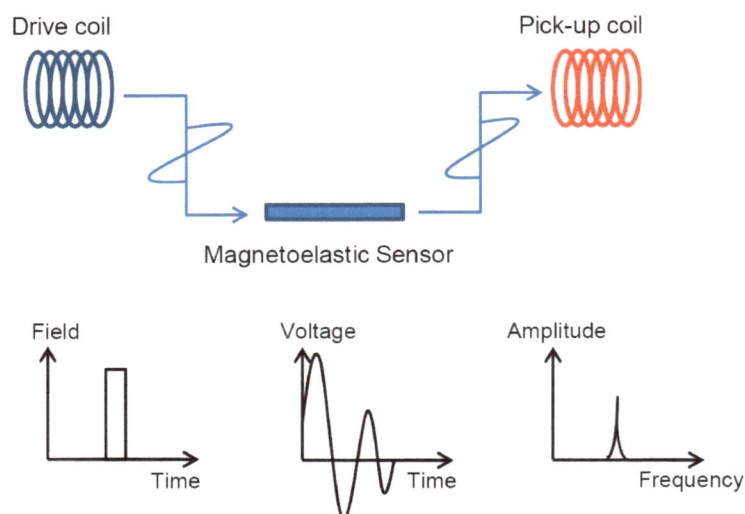

Fig. (7). Schematic representation of the principle behind a magnetoelastic sensor (adapted from [175]). A magnetic pulse is generated when an analyte makes contact with the probe. This impulse is converted by the sensor transducer to a frequency and provides information for analysis of the interaction between the probe:analyte. Reprinted with permission from Ref. [75].

To detect *E. coli* O157:H7, specific antibodies were covalently attached to a 370 kHz magnetoelastic sensor surface (dimensions 6 mm x 1 mm x 28 μm), followed by pathogen introduction and a secondary alkaline phosphatase (AP) labeled anti-*E. coli* O157:H7 antibody. The resulting resonance frequency was then measured [175]. The time-to-result was approximately 2 hours, with a limit of detection of 100 *E. coli* O157:H7 cells mL^{-1} and a log-linear dose-response relationship across the range of 10^2–10^6 bacterial cells mL^{-1}. To detect staphylococcal enterotoxin Type B [197], anti-SEB antibody was covalently attached to the magnetoelastic sensor surface, followed by toxin introduction, secondary biotin-labeled anti-SEB antibody, and AP-labeled avidin [176]. The time-to-result was approximately 3 hours, with a limit of detection of 0.5 ng mL^{-1} and a linear dose-response relationship across the range of 0.5 to 5 ng mL^{-1} of SEB. To detect *B. anthracis* spores, filamentous landscape phage probes were adsorbed onto the surface of an iron-boron alloy-based magnetoelastic sensor [177], followed by increasing concentrations of spore injection. The time-to-result was approximately 15 minutes, with a limit of detection of 1000 Colony Forming Units (CFU) mL^{-1} and a log-linear dose-response relationship across the range of 10^3–10^7 CFU mL^{-1}

4.2. Electrical Perturbance Biosensors

Biosensors that detect electrical perturbances include amperometric, potentiometric, and impedance-based platforms, which measure changes in current, voltage, impedance and/or capacitance, respectively. For all of these platform types, a probe:analyte interaction results in a perturbance at the sensing interface, which is measured by a transducer.

4.2.1. Amperometric Devices

Amperometric devices operate on the principle of analyte-induced current changes while keeping the transducer potential constant [191,198]. They are commonly used to detect blood sugar levels [199, 200], though they also possess the potential to detect disease causing microbiological agents [178,179, 201-203]. For example, Abdel-Hamid *et al.* [178], detected *E. coli* O157:H7 using an amperometric immunofiltration sensor that was coated with primary antibody on a disposable filter [178]. Cells were captured by the primary antibody as the bacterial sample passed through the filter. Next, an enzyme-conjugated secondary antibody was added, giving rise to a chemical reaction that produced a shift in current that increased monotonically with conjugate concentration. This amperometric immunofiltration sensor is simple and rapid. The time-to-result was under 30 minutes with a limit of detection of 100 cells mL^{-1} and a working range up to 600 cells mL^{-1}. Further, Sippy *et al.* used a similar amperometric immunofiltration sensor to measure *E. coli* O55 [179]. They were able to reduce the time-to-result to 10 minutes by using a lateral flow immunoassay rather than a filter membrane during the capture step [179]. Comparable to the previous work by Abdel-Hamid *et al.* [178], Sippy *et al.* also determined that the limit of detection was 100 cells mL^{-1}. Overall, these amperometric immune-biosensors are potentially portable and could be used to identify other important infectious agents in the field. Nonetheless, a limiting factor for this type of biosensor platform is the availability of primary antibodies for the target agents.

4.2.2. Potentiometric Devices

Potentiometric sensors are typically able to make sensitive measurements of low analyte concentrations due to their logarithmic dose-response curves [191]. One particular type, the Light Addressable Potentiometric Sensor (LAPS), initially described by Hafeman *et al.* in 1988 is highly sensitive (1 amol) and rapid (< 2 min) [204]. This high sensitivity is due in part to the relative uniformity of its surface potential which results in signal stability and the ability of the sensor to detect small concentrations of the analyte. A commercially available LAPS instrument (Molecular Devices; [205]) has successfully detected *Y. pestis* and *B. globigii* using an antibody-mediated capture filtration method [180]. Here, immunocomplexes were formed on a nitrocellulose filter comprising biotinylated primary antibodies, the analytes and secondary antibodies. A pH change that takes place in the presence of urea is monitored as a function of time and expressed as a rate ($\mu V\ s^{-1}$). Thus, the signal generated is directly proportional to the quantity of immunocomplex (hence analyte) that is formed and captured. The time-to-result was not reported. The sensor's limit of detection was 10 cells for *Y. pestis* and 15 spores for *B. globigii*. Using a similar approach, Uithoven *et al.* reported a time-to-result in under 15 minutes with a limit of detection of 3×10^{3} spores mL^{-1} for *B. subtilis* [118]. Lastly, to detect Venezuelan equine encephalitis virus, Hu *et al.* successfully employed biotinylated scFv using the same platform. The time-to-result was under 90 minutes with a detection limit of 30 ng mL^{-1} [181].

4.2.3. Impedance Devices

Impedance-based platforms operate on the concept of Electrochemical Impedance Spectroscopy (EIS). This technique monitors changes in the electrochemical property (*i.e.* impedance) of the sample during the application of an externally applied Alternating Current (AC). The impedance can be determined from measuring the electrochemical current at the electrode upon application of the external AC potential *e.g.* 5 mV, at a set of frequencies *e.g.* 1-100 KHz [182]. In the context of a biosensor, the probe would be attached to an electrode, and any sustained changes would occur in response to an analyte binding event. To detect *S. enterica* serovar Typhimurium using EIS, a mass-fabricated gold-electrode was covalently immobilized using monoclonal antibodies specific for the surface exposed lipopolysaccharide of *Salmonella*. The time-to-result was under 90 seconds, with a limit of detection of 10 CFU [182]. To expand on the throughput of EIS, another research group developed a method to fabricate an array of ten electrodes and to functionalize two different types of peptides onto the electrode array [206]. Preliminary results measured from proteins in whole cell lysates suggest there is promise for EIS to be a label-free, scalable, and affordable biosensor platform. However, more research is needed to understand the underlying mechanisms that give rise to binding-induced impedance changes.

4.3. Optical

Biosensors that monitor optical perturbations include label-free and label-based detection techniques. The term "label" here refers to the use of visualizable molecules that are attached to either the analyte or to the probe, and provide information on the status of probe:analyte binding. Label-free detection techniques directly measure the optical parameters that change upon analyte binding, and are therefore not reliant on analyte or probe labeling. Popular label-free adaptations monitor changes in the index of refraction induced by analyte binding at a sensor surface (*e.g.* surface plasmon resonance), or changes in the height of a biological layer situated on top of the sensor surface (*e.g.* spectral reflectance interferometric imaging). Label-based detection techniques commonly rely on the attachment of fluorescent molecules to probes. If the label is attached to a secondary probe, then analyte may be indirectly measured *via* the fluorescence levels of secondary labelled molecules that have bound to the antigen(s) of interest. The normal setup involves an antigen-sandwich configuration with an unlabeled primary probe bound to the sensor surface and the secondary labeled probe binding to the analyte. Although label-based detection is extremely sensitive, it requires additional preparation steps, expensive reagents, and there is a capacity for potential functional interference upon the addition of a label to the probe. Indeed, the need to use labeled probe-based technologies to achieve adequate sensitivity is creating some of the greatest challenges in quantitative clinical biological analysis today [207]. In the following subsection, we will focus on two types of label-free detection techniques that we believe have the greatest promise for achieving the required sensitivity in massively parallel clinical diagnosis.

4.3.1. Surface Plasmon Resonance

Surface Plasmon Resonance (SPR) is the most popular label-free optical analyte detection technique used in many research laboratories that was first conceptualized in 1983 [208]. Surface Plasmons (SPs) are electron density waves formed at the interface of a metal (*e.g.* a thin layer of gold) and a dielectric material (*e.g.* glass). The electron density wave interacts with an electromagnetic wave and together they form a plasmonic standing wave at this interface which decays exponentially into both materials. The penetration depth refers to the distance that the plasmon wave decays into the material.

Here we consider only the penetration depth of the plasmon wave into the dielectric material (*i.e.* towards analytes in solution). Typically, SPs are characterized by using polarized light to optically measure changes in the refractive index that arise from analyte binding at the liquid and metal-coated interface of a prism [209, 210]. The penetration depth is a function of the illumination wavelength and material properties. For example, the depth into the dielectric for gold is under 160 nm or 400 nm for an excitation of 630 or 850 nm, respectively [211]. There are two common methods to excite and monitor SPs in biosensing: i) wavelength interrogation, in which the excitation angle of incidence is fixed and the reflected photons are monitored across a set of excitation wavelengths; and ii) angle interrogation, in which the illumination wavelength is fixed and the reflected photons are measured across a set of reflectance angles along the optical receiver path. The most common SPR method uses the prism-based Kretschmann-Raether geometry (Fig. **8**) [212], wherein fluidics channels are commonly constructed to abut the thin gold layer where probe molecules for the target analytes are anchored (illustrated as antibodies in Fig. **8** inset). Perturbations in the refractive index occur when the analytes introduced into the fluidics channel bind to the fixed layer of receptors within the penetration depth at the metal and dielectric interface. These refractive index perturbations give rise to a shift in the SPR wavelength (or a shift in the reflected light as a function of incidence angle). The magnitude of the SPR shift can be correlated to the number of analytes bound.

Although the advantages of direct, label-free, SPR measurements are substantial, some groups have reported on the use of secondary antibodies [183, 184], whilst others have even coupled secondary antibodies to latex spheres or gold beads in order to further amplify the SPR signal [209]. To measure SEB, ricin, and *B. globigii* spores, Anderson *et al.* employed a wavelength-interrogation, prism-based, SPR system in conjunction with antibodies as probes and secondary antibodies to amplify the SPR signal [183]. The time-to-result was approximately 20 minutes, with limits of detection for SEB, ricin, and *B. globigii* of 25 ng mL^{-1}, 100 ng mL^{-1}, and 10^6 spores mL^{-1}, respectively. The investigators further reported that they were able to obtain up to 5 regenerations for each gold surface without any loss of function. Similarly,

Chinowsky *et al.* employed a 24-analyte prism-based SPR sensor to measure *B. subtilis* [80]. The time-to-result was under 20 minutes including the secondary antibody incubation period, with a limit of detection of 9×10^4 CFU mL^{-1}. More recently, Feltis *et al.* [184] utilized a portable, wireless prism-based SPR system to detect ricin with antibody probes and secondary anti -ricin antibodies. The time-to-result was 10 minutes with a detection limit of 200ng mL^{-1}.

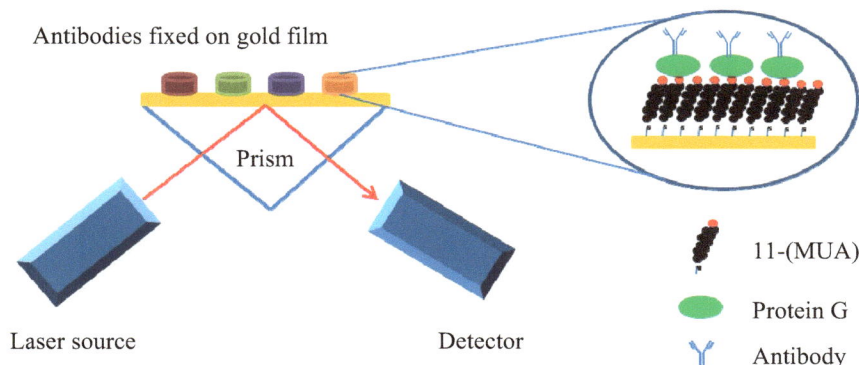

Fig. (8). Schematic representation of a prism-based Surface Plasmon Resonance (SPR) sensor (adapted from [84]). A typical SPR schematic consists of a prism with one side coated with a thin layer of gold (<100 nm), to which probes such as antibodies are bound. The prism is illuminated at an oblique angle through one of the uncoated sides. Reflected photons are monitored by a photo detector that collects the photons emitted from the uncoated side of the prism. Binding of an analyte leads to a change in the refractive index within the penetration depth, which results in a shift in the reflected light measured as a function of the incidence angle. Reprinted with permission from [75].

To develop a multiplex prism-based SPR system, Oh *et al.* [84], attached monoclonal antibody probes to separate patches of a gold sensing surface and simultaneously monitored the binding of *E. coli* O157:H7, *S. enterica* serovar Typhimurium, *L. pneumophila*, and *Y. enterocolitica*. The chips were exposed to approximately 10^5 CFU mL^{-1} of the various pathogens and the refractive SPR angles were measured. Based on the shift in the SPR angle that resulted from binding of a particular pathogen to its cognate antibody, the investigators were able to differentiate the interaction of specific probe:analyte pairs. To detect *S. aureus*, Balasubramanian *et al.* [185] used a lytic phage (bacteriophage ATCC 12600) adsorbed to a prism-based SPR system (SPREETA^{TM}). The time-to-result was approximately 30 minutes, with a limit of detection of 10^4 CFU mL^{-1} and a log-linear dose-response relationship ranging across 10^4 to 10^7 CFU mL^{-1}. Moreover, because the probe used was a natural *S. aureus* phage, the interactions were very specific and suggested the potential of this biosensor for real-world applications.

To increase sensitivity and multiplexity, Endo *et al.* developed a localized SPR (LSPR) nano-scale microarray chip, containing 300 spots, that can be deposited with an assortment of antibodies for multiplexing capabilities [186]. The time-to-result was just over 30 minutes with a limit of detection of 100 pg mL^{-1} and a linear dose-response relationship up to 100 µg mL^{-1}. This highly sensitive biosensing platform is both affordable and has a small packaging footprint. Further, it only requires small amount of reagent fluid, which is critical to field deployment. The continued development of direct label-free LSPR substrates will likely make hand-portable sensor devices possible for both biosecurity applications and point-of-care diagnostics. Moreover, recent advances in nanofabrication techniques have made it possible to excite surface plasmons using metallic subwavelength structures and nanoparticles instead of conventional metal-coated prism couplings [188, 209, 213, 214]. Extraordinary optical transmission through sub-wavelength nanohole arrays also has the potential for high-throughput biosensing [188, 215-221], and an example schematic from the Fainman lab at the University of California, San Diego is shown in Fig. **9**. Hwang *et al.* demonstrated rapid protein-carbohydrate (ovomucoid:concanavalin A) and protein:protein (BSA:anti-BSA) binding at the Fainman lab [218]. The time-to-result was under 10 minutes with a limit of detection of 5.3 µM and 190 nM, respectively. More recently, Fainman's group demonstrated the potential of a variant of the nanohole array termed the "composite mushroom-like metallo-dielectric nanostructure" (MMN) [187]. The time-to-result for Fainman's laboratory set-up was under 30 minutes with a limit of detection of 0.3 nM for the model protein avidin. To demonstrate multi-spot SPR-imaging using a model probe:analyte pair, yet another research group covalently attached S-glutathione-S-transferase (GST) to a self-assembled monolayer situated on top of their nanohole array [188]. Using antibodies for GST, Ji *et al.* reported a time-to-result in under 10 minutes with a limit of detection of 13 nM. In fact, several companies already sell multi-analyte prism-based SPR instruments [212, 222-225], each with varying performance and limited throughput. The authors anticipate that further biosensor research into two-dimensional grating coupler SPR and LSPR systems will be readily miniaturizable, allowing massively parallel processing that will reduce time-to-result, improve the limit of detection, and increase the dynamic range of analyte concentrations that are measureable for quantitative clinical applications.

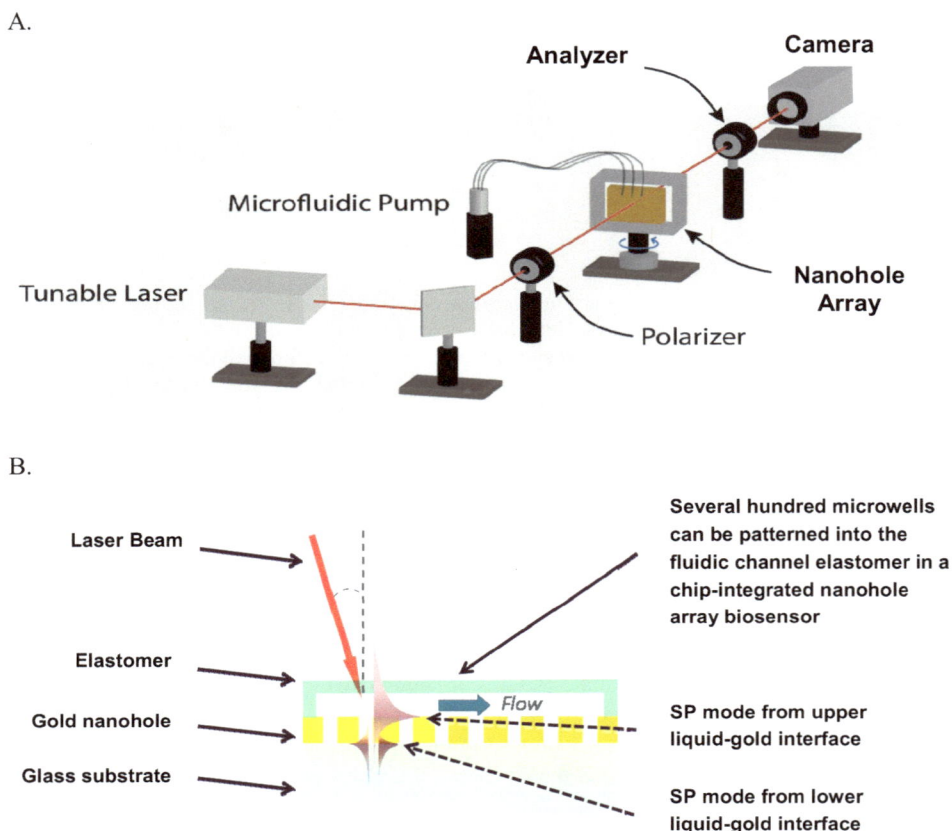

Fig. (9). Schematic representation of a nanohole SPR system. A. A nanohole sample is inserted between a polarizer-analyzer pair. A collimated tunable infrared laser beam, matched to the periodicity of the nanohole substrate, is used to illuminate the sample. Transmitted photons are measured by an InGaAs photodiode or camera. The optical setup can be integrated into an on-chip portable instrument to perform for example, multi-analyte, label-free, lectin screening or influenza typing. B. A side schematic of the gold nanohole array. Spacing of nanoholes on glass ~ 1.5 μm. Nanohole diameter ~300 nm. Gold film thickness ranges between 150 and 200 nm. Figures are illustrated by Joe Monaco (A) and Elaine Mullen (B).

4.3.2. Interferometric Biosensors

Optical interferometric biosensing is a detection technique that relies on a phase shift, or optical path-length difference, that occurs as a result of analyte binding. Several types of optical interferometer biosensors have been investigated including Mach-Zehnder, Young's, and Hartman [226]. In this respect, some of the affordable and readily scalable optical path-length interferometric biosensors that utilize label-free detection will now be discussed.

A.

B.

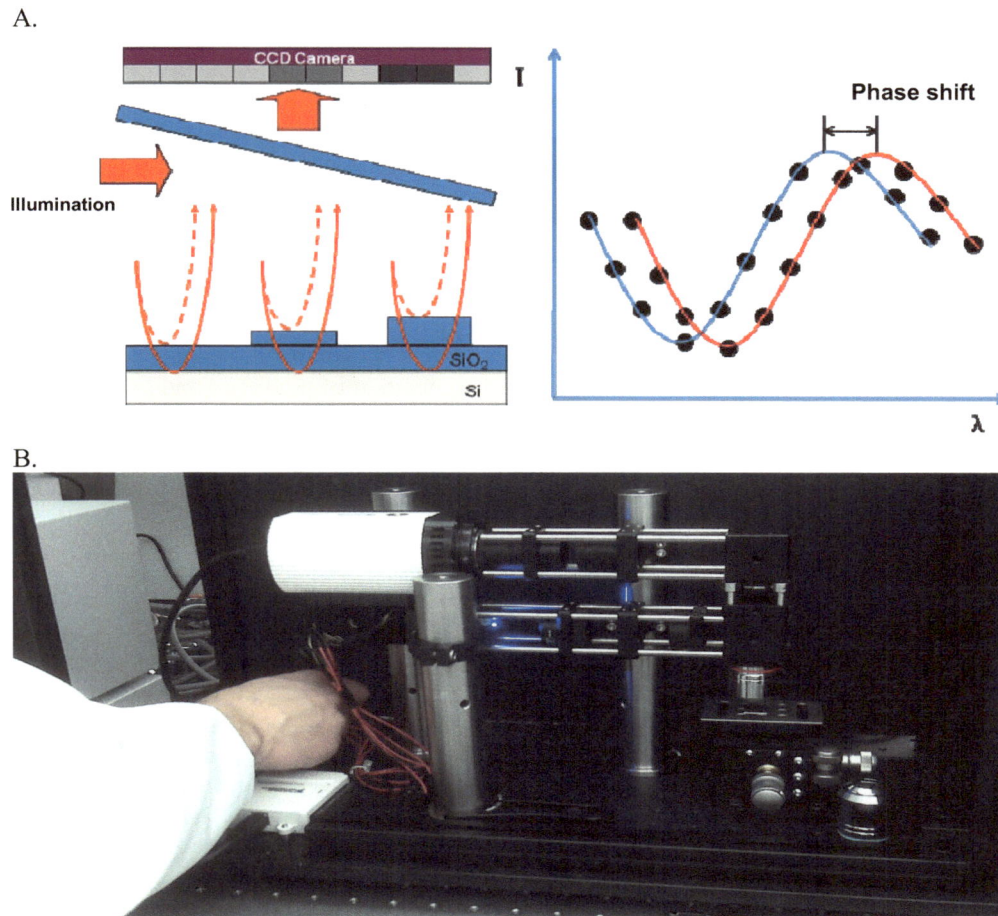

Fig. (10). A. Principle of the IRIS technology: light reflected off a Si/SiO_2 surface is imaged by a CCD. The interference pattern is created using 3 or more spectrally separated LED wavelengths in the blue through red region. A shift in phase of the interference pattern indicates an accumulation of biomass on the surface. Figures are adapted with permission from [190]. "Label-free and dynamic detection of biomolecular interactions for high-throughput microarray applications" by Ozkumur *et al.*, Proc Natl Acad Sci U S A. 2008;105 (23): 7988-7992. © Copyright 2008 National Academy of Sciences U.S.A. B. Photograph of IRIS prototype by G. Hwang.

The MITRE Corporation is currently working with Boston University to adapt an LED-based Interferometric Reflectance Imaging Sensor (IRIS) for intact virus and antigen detection [189, 227, 228]. As shown in the schematic in Fig. **10A**, a silicon (Si) chip with a Silicon Dioxide (SiO_2) layer is serially illuminated by a set of 3 or more spectrally separated LED's to allow accurate sampling of the interference curve. Interference from the layered substrate is imaged as a modulation in the acquired intensity at each pixel on the CCD camera for each of the different LEDs. The reflected intensity images of the Si/SiO_2 chip for each pixel are fitted to a formula based on the Fresnel reflection coefficients to calculate the optical path length through the top of the SiO_2 surface [190]. If a layer of biomass accumulates on the surface, the interference curve shifts due to the added optical path length of the top layer. Using a calibrated system, the shift in phase can be used to estimate the amount of accumulated biomass. A photograph of the IRIS prototype is presented in Fig. **10B**. There are several advantages of the IRIS device. First, unlike SPR or other waveguide sensors, which are sensitive to variations in temperature or buffer refractive indices (referred to as bulk effect), IRIS is insensitive to these factors because the reflected rays that give rise to the phase-shift are co-propagating. Second, the device can operate in high and low magnification to achieve label-free, sub-diffraction limited, single pathogen detection, or protein, quantification [190]. This results in a larger overall system dynamic range and a lower limit of detection per spot. The time-to-result for acquiring and processing data for virus detection and protein detection are both under 10 minutes. The limits of detection in high and low magnification are a single 100-nm virus particle and 26 pg mm^{-2}, respectively. In single particle detection modality, the IRIS system is capable of distinguishing particles of 70, 100, 150, and 200nm in diameter. This is based on an experimental demonstration using a mixture of different sized polystyrene spheres [227]. Third, the Si/SiO_2 chip can be spotted with an array of different biological receptors, whereby the system can simultaneously measure the detection of multiple analytes, or alternatively may make control measurements with respect to the detection of a single analyte. To date, up to 1000 spots have been measured simultaneously, yet calculations indicate that approximately 10,000 spots can be Imaged, based on a 10 mega-pixel camera [190].

In addition to the work on single particle detection for influenza viruses, Boston University has demonstrated IRIS detection of: i) single-nucleotide DNA polymorphisms from strand denaturation kinetics; ii) transcription factor (TATA binding protein) recognition of consensus binding sequences in a microarray format; and iii) viral antigen- and whole virion-detection of vesicular stomatitis virus [229, 230]. Currently, prototype instruments of the IRIS can be acquired from Zoiray Technologies Inc. [231]. However, 510(k) FDA approval has not yet been obtained.

5. POINT-OF-CARE TESTING (POCT) IN MEDICAL MICROBIAL DIAGNOSIS

Peptide-based probes already play an essential role in rapid POCT in clinical settings, most commonly in the form of either immunochromatographic tests or enzyme-linked immunosorbent assays that provide results in under 30 minutes [47]. POCT solutions already exist for a variety of diseases, including HIV, *Legionella, Streptococci, Plasmodium falciparum* (malaria), and influenza [74]. In this section, POCT sensors are considered to be a class of biosensors that operate on visual inspection and this section focuses on the utility of POCTs for rapid diagnosis of influenza from human samples. Until now, biosensors have been characterized based on sensitivity, specificity, speed of analysis and other parameters listed in Table **4**. Here, clinically relevant terms to characterize POCTs are employed including sensitivity, specificity, Positive Predictive Value (PPV) and Negative Predictive Value (NPV). Sensitivity refers to the percentage of true influenza cases detected by the POCT. Specificity refers to the percentage of true negative cases that actually test negative (usually in comparison with a "gold" standard). PPV is a measure of the percentage of positive tests in which the identified disease-causing agent is actually present in the sample. NPV is a measure of the percentage of negative test results in which no identified disease-causing agent is actually present in the sample. PPVs and NPVs are values that change with disease prevalence across time and are useful to clinicians in interpreting results and informing their diagnostic decision making. However, because PPVs and NPVs are unique to the particular disease outbreak, one should be cautious in using PPVs and NPVs to evaluate POCT across different studies unless the different studies have comparable disease prevalence and severity [74]. Studies have shown that PPV improves for rapid influenza POCT testing with higher actual prevalences of circulating influenza in the population [74, 232]. Thus, POCT for influenza should have a higher probability of improving patient care during the flu season, although this is still a matter of debate among clinical practitioners [232]. Nevertheless, the World Health Organization recommends POCT to complement the rapid distribution of antiviral medication for treatment purposes [233].

As shown in Table **5**, POCT testing for Influenza A is reported to yield sensitivities as low as 11.1%. However, specificity is generally quite good with most studies reporting values between 82% and 100% (despite one anomalous study reporting a surprisingly poor test specificity of 2.7% [234]). Variability in sample quality and user experience can give rise to anomalous findings on POCT performance. In addition, POCT has been shown to be more effective for tests of nasal aspirate samples than throat swab samples [235, 236], indicating that the origin of a sample could give rise to a large variance in both sensitivity and specificity. In spite of ongoing debate on when POCT should be employed in light of the lessons learned from the 2009 H1N1 influenza outbreak [237, 238], the authors expect peptide-based biosensor-related POCT testing to become more commonplace in the clinical setting. Furthermore, given that most hospitals cannot afford to have real-time PCR on-site, POCT (at least for influenza diagnosis) should eventually provide a more cost-effective alternative. However, currently, most influenza POCT test kit vendors suggest that all negative POCT results should be confirmed by cell culture and/or other gold standard techniques.

6. DETERMINATION OF THE LIMIT OF DETECTION

Scientists who develop biosensors frequently report the Limit of Detection (LoD) of their technical platforms in a variety of units of measurements (*i.e.* concentration, absolute number counts, surface number density). There is no universally accepted figure-of-merit or standard that all scientists follow to quantify their instrument's LoD for a variety of factors, including how the sample is actually processed after it enters the biosensor. Some biosensors do not require fluidic manipulations, so their LoD determination can be based on the concentration of the analyte during the initial stages of biosensor-processing.

Table 5: Summary of POCT for Influenza A.

POCT Name	Sens (%)	Spec (%)	PPV (%)	NPV (%)	Comments
BinaxNOW Inf A+B [239]	59-71	98-99	91-93	88-92	Study size=521. 338 nasopharyngeal swabs, 162 throat swabs, 19 nasal washes, 2 unspecified [236]. Gold standard = cell culture.
			97-100	83-93	
Directigen Flu A+B [240]	53-67	99.7-100	86-89	89-99	
		97-98			
Direct Immunofluorescence (DFA) [241]	80-97				
Remel Xpert Flu A+B	47	86	92	32	Study size = 63 patients [242].
BinaxNOW or 3M Rapid Detection A&B	17.8	93.6	77.4	47.9	Study size = 6090 patients between the age of 4 and 98 years. 4369 samples submitted for POCT. This study was part of a New York city study during a 5-week period in response to the novel H1N1 outbreak [245]. R-Mix culture and Luminex xTAG Respiratory Panel served as gold standards in this study.
DFA	46.7	94.5	91.3	58.9	
R-Mix culture [41, 243]	88.9	100	100	87.9	
Luminex xTAG Respiratory Panel [244]	97.8	100	100	97.3	
R-Mix Culture	96.9	100	100	99.3	Study size = 500 patients between the age of 5 and 99 years [247].
DFA	80.4	99.2	96.1	95.3	
3M Influenza A+B [246]	70.1	99.8	98.6	93	
BinaxNOW Influenza A+B	46.4	100	100	88.6	
3M Influenza A+B	75	98	88	95	Study size = 249 patients [248].
Quidel QuickVue Influenza A+B	73	99.5	96.7	95	
BinaxNOW Influenza A+B	55	100	100	92	
SD Bioline Influenza Ag Test Kit [249]	63	100	99	78	Study size = 561 patients between the age of 2 and 83 years [250].
BinaxNOW Influenza A+B	47	95	NR	NR	Study size = 135 patients between the age of 0 and 81 years [251].
BinaxNOW Influenza A+B	11.1	NR	NR	NR	Retrospective - Study size. 144 clinical samples in patients with pandemic H1N1 2009 virus [252].
Binax Now Influenza A+B	73	99	97	91	Study size = 177 patients [235]. Gold standards = immunofluorescence, cell culture and real-time RT-PCR.
Directigen EZ Flu A+B	69	100	100	90	
Denka Seiken Quick Ex-Flu	71	100	100	90	
Fujirebio Espline Influenza A+B-N [253]	67	100	100	89	
Rockeby Influenza A Antigen Test [254]	10	100	100	74	
QuidelQuickVue Influenza A+B [255]	67	100	100	89	
Quidel QuickVue Influenza A+B	48.7	96.5	88.6	77.3	Study size = 231 clinical nasopharyngeal wash samples. Gold standard = RT-PCR [256].
Quidel QuickVue Influenza A+B	53.4-77.2	100	100	76.2-92	Study size = 500 specimens from patients with influenza like illness [257].
Quidel QuickVue Influenza A+B	66	84	84	64	Study size = 703 patients between the age of 0 and 80 years [258].

Table 5: cont....

	Sens.	Spec.	PPV	NPV	
Quidel QuickVue Influenza A+B	93	100	100	92	Study size = 102 respiratory samples [259]. Values shown are for cell culture as gold standard.
Z Stat Flu	70.1	92.4	76.3	89.9	Study size = 479 samples [260].
Directigen Flu A	95	84	86	94	Study size = 116 samples [262].
Z Stat Flu	72	83	80	75	
Quidel Quickvue Influenza A+B	95	76	81	93	
Flu OIA [261]	93	82	84	92	
Directigen Flu A	86	94	89	92	Study size = 192 patients [263]. Values shown are for cell culture as gold standard.
Quickvue Influenza A+B	91	86	78	95	
BinaxNOW Influenza A+B	93.9	65	43.1	97.4	Study size = 336 patients between the age of 0 and 88 years during the first five weeks of the 2009 H1N1 outbreak. Gold standard = Luminex xTAG Respiratory Viral Panel [234].
Truflu	100	37.5	57.1	100	
Xpect [264]	92.3	2.7	25	50	
Quidel QuickVue Influenza A+B	100	46.4	81	100	
Directigen EZ Flu A+B	46.7	100	100	89.6	Study size = 84 nasopharyngeal samples collected during the first five weeks of the 2009 H1N1 outbreak. Gold standard = Luminex xTAG Respiratory Viral Panel [265].
BinaxNOW Influenza A+B	38.3	100	100	88.2	
Quidel QuickVue Influenza A+B	53.3	100	100	90.8	
Directigen Flu A+B	66	99	93	85	Study size = 178 respiratory samples [266].
Directigen EZ Flu A+B	41	97	56	89	
BinaxNOW Influenza A+B	73	95	93	81	
Quidel QuickVue Influenza A+B	30.9	92.2	48.6	84.9	Study size = 287 specimens. Gold standard = RT-PCR. Note: Only information from Site #3 of this study is summarised [267].

Legend: Sens. refers to sensitivity - the percentage of true influenza cases detected by the test. Spec. refers to pecificity – the percentage of true negative cases that actually test negative (usually in comparison with a "gold" standard). Positive Predictive Value (PPV) refers to the percentage of positive test results that correctly corroborates the patient's disease state. Negative Predictive Value (NPV) refers to the percentage of negative cases that correctly corroborates the patient's disease state. NR represents values not reported.

This assumption does not hold in every case. In some cases, a starting analyte concentration can be altered before it is actually exposed to the sensing element. Further, dependant on the fluidics construction of the biosensor platform, some analytes may also be lost. Other analytes may be exposed to the sensing surface but do not come into close enough contact with the sensing element to be captured by the probe for detection. The probability that analytes will contact the sensing surface is a function of time and mixing. This is complicated by the fact that neither sample incubation/mixing time nor the time-to-result are standardized across label-free biosensors. Another inherent variable is the signal-to-noise ratio of the detection system which additionally determines how much of the analyte needs to be deposited on the sensing element, mediated by the probe, before a statistically significant signal can be measured. Here, we do not try to resolve the issues surrounding the ambiguity in LoD determinations, but in this section, we present an established method for determining the LoD in the clinical laboratory in the hopes that scientists and engineers who develop biosensors will start to adhere to a standard method. Until standardized methods are used, it will be difficult to compare biosensor performance across different detection platforms. The method presented is taken from the Clinical and Laboratory Standards Institute's guidance EP17-A [268]. In statistics, the probability of a false positive occurring is referred to as the Alpha (α) or Type I error rate. The probability of a false negative occurring is called the Beta (β) or Type II error rate. In order to determine the LoD for a biosensor, we must first establish acceptable values for these error rates. We then determine the Limit of the Blank (LoB), which is a detection threshold for the distribution of results from a series of blank samples devoid of any analyte (*i.e.* 0% concentration), such that the resultant false positive rate matches the acceptable α value. The LoD is then computed as the lowest amount of analyte that the instrument reads such that the probability of results less than the LoB matches the acceptable β value. It follows that any measurements of a blank that result in a value that exceeds the LoB are considered to be false positives (Type I error). In fact, EP17-A recommends using a minimum of 60 measurements to determine the LoB and 60 sample measurements to determine the LoD.

Fig. **11A**, shows examples of LoB and LoD measurements for Gaussian distributions of blanks and sample measurements, where the false negative error is set to 5% and the false positive error is also set to 5% (α = β = 5%). The LoB is set to a value above which only 5% of blank measurements will produce a result. The LoD is chosen as the smallest measured analyte concentration that will lead to 5% of the results being less than the LoB. In contrast, if measurements are made on an analyte amount equal to the LoB, as shown in Fig. **11B**, then 50% of the measurements of the sample will result in false negative results.

For the rest of this section we will assume α = β = 5%, values that the International Organization for Standardization recommends as the defaults in their definition of minimum LoD.

The specific method for determining the LoB and LoD of a system depends on whether or not the measurements produce a Gaussian distribution of results. For a Gaussian distribution, the method to determine the LoB using the parameters of the distribution curve is shown in equation 6-1 [268]:

$$LoB = u_B + 1.645\sigma_B \qquad\qquad (6\text{-}1)$$

where u_B is the mean of the distribution of blank measurements and σ_B is the standard deviation of the distribution. LoB is the threshold value above which 5% of the blank measurement result in detection. The value 1.645 is derived from the x component of the standard Gaussian distribution at the 95th percentile. This value will vary slightly depending on the number of measurements used to determine the LoB.

A similar method is used to determine the LoD for a Gaussian distribution as shown in equation 6-2 [268]:

$$LoD = LoB + 1.645\sigma_S = u_B + 1.645\sigma_B + 1.645\sigma_S \qquad\qquad (6\text{-}2)$$

where σ_S is the standard deviation of the measurements of a small amount of sample.

For example, using the data shown in Fig. **11A**, the blank measurements have a distribution with u_B =0 and a σ_B=1 yielding an LoB = 0 + 1.645*1 = 1.645. The sample measurements possess a σ_S = 1.5, yielding an LoD = 1.645 + 1.645*1.5 = 4.113. It is important to note that the standard deviation is not required for a measurement from a sample exactly at the LoD, provided that the standard deviation is relatively constant for measurements made at low levels.

A non-Gaussian distribution of the blank may occur in instruments that, for example, discard negative results. Fig. **12** presents two example distributions from blanks and sample measurements that deviate from a Gaussian distribution. To determine the LOB, one needs to rank the blank measurements in order of descending magnitude. The LoB can be calculated from the result of the values at at the 95th percentile, as described by equation 6-3 [268]:

$$LoB = \text{Result at position } [Nb(p/100) + 0.5\,] = \text{Result at position } [Nb*0.95 + 0.5] \qquad (6\text{-}3)$$

where Nb is the number of samples measured and

$$p = 100 - \alpha = 95.$$

A)

B)

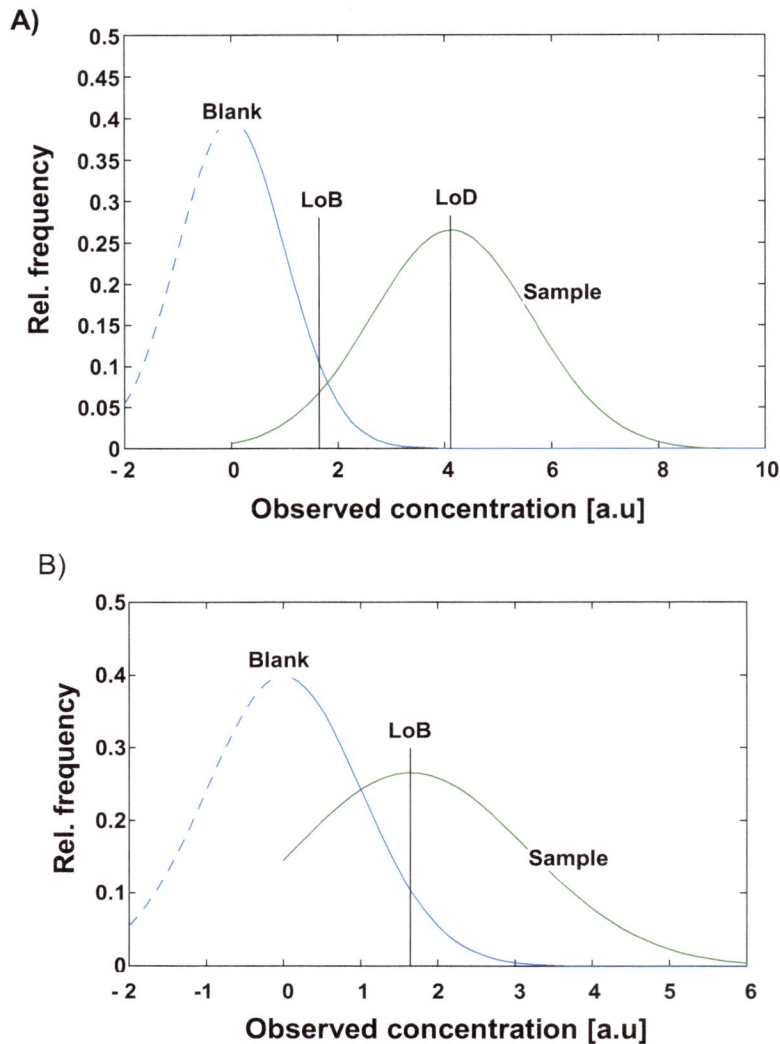

Fig. (11). Example distributions of blank samples and low level samples based on arbitrary units (x-axis) for A) where the actual sample amount is equal to the LoD for $\beta = 5\%$, and for B) where the actual sample amount is equal to the LoB so that 50% of the resulting measurements result in false negatives. Adapted from Ref. [268] with permission from the Clinical and Laboratory Standards Institute's (CLSI) internationally copyrighted EP17-A: Protocols for Determination of Limits of Detection and Limits of Quantitation; Approved Guideline.

Table **6** shows the last 15 data points of those that are plotted in Fig. **12** for the blank. In this example, the $N_b = 100$, therefore the LoB is the result at the position 95.5 which is the average of the 95th and 96th ranked values, *i.e.* 2.839.

A similar method is used to determine the LoD using nonparametric measurements. First, the difference between the reference value, or known amount of analyte being measured, and the value of the distribution of measurements at the 5th percentile is calculated following equation 6-4 [268].

$$D_{s,\beta} = AV^* - p_\beta \tag{6-4}$$

where AV* stands for assigned value of the substance being measured and p_β represents the value at the 5th percentile. Then, $D_{s,\beta}$ is added to the LoB to calculate the LoD as shown in equation 6-5 [268].

$$LoD = LoB + D_{s,\beta} \tag{6-5}$$

Table 6: Example of ranked blank values.

Ranks	Blank values
100	3.000
99	2.964
98	2.929
97	2.893
96	**2.857**
95	**2.821**
94	2.786
93	2.750
92	2.714
91	2.679
90	2.643
89	2.607
88	2.571
87	2.536
86	2.500
85	2.464

The method described in this subsection will only work in situations where the standard deviation is relatively constant at low level sample concentrations. If this is not the case, a trial and error method must be undertaken by taking measurements of varying sample amounts until one is found that produces measurements with a 5th percentile equal to the LoB.

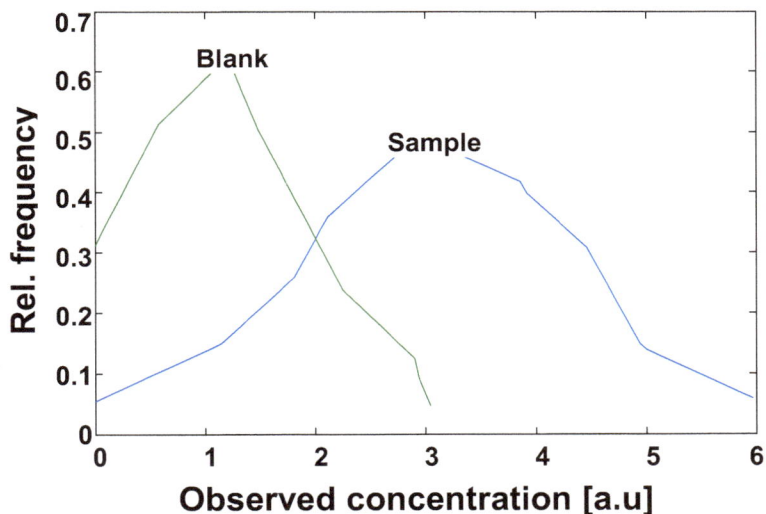

Fig. (12). Example of non-Gaussian blank and sample data. Adapted from Ref. [268] with permission from the Clinical and Laboratory Standards Institute's (CLSI) internationally copyrighted EP17-A: Protocols for Determination of Limits of Detection and Limits of Quantitation; Approved Guideline.

The EP17-A standard may be applied to assays in a platform independent fashion. As an example, the determination of the LoD for the Interferometric Reflectance Imaging Sensor (IRIS) device (previously described in section 4.3.2 above) is now explained. In the IRIS method, a blank (zero analyte concentration) sample is prepared by depositing an array of a uniform layer of probe molecules (*e.g.* antibodies), on top of the silicon dioxide layer (Fig. **10A**). The IRIS is adjusted so that the field of view is able to image more than 100 spots simultaneously. Since the EP-17A standard recommends 60 blank measurements, it is assumed that at least three different Si/SiO_2 chips will be imaged, each with at least 20 usable spots recorded per recordable image. The interference curve associated with each spot can be calculated based on the optical path length increase that results from capture probe molecule deposition. The distribution of these values across all the measurements will allow the LoB to be determined as described in equation (6-1). In a calibrated system, this estimated LoB is correlated with accumulated biomass.

Once the LoB is determined, the LoD can be calculated by taking at least 60 measurements of multiple samples of low analyte concentrations that have been applied to the Si/SiO_2 chip. Assuming the sampledistribution is Gaussian, the standard deviation of the increase in path length can be used to determine the LoD *via* equation (6-2). In a calibrated system, this estimated LoD can be used to predict the sample analyte concentration. However, if the distribution of results is non-Gaussian, then the actual concentrations of analytes being applied to the Si/SiO_2 chip must be known in order to calculate the LoD (equations (6-3) - (6-5)).

7. FUTURE OUTLOOK

In this chapter, the authors have focused on peptide-based probes without giving consideration to other promising approaches that are likely to become popular in the clinical microbial environment such as the rapidly growing field of genomic sequencing [269]. However, the genomic approach has many potential pitfalls and is unlikely to yield fast and near real time detection capabilities. In theory, any probe that can be affordably mass-produced, with reproducible binding characteristics, could be bound to an array surface to make a platform for label-free, massively parallel, infectious agent quantification and analysis. One key advantage of employing peptide-based probes is that they use phenotypic characteristics, unlike DNA-based approaches that rely on genotypic characteristics. Thus, the detection of a given nucleic acid sequence *via* the use of a genotypic test does not necessarily indicate the presence of a pathogen that can cause infections because the DNA approach does not distinguish whether a given gene is actually expressed, nor does it differentiate between living and dead organisms. In contrast, peptide probes can be designed to recognize an expressed gene product (including toxins), living cells or virus particles. Interestingly, several other classes of phenotypic receptors may be used in biosensor technologies (either in conjunction or *in lieu* of peptide-based probes). These include glycan, lectin [270], aptamer [271], and peptide nucleic acid probe classes [272].

Observing the collective signature from a combination of probe types simultaneously on one array is likely to become an effective strategy for minimizing false positive errors. Several label-free technologies can be spotted with >100 spots, which may give rise to massively parallel bio-detection (see Table **4** and [207, 273]). However, a few key challenges must be solved before multiplex-receptor arrays can become a reality as summarized below.

The development of biochemical methods that facilitate the attachment of different probe classes *e.g.* lectin, glycan, peptide, synthetics etc, to different substrate types *e.g.* glass, gold, polymer need to be perfected. Interesting work on the development of non-fouling materials that resist non-specific adsorption is being conducted by Semprus BioSciences (Cambridge, MA, USA) [274-276], and is likely to influence the development of the label-free biosensor field if the non-fouling material can be applied in an affordable and scalable fashion. A competing approach is being explored at the Mirkin lab at Northwestern University [277-280], this research appears to have promise for the functional attachment of large amounts of probes (11 million pyramidal inking-pens per wafer; <150,000 sub-100 nm features per second) onto an array in a scalable and affordable fashion.

In order for label-free techniques to compete with label-based techniques, it will be necessary to create and implement robust and rapid methods for directing analytes to the array sensing elements and washing away near-neighbor pathogens and contaminants. Digital fluidics - the application of an electrical potential (to form small mixing vessels that can be steered or used to form virtual microchannels dynamically), is one such technology that offers promise in the future [271-272]

Another key limitation is that peptide-based assays and biosensors can only identify known sequences or motifs (as with most molecular approaches). Therefore, in spite of the promise of label-free parallel bio-detection, it is currently still necessary to base clinical patient management decisions on the results obtained from a range of clinical assays in order to accurately arrive at the correct medical microbiological diagnosis.

ACKNOWLEDGEMENTS

G.M. Hwang thanks M. Keybl for advice on epidemiology, R. Graef and E. Mullen for research on section 2.2, A. Steinberg for initial clinical literature contributions, and A. Moore for financial support. This research was funded in part by The MITRE Corporation and S.-J. Suh was supported by the Auburn University Detection and Food Safety Peaks of Excellence program (USDA grant 2005-3439415674A). Approved for Public Release; Case # 10-2302, 10-2399, 10-3077. ©2010 The MITRE Corporation.

REFERENCES

[1]   Cunliffe NA, Gentsch JR, Kirkwood CD, *et al.* Molecular and Serologic Characterization of Novel Serotype G8 Human Rotavirus Strains Detected in Blantyre, Malawi. Virology 2000; 274(2): 309-20.

[2]   Bwaka MA, Bonnet MJ, Calain P, *et al.* Ebola hemorrhagic fever in Kikwit, Democratic Republic of the Congo: clinical observations in 103 patients. J Infect Dis 1999; 179 Suppl 1: 1-7.

[3]   Diederen BM. Legionella spp. and Legionnaires' disease. J Infect 2008; 56(1): 1-12.

[4]   Klevens RM, Morrison MA, Nadle J, *et al.* Invasive methicillin-resistant Staphylococcus aureus infections in the United States. JAMA 2007; 298(15): 1763-71.

[5]   Rota PA, Oberste MS, Monroe SS, *et al.* Characterization of a Novel Coronavirus Associated with Severe Acute Respiratory Syndrome. Science 2003; 300(5624) : 1394-9.

[6]   Berkelman RL. Emerging Infectious Diseases in the United States1993.J Infect Dis 1994; 170(2): 272-7.

[7]   Johnson RC, Schmid GP, Hyde FW, Steigerwalt AG, Brenner DJ. Borrelia burgdorferi sp. nov.: Etiologic Agent of Lyme Disease. Int J Syst Bacteriol 1984; 34(4): 496-7.

[8]   Gallo R, Salahuddin S, Popovic M, *et al.* Frequent detection and isolation of cytopathic retroviruses (HTLV-III) from patients with AIDS and at risk for AIDS. Science 1984; 224(4648): 500-3.

[9]   Parsonnet J, Friedman GD, Vandersteen DP, *et al.* Helicobacter pylori infection and the risk of gastric carcinoma. N Engl J Med 1991; 325(16): 1127-31.

[10]   Faruque SM, Mekalanos JJ. Pathogenicity islands and phages in Vibrio cholerae evolution. Trends Microbiol 2003; 11(11): 505-10.

[11]   Chizhikov V, Spiropoulou C, Morzunov S, Monroe M, Peters C, Nichol S. Complete genetic characterization and analysis of isolation of Sin Nombre virus. J Virol 1995; 69(12): 8132-6.

[12]   Wong KT, Shieh W-J, Kumar S, *et al.* Nipah Virus Infection: Pathology and Pathogenesis of an Emerging Paramyxoviral Zoonosis. Am J Pathol 2002; 161(6): 2153-67.

[13]   Daniels P, Ksiazek T, Eaton BT. Laboratory diagnosis of Nipah and Hendra virus infections. Microbes Infect 2001; 3(4): 289-95.

[14]   Ambrosio AM, Enria DA, Maiztegui JI. Junin virus isolation from lympho-mononuclear cells of patients with Argentine hemorrhagic fever. Intervirology 1986; 25(2): 97-9102.

[15]   Bowen MD, Peters CJ, Nichol ST. The Phylogeny of New World (Tacaribe Complex) Arenaviruses. Virology 1996; 219(1): 285-90.

[16]   Bowen MD, Peters CJ, Nichol ST. Phylogenetic analysis of the Arenaviridae: Patterns of virus evolution and evidence for cospeciation between Arenaviruses and their rodent hosts. Mol Phylogenet Evol 1997; 8(3): 301-16.

[17]   Fraser C, Donnelly CA, Cauchemez S, *et al.* Pandemic potential of a strain of influenza A (H1N1): early findings. Science 2009; 324(5934): 1557-61.

[18]   Chan PKS. Outbreak of avian influenza A(H5N1) virus infection in Hong Kong in 1997. Clin Infec Dis 2002 May; 34: S58-S64.

[19]   Fennelly KP, Davidow AL, Miller SL, N. C, J.J. E. Airborne infection with Bacillus anthracis-from mills to mail. Emerg Infect Dis 2004; 10(6): 996-1002.

[20]   Christopher LGW, Cieslak LTJ, Pavlin JA, Eitzen EM, Jr. Biological Warfare: A Historical Perspective. JAMA 1997; 278(5): 412-7.

[21]   Lim DV, Simpson JM, Kearns EA, Kramer MF. Current and developing technologies for monitoring agents of bioterrorism and biowarfare. Clin Microbiol Rev 2005; 18(4): 583-607.

[22]   Morse SA, Kellogg RB, Perry S, *et al.* Detecting Biothreat Agents: the Laboratory Response Network. ASM News 2003; 69(9): 433.

[23]   http: //www.who.int/csr/outbreaknetwork/en/. Accessed on 5/21/2010.

[24]   http: //www.afrims.org/geis.html. Accessed on 5/20/2010.

[25]   http: //www.phac-aspc.gc.ca/surveillance-eng.php. Accessed on 5/21/2010.

[26]   http: //www.cdc.gov/phin/activities/applications-services/nedss/index.html. Accessed on 5/21/2010.

[27]   http: //www.cdc.gov/phin/. Accessed on 5/21/2010.

[28]   https: //www.rods.pitt.edu/site/. Accessed on 5/21/2010.

[29]   Committee on Effectiveness of National Biosurveillance Systems: Biowatch and the Public Health System NRC. BioWatch and the Public Health Surveillance: Evaluating Systems for the Early Detection of Biological Threats. Washington DC: The National Academies Press; 2009.

[30]   http: //www.bt.cdc.gov/lrn/factsheet.asp. Accessed on 4/3/2010.

[31]   Klietmann WF, Ruoff KL. Bioterrorism: Implications for the Clinical Microbiologist. Clin Microbiol Rev 2001; 14(2): 364-81.

[32]   Committee on Materials and Manufacturing Processes for Advanced Sensors NRC. Sensor Systems for Biological Agent Attacks: Protecting Buildings and Military Bases. Washington DC: The National Academies Press; 2005.

[33]   Kaufmann AF, Meltzer MI, Schmid GP. The economic impact of a bioterrorist attack: are prevention and postattack intervention programs justifiable? Emerg Infect Dis 1997; (2): 83-94.

[34]   Rothel JS, Andersen P. Diagnosis of latent Mycobacterium tuberculosis infection: is the demise of the Mantoux test imminent? Expert Rev Anti Infect Ther 2005; 3(6): 981-93.

[35]   Espy MJ, Smith TF, Harmon MW, Kendal AP. Rapid detection of influenza virus by shell vial assay with monoclonal antibodies. J Clin Microbiol 1986; 24(4): 677-9.

[36]   Deisingh AK, Thompson M. Detection of infectious and toxigenic bacteria. Analyst 2002; 127(5): 567-81.

[37]   Takahashi H, Otsuka Y, Patterson BK. Diagnostic tests for influenza and other respiratory viruses: determining performance specifications based on clinical setting. J Infect Chemother 2010; 16(3): 155-61.

[38]   Balish A, Warnes CM, Wu K, *et al.* Evaluation of rapid influenza diagnostic tests for detection of novel Influenza A (H1N1) virus-United States, 2009 (Reprinted from MMWR, vol 58, pg 826-829, 2009). JAMA 2009; 302(11): 1163-4.

[39]   Cao B, Li X-W, Mao Y, *et al.* Clinical features of the initial cases of 2009 pandemic Influenza A (H1N1) virus infection in China. N Engl J Med 2009; 361(26): 2507-17.

[40]   Kim JS, Kim SH, Bae SY, *et al.* Enhanced detection of respiratory viruses using cryopreserved R-Mix ReadyCells. J Clin Virol 2008; 42(3): 264-7.

[41]   St George K, Patel NM, Hartwig RA, *et al.* Rapid and sensitive detection of respiratory virus infections for directed antiviral treatment using R-Mix cultures. J Clin Virol 2002; 24(1-2): 107-15.

[42]   Taggart EW, Crist G, Billetdeaux E, Langer J, Petti CA. Utility of terminal hemadsorption for detection of hemadsorbing respiratory viruses from conventional shell vial cultures for laboratories using R-Mix cultures. J Clinical Virol 2009; 44(1): 86-7.

[43]   Lequin RM. Enzyme immunoassay (EIA)/enzyme-linked immunosorbent assay (ELISA). Clin Chem 2005; 51(12): 2415-8.

[44]   Branton D, Deamer DW, Marziali A, *et al.* The potential and challenges of nanopore sequencing. Nat Biotech 2008; 26(10): 1146-53.

[45]   Engvall E, Perlmann P. Enzyme-linked immunosorbent assay (ELISA). Quantitative assay of immunoglobulin G. Immunochemistry 1971; 8(9): 871-4.

[46]   Van Weemen BK, Schuurs AHWM. Immunoassay using antigen-enzyme conjugates. FEBS Lett 1971; 15(9): 232-6.

[47]   Crowther JR. ELISA Theory and Practice. Totowa, N.J.: Humana Press Inc; 1995.

[48]   http: //www.biocompare.com/ProductListings/2298/Microplate-Reader-ELISA-Plate-Reader.html. Accessed on 7/20/2010.

[49]   http: //www.authorstream.com/Presentation/Mertice -15284-lecture001-BMS-631-LECTURE-1Flow-Cytometry -TheoryJ-Paul-RobinsonProfessor-ImmunopharmacologyPr-ofessor-Biome-2007-2008proposal-Entertainment-ppt-powerpoint/. Accessed on 4/4/2010..

[50]   Crosland-Taylor PJ. A device for counting small particles suspended in a fluid through a tube. Nature 1953; 171(4340): 37-8.

[51]   McBride MT, Masquelier D, Hindson BJ, *et al.* Autonomous detection of aerosolized Bacillus anthracis and Yersinia pestis. Anal Chem 2003; 75(20): 5293-9.

[52]   Lee WM, Grindle K, Pappas T, *et al.* High-throughput, sensitive, and accurate multiplex PCR-microsphere flow cytometry system for large-scale comprehensive detection of respiratory viruses. J Clin Microbiol 2007; 45(8): 2626-34.

[53]   Baker HN. A Method to Rapidly Evaluate and Identify Antibody Pairs for use in Sandwich Immunoassays.Personal Communication. American Association for Clinical Chemistry (AACC) Poster. Chicago, IL: USA 2009.

[54]   http: //www.accessdata.fda.gov/scripts/cdrh/cfdocs/cfPMN/pmn.cfm. Accessed on 04/04/2010.

[55]   Ateya DA, Erickson JS, Howell PB, Hilliard LR, Golden JP, Ligler FS. The good, the bad, and the tiny: a review of microflow cytometry. Anal Bioanal Chem 2008; 391(5): 1485-98.

[56]   Golden JP, Kim JS, Erickson JS, *et al.* Multi-wavelength microflow cytometer using groove-generated sheath flow. Lab Chip 2009; 9(13): 1942-50.

[57]   Kim JS, Anderson GP, Erickson JS, Golden JP, Nasir M, Ligler FS. Multiplexed Detection of Bacteria and Toxins Using a Microflow Cytometer. Anal Chem 2009; 81(13): 5426-32.

[58]   Mullis K, Faloona F, Scharf S, Saiki R, Horn G, Erlich H. Specific enzymatic amplification of DNA *in vitro*: the polymerase chain reaction. Cold Spring Harb Symp Quant Biol 1986; 51 Pt 1: 263-73.

[59]   http: //www.cepheid.com/systems-and software/genexpert-system/. Accessed on 5/23/2010.

[60]   http: //www.idahotech.com/RAPID/index.html. Accessed on 5/23/2010.

[61]   Rossney AS, Herra CM, Brennan GI, Morgan PM, O'Connell B. Evaluation of the XpertTM MRSA assay on the GeneXpert real-time PCR platform for rapid detection of MRSA from screening specimens. J Clin Microbiol 2008; 46(10): 3285-90.

[62]   Ulrich MP, Christensen DR, Coyne SR, *et al.* Evaluation of the Cepheid GeneXpert[(R)] system for detecting Bacillus anthracis. J Appl Microbiol 2006; 100(5): 1011-6.

[63]   Sails AD, Saunders D, Airs S, Roberts D, Eltringham G, Magee JG. Evaluation of the Cepheid respiratory syncytial virus and Influenza virus A/B real-time PCR analyte specific reagent. J Virol Methods 2009; 162(1-2): 88-90.

[64]   Lyon E, Wittwer CT. LightCycler technology in molecular diagnostics. J Mol Diagn 2009; 11(2): 93-101.

[65]   Christensen DR, Hartman LJ, Loveless BM, *et al.* Detection of Biological Threat Agents by Real-Time PCR: Comparison of Assay Performance on the R.A.P.I.D., the LightCycler, and the Smart Cycler Platforms. Clin Chem 2006; 52(1): 141-5.

[66]   http: //www.idahotech.com/FilmArray/. Accessed on 07/21/2010.

[67]   Bryant PA, Venter D, Robins-Browne R, Curtis N. Chips with everything: DNA microarrays in infectious diseases. Lancet Infect Dis 2004; 4(2): 100-11.

[68]   Mikhailovich V, Gryadunov D, Kolchinsky A, Makarov AA, Zasedatelev A. DNA microarrays in the clinic: infectious diseases. Bioessays 2008; 30(7): 673-82.

[69]   Ecker DJ, Sampath R, Blyn LB, *et al.* Rapid identification and strain-typing of respiratory pathogens for epidemic surveillance. Proc of the Natl Acad Sci USA 2005; 102(22): 8012-7.

[70]   Hofstadler SA, Sampath R, Blyn LB, *et al.* TIGER: the universal biosensor. Inter J Mass Spectrom 2005; 242(1): 23-41.

[71]   Wolk DM, Blyn LB, Hall TA, *et al.* Pathogen profiling: Rapid molecular characterization of Staphylococcus aureus by PCR/ESI-MS and correlation with phenotype. J Clin Microbiol 2009; 47(10): 3129-37.

[72]   Ecker DJ, Drader JJ, Gutierrez J, *et al.* The Ibis T5000 Universal Biosensor: An Automated Platform for Pathogen Identification and Strain Typing. J Assoc Lab Automation 2006; 11(6): 341-51.

[73]   Gavin PJ, Thomson RB. Review of Rapid Diagnostic Tests for Influenza. Clin Appl Immunol Rev 2004; 4(3): 151-72.

[74]   Sturenburg E, Junker R. Point-of-care testing in microbiology: the advantages and disadvantages of immunochromatographic test strips. Dtsch Arztebl Int 2009; 106(4): 48-54.

[75] Dover JE, Hwang GM, Mullen EH, Prorok BC, Suh SJ. Recent advances in peptide probe-based biosensors for detection of infectious agents. J Microbiol Methods 2009 78(1): 10-9.

[76] Abbas AK, Lichtman AH. Cellular and Molecular Immunology. Fifth ed. Philadephia: Elsevier Saunders; 2005.

[77] Conroy PJ, Hearty S, Leonard P, O'Kennedy RJ. Antibody production, design and use for biosensor-based applications. Semin Cell Dev Biol 2009; 20(1): 10-26.

[78] Donohue AC, Albitar M. Antibodies in biosensing. In: Zourob M, editor. Recognition Receptors in Biosensors. New York: Springer; 2009. p 221-48.

[79] Zhang A, Jin M, Liu F, *et al.* Development and evaluation of a DAS-ELISA for rapid detection of avian Influenza viruses. Avian Dis 2006; 50(3): 325-30.

[80] Chinowsky TM, Soelberg SD, Baker P, *et al.* Portable 24-analyte surface plasmon resonance instruments for rapid, versatile biodetection. Biosensors Bioelectron 2007; 22(9-10): 2268-75.

[81] Tully E, Higson SP, O'Kennedy R. The development of a labeless immunosensor for the detection of Listeria monocytogenes cell surface protein, Internalin B. Biosens Bioelectron 2008; 23(6): 906-12.

[82] Saerens D, Huang L, Bonroy K, Muyldermans S. Antibody Fragments as probe in biosensor development. Sensors 2008; 8(8): 4669-86.

[83] Swiecki MK, Lisanby MW, Shu F, Turnbough CL, Jr., Kearney JF. Monoclonal antibodies for Bacillus anthracis spore detection and functional analyses of spore germination and outgrowth. J Immunol 2006; 176(10): 6076-84.

[84] Oh B-K, Lee W, Chun BS, Bae YM, Lee WH, Choi J-W. The fabrication of protein chip based on surface plasmon resonance for detection of pathogens. Biosens Bioelectron 2005; 20(9): 1847.

[85] Vermeer AWP, Norde W. The thermal stability of immunoglobulin: unfolding and aggregation of a multi-domain protein. Biophys J 2000; 78(1): 394-404.

[86] Goldman ER, Anderson GP, Liu JL, *et al.* Facile generation of heat-stable antiviral and antitoxin single domain antibodies from a semisynthetic llama library. Anal Chem 2006; 78: 8245-55.

[87] Pancrazio JJ, Whelan JP, Borkholder DA, Ma W, Stenger DA. Development and application of cell-based biosensors. Ann Biomed Eng 1999; 27(6): 697-711.

[88.] Greenberg AS, Avila D, Hughes M, Hughes A, McKinney EC, Flajnik MF. A new antigen receptor gene family that undergoes rearrangement and extensive somatic diversification in sharks. Nature 1995; 374: 168-73.

[89] Hamers-Casterman C, Atarhouch T, Muyldermans S, *et al.* Naturally occurring antibodies devoid of light chains. Nature 1993; 363: 446-8.

[90] Muyldermans S. Single domain camel antibodies: current status. Rev Mol Biotechnol 2001; 74(4): 277-302.

[91] Dumoulin M CK, Van Meirhaeghe A, Meersman F, Heremans K, Frenken LG, Muyldermans S, Wyns L, Matagne A. Single-domain antibody fragments with high conformational stability. Protein Sci 2002; 11(3): 500-15.

[92] van der Linden RHJ, Frenken LGJ, de Geus B, *et al.* Comparison of physical chemical properties of llama V_{HH} antibody fragments and mouse monoclonal antibodies. Biochim Biophys Acta, Protein Struct Mol Enzymol 1999; 1431(1): 37-46.

[93] Harmsen MM, De Haard HJ. Properties, production, and applications of camelid single-domain antibody fragments. Appl Microbiol Biotechnol 2007; 77(1): 13-22.

[94] Conway JO, Sherwood LJ, Collazo MT, Garza JA, Hayhurst A. Llama single domain antibodies specific for the 7 botulinum neurotoxin serotypes as heptaplex immunoreagents. PLoS One 2010; 5(1): e8818.

[95] Goldman ER, Anderson GP, Conway J, *et al.* Thermostable llama single domain antibodies for the detection of botulinum A neurotoxin complex. Anal Chem 2008; 80(22): 8583-91.

[96] Liu J, Anderson G, Goldman E. Isolation of anti-toxin single domain antibodies from a semi-synthetic spiny dogfish shark display library. BMC Biotechnol 2007; 7(1): 78.

[97] Sherwood LJ, Osborn LE, Carrion J, R., Patterson JL, Hayburst A. Rapid assembly of sensitive antigen-capture assays for marburg virus, using *in vitro* selection of llama single-domain antibodies, at biosafety level 4. J Infect Dis 2007; 196: S213-S9.

[98] Goldman ER, Liu JL, Bernstein RD, Swain MD, Mitchell SQ, Anderson GP. Ricin detection using phage displayed single domain antibodies. Sensors 2009; 9(1): 542-55.

[99] Conrad U, Scheller J. Considerations on antibody-phage display methodology. Comb Chem High Throughput Screen 2005; 8: 117-26.

[100] Marks JD, Hoogenboom HR, Bonnert TP, McCafferty J, Griffiths AD, Winter G. By-passing immunization: Human antibodies from V-gene libraries displayed on phage. J Mol Biol 1991; 222: 581-97.

[101] McCafferty J, Griffiths AD, Winter G, Chiswell DJ. Phage antibodies: filamentous phage displaying antibody variable domains. Nature 1990; 348: 552-4.

[102] Iqbal SS, Mayo MW, Bruno JG, Bronk BV, Batt CA, Chambers JP. A review of molecular recognition technologies for detection of biological threat agents. Biosens Bioelectron 2000; 15(11-12): 549-78.

[103] Petrenko VA, Vodyanoy VJ. Phage display for detection of biological threat agents. J Microbiol Methods 2003; 53(2): 253-62.

[104] Brigati JR, Petrenko VA. Thermostability of landscape phage probes. Anal Bioanal Chem 2005; 382(6): 1346-50.

[105] Petrenko VA, Sorokulova IB. Detection of biological threats. A challenge for directed molecular evolution. J Microbiol Methods 2004; 58(2): 147-68.

[106] Byrne B, Stack E, Gilmartin N, O'Kennedy R. Antibody-based sensors: principles, problems and potential for detection of pathogens and associated toxins. Sensors 2009; 9(6): 4407-45.

[107] Hust M, Jostock T, Menzel C, et al. Single chain Fab (scFab) fragment. BMC Biotechnology 2007; 7(14).

[108] Teerinen T, Valjakka J, Rouvinen J, Takkinen K. Structure-based stability engineering of the mouse IgG1 Fab fragment by modifying constant domains. J Mol Biol 2006; 361(4): 687.

[109] Benhar I, Eshkenazi I, Neufeld T, Opatowsky J, Shaky S, Rishpon J. Recombinant single chain antibodies in bioelectrochemical sensors. Talanta 2001; 55(5): 899-907.

[110] Goldman ER, Anderson GP, Bernstein RD, Swain MD. Amplification of immunoassays using phage-displayed single domain antibodies. J Immunol Methods 2010; 352(1-2): 182-5.

[111] Mao C, Liu A, Cao B. Virus-based chemical and biological sensing. Angew Chem Int Ed 2009; 48(37): 6790-810.

[112] Petrenko VA, Smith GP. Phages from landscape libraries as substitute antibodies. Protein Eng 2000; 13(8): 589-92.

[113] Smith GP, Petrenko VA. Phage display. Chem Rev 1997; 97(2): 391-410.

[114] Szardenings M. Phage display of random peptide libraries: applications, limits, and potential. J Recept Signal Transduct Res 2003; 23(4): 307-49.

[115] Turnbough CL, Jr. Discovery of phage display peptide ligands for species-specific detection of Bacillus spores. J Microbiol Methods 2003; 53(2): 263-71.

[116] Tothill I. Peptides as Molecular Receptors. In: Zourob M, editor. Recognition receptors in biosensors. New York: Springer; 2010. p 249-74.

[117] Brigati J, Williams DD, Sorokulova IB, et al. Diagnostic probes for Bacillus anthracis spores selected from a landscape phage library. Clin Chem 2004; 50(10): 1899-906.

[118] Uithoven KA, Schmidt JC, Ballman ME. Rapid identification of biological warfare agents using an instrument employing a light addressable potentiometric sensor and a flow-through immunofiltration-enzyme assay system. Biosens Bioelectron 2000; 14(10-11): 761-70.

[119] Williams DD, Benedek O, Turnbough CL, Jr. Species-specific peptide ligands for the detection of Bacillus anthracis spores. Appl Environ Microbiol 2003; 69(10): 6288-93.

[120] Nanduri V, Sorokulova IB, Samoylov AM, Simonian AL, Petrenko VA, Vodyanoy V. Phage as a molecular recognition element in biosensors immobilized by physical adsorption. Biosens Bioelectron 2007; 22(6): 986-92.

[121] Goldman ER, Pazirandeh MP, Mauro JM, King KD, Frey JC, Anderson GP. Phage-displayed peptides as biosensor reagents. J Mol Recognit 2000; 13(6): 382-7.

[122] Binz HK, Amstutz P, Pluckthun A. Engineering novel binding proteins from nonimmunoglobulin domains. Nat Biotech 2005; 23(10): 1257-68.

[123] Grönwall C, Ståhl S. Engineered affinity proteins-Generation and applications. J Biotechnol 2009; 140(3-4): 254-69.

[124] Hosse RJ, Rothe A, Power BE. A new generation of protein display scaffolds for molecular recognition. Protein Sci 2006; 15(1): 14-27.

[125] Skerra A. Alternative non-antibody scaffolds for molecular recognition. Curr Opin Biotechnol 2007; 18(4): 295-304.

[126] Wikman M, Rocliffe E, finish. Selection and characterization of an HIV-1 gp120-binding affibody ligand. Biotechnol Appl Biochem 2006; 45(Pt 2): 92-105.

[127] Jung CC, Saaski EW, McCrae DA, Lingerfelt BM, Anderson GP. RAPTOR: a fluoroimmunoassay-based fiber optic sensor for detection of biological threats. IEEE Sensors Journal 2003; 3(4): 352-60.

[128] Hao R, Wang D, Zhang Xe, *et al.* Rapid detection of Bacillus anthracis using monoclonal antibody functionalized QCM sensor 2009; 24(5): 1330-5.

[129] Campbell GA, Mutharasan R. Method of Measuring Bacillus anthracis Spores in the Presence of Copious Amounts of Bacillus thuringiensis and Bacillus cereus. Anal Chem 2007; 79(3): 1145-52.

[130] Love TE, Redmond C, Mayers CN. Real time detection of anthrax spores using highly specific anti-EA1 recombinant antibodies produced by competitive panning. J Immunol Methods 2008; 334(1-2): 1-10.

[131] Mechaly A, Zahavy E, Fisher M. Development and implementation of a single-chain Fv antibody for specific detection of Bacillus anthracis spores. Appl Environ Microbiol 2008; 74(3): 818-22.

[132] Zhou B, Wirsching P, Janda KD. Human antibodies against spores of the genus Bacillus: A model study for detection of and protection against anthrax and the bioterrorist threat. Proc Natl Acad Sci U S A 2002; 99(8): 5241-6.

[133] Hayhurst A, Happe S, Mabry R, Koch Z, Iverson BL, Georgiou G. Isolation and expression of recombinant antibody fragments to the biological warfare pathogen Brucella melitensis. J Immunol Methods 2003; 276(1-2): 185.

[134] Wei D, Oyarzabal OA, Huang T-S, Balasubramanian S, Sista S, Simonian AL. Development of a surface plasmon resonance biosensor for the identification of Campylobacter jejuni. J Microbiol Methods 2007; 69(1): 78-85.

[135] Lindquist EA, Marks JD, Kleba BJ, Stephens RS. Phage-display antibody detection of Chlamydia trachomatis-associated antigens. Microbiology 2002; 148(2): 443-51.

[136] Yang L, Li Y. Simultaneous detection of Escherichia coli O157H7 and Salmonella Typhimurium using quantum dots as fluorescence labels. Analyst 2006; 131: 394-401.

[137] Anderson GP, King KD, Gaffney KL, Johnson LH. Multi-analyte interrogation using the fiber optic biosensor. Biosens Bioelectron 2000; 14(10-11): 771-7.

[138] Meyer MHF, Krause HJ, Hartmann M, Miethe P, Oster J, Keusgen M. Francisella tularensis detection using magnetic labels and a magnetic biosensor based on frequency mixing. J Magn Magn Materials 2007; 311(1): 259-63.

[139] Lathrop AA, Jaradat ZW, Haley T, Bhunia AK. Characterization and application of a Listeria monocytogenes reactive monoclonal antibody C11E9 in a resonant mirror biosensor. J Immunol Methods 2003; 281(1-2): 119-28.

[140] Nanduri V, Bhunia AK, Tu S-I, Paoli GC, Brewster JD. SPR biosensor for the detection of L. monocytogenes using phage-displayed antibody. Biosens Bioelectron 2007; 23(2): 248-52.

[141] He FJ, Zhang LD. Rapid diagnosis of M. tuberculosis using a piezoelectric immunosensor. Anal Sci 2002; 18(4): 397-401.

[142] Diaz-Gonzalez M, Gonzalez-Garcia MB, Costa-Garcia A. Immunosensor for Mycobacterium tuberculosis on screen-printed carbon electrodes. Biosens Bioelectron 2005; 20(10): 2035-43.

[143] Oh B-K, Kim Y-K, Park KW, Lee WH, Choi J-W. Surface plasmon resonance immunosensor for the detection of Salmonella typhimurium. Biosens Bioelectron 2004; 19(11): 1497-504.

[144] Olsen EV, Sorokulova IB, Petrenko VA, Chen IH, Barbaree JM, Vodyanoy VJ. Affinity-selected filamentous bacteriophage as a probe for acoustic wave biodetectors of Salmonella typhimurium. Biosens Bioelectron 2006; 21(8): 1434-42.

[145] Sorokulova IB, Olsen EV, Chen IH, *et al.* Landscape phage probes for Salmonella typhimurium. J Microbiol Methods 2005; 63(1): 55-72.

[146] Rao VK, Sharma MK, Goel AK, Singh L, Sekhar K. Amperometric immunosensor for the detection of Vibrio cholerae O1 using disposable screen-printed electrodes. Anal Sci 2006; 22(9): 1207-11.

[147] Jyoung JY, Hong SH, Lee W, Choi JW. Immunosensor for the detection of Vibrio cholerae O1 using surface plasmon resonance. Biosens Bioelectron 2006; 21(12): 2315-9.

[148] Cao LK, Anderson GP, Ligler FS, Ezzell J. Detection of Yersinia pestis fraction 1 antigen with a fiber optic biosensor. J Clin Microbiol 1995; 33(2): 336-41.

[149] Nuttall SD, Humberstone KS, Krishnan UV, *et al.* Selection and affinity maturation of IgNAR variable domains targeting Plasmodium falciparum AMA1. Proteins Struct Funct Bioinf 2004; 55(1): 187-97.

[150] Yu J-S, Liao H-X, Gerdon AE, *et al.* Detection of Ebola virus envelope using monoclonal and polyclonal antibodies in ELISA, surface plasmon resonance and a quartz crystal microbalance immunosensor. J Virol Methods 2006; 137(2): 219-28.

[151] Maruyama T, Parren Paul WHI, *et al.* Recombinant Human Monoclonal Antibodies to Ebola Virus. J Infect Dis 1999; 179(S1): S235-S9.

[152] Konig B, Gratzel M. A novel immunosensor for HERPES viruses. Anal Chem 1994; 66(3): 341-4.

[153] Zebedee SL, Barbas CF, Hom Y-L, *et al.* Human Combinatorial Antibody Libraries to Hepatitis B Surface Antigen. Proc Natl Acad Sci U S A 1992; 89(8): 3175-9.

[154] Tan WS, Tan GH, Yusoff K, Seow HF. A phage-displayed cyclic peptide that interacts tightly with the immunodominant region of hepatitis B surface antigen. J Clin Virol 2005; 34(1): 35-41.

[155] Lu X, Weiss P, Block T. A phage with high affinity for hepatitis B surface antigen for the detection of HBsAg. J Virol Methods 2004; 119(1): 51-4.

[156] Chan S-W, Bye JM, Jackson P, Allain J-P. Human recombinant antibodies specific for hepatitis C virus core and envelope E2 peptides from an immune phage display library. J Gen Virol 1996; 77(10): 2531-9.

[157] Plaisant P, Burioni R, Manzin A, *et al.* Human monoclonal recombinant Fabs specific for HCV antigens obtained by repertoire cloning in phage display combinatorial vectors. Res Virol 1997; 148(2): 165-9.

[158] Sanna PP, Williamson RA, De Logu A, Bloom FE, Burton DR. Directed selection of recombinant human monoclonal antibodies to herpes simplex virus glycoproteins from phage display libraries. Proc Natl Acad Sci U S A 1995; 92(14): 6439-43.

[159] Zhao XL, Chen WQ, Yang ZH, Li JM, Zhang SJ, Tian LF. Selection and affinity maturation of human antibodies against rabies virus from a scFv gene library using ribosome display. J Biotechnol 2009; 144(4): 253-8.

[160] Muller BH, Lafay F, Demangel C, *et al.* Phage-displayed and soluble mouse scFv fragments neutralize rabies virus. J Virol Methods 1997; 67(2): 221-33.

[161] Zuo B, Li S, Guo Z, Zhang J, Chen C. Piezoelectric Immunosensor for SARS-associated Coronavirus in sputum. Anal Chem 2004; 76(13): 3536-40.

[162] Liu ZX, Yi GH, Qi YP, *et al.* Identification of single-chain antibody fragments specific against SARS-associated coronavirus from phage-displayed antibody library. Biochem Biophys Res Commun 2005; 329(2): 437-44.

[163] Schmaljohn C, Cui YC, Kerby S, Pennock D, Spik K. Production and characterization of human monoclonal antibody Fab fragments to vaccinia virus from a phage-display combinatorial library. Virology 1999; 258(1): 189-200.

[164] Hu WG, Alvi AZ, Fulton RE, Suresh MR, Nagata LP. Genetic engineering of streptavidin-binding peptide tagged single-chain variable fragment antibody to Venezuelan equine encephalitis virus. Hybridoma and Hybridomics 2002; 21(6): 415-20.

[165] Ma H, Zhou B, Kim Y, Janda KD. A cyclic peptide-polymer probe for the detection of Clostridium botulinum neurotoxin serotype A. Toxicon 2006; 47(8): 901-8.

[166] Deng XK, Nesbit LA, Morrow KJ, Jr. Recombinant single-chain variable fragment antibodies directed against Clostridium difficile toxin B produced by use of an optimized phage display system. Clin Diagn Lab Immunol 2003; 10(4): 587-95.

[167] Lian W, Wu D, Lim DV, Jin S. Sensitive detection of multiplex toxins using antibody microarray. Anal Biochem 2010; 401(2): 271-9.

[168] Liu JL, Anderson GP, Delehanty JB, Baumann R, Hayhurst A, Goldman ER. Selection of cholera toxin specific IgNAR single-domain antibodies from a naïve shark library. Mol Immunol 2007; 44(7): 1775-83.

[169] Tang D, Ren J. Direct and Rapid Detection of Diphtherotoxin via Potentiometric Immunosensor Based on Nanoparticles Mixture and Polyvinyl Butyral as Matrixes. Electroanalysis 2005; 17(24): 2208-16.

[170] Anderson GP, Liu JL, Hale ML, *et al.* Development of Antiricin Single Domain Antibodies Toward Detection and Therapeutic Reagents. Anal Chem 2008; 80(24): 9604-11.

[171] Soykut EA, Dudak FC, Boyaci IH. Selection of staphylococcal enterotoxin B (SEB)-binding peptide using phage display technology. Biochem Biophys Res Commun 2008; 370(1): 104-8.

[172] Bisoffi M, Hjelle B, Brown DC, *et al.* Detection of viral bioagents using a shear horizontal surface acoustic wave biosensor. Biosens Bioelectron 2008; 23: 1397-403.

[173] Campbell GA, Mutharasan R. Piezoelectric-excited millimeter-sized cantilever (PEMC) sensors detect Bacillus anthracis at 300 spores/mL. Biosens Bioelectron 2006; 21(9): 1684.

[174] Campbell GA, Mutharasan R. Near real-time detection of Cryptosporidium parvum oocyst by IgM-functionalized piezoelectric-excited millimeter-sized cantilever biosensor. Biosens Bioelectron 2008; 23(7): 1039-45.

[175] Ruan C, Zeng K, Varghese OK, Grimes CA. Magnetoelastic immunosensors: amplified mass immunosorbent assay for detection of Escherichia coli O157: H7. Anal Chem 2003; 75(23): 6494-8.

[176] Ruan C, Zeng K, Varghese OK, Grimes CA. A staphylococcal enterotoxin B magnetoelastic immunosensor. Biosens Bioelectron 2004; 20(3): 585.

[177] Wan J, Shu H, Huang S, *et al*. Phage-based magnetoelastic wireless biosensors for detecting Bacillus anthracis spores. IEEE Sensors Journal 2007; 7(3): 470-7.

[178] Abdel-Hamid I, Ivnitski D, Atanasov P, Wilkins E. Flow-through immunofiltration assay system for rapid detection of E. coli O157: H7. Biosens Bioelectron 1999; 14(3): 309.

[179] Sippy N, Luxton R, Lewis RJ, Cowell DC. Rapid electrochemical detection and identification of catalase positive micro-organisms. Biosens Bioelectron 2003; 18(5-6): 741-9.

[180] Dill K, Song JH, Blomdahl JA, D. Olson J. Rapid, sensitive and specific detection of whole cells and spores using the light-addressable potentiometric sensor. J Biochem Biophys Methods 1997; 34(2): 161-6.

[181] Hu W-G, Thompson HG, Alvi AZ, Nagata LP, Suresh MR, Fulton RE. Development of immunofiltration assay by light addressable potentiometric sensor with genetically biotinylated recombinant antibody for rapid identification of Venezuelan equine encephalitis virus. J Immunol Methods 2004; 289(1-2): 27.

[182] La Belle JT, Shah M, Reed J, *et al*. Label-free and ultra-low level detection of Salmonella enterica serovar Typhimurium using electrochemical impedance spectroscopy. Electroanalysis 2009; 21(20): 2267-71.

[183] Anderson GP, Merrick EC, Trammell SA, Chinowsky TM, Shenoy DK. Simplified avidin-biotin mediated antibody attachment for a surface plasmon resonance biosensor. Sens Lett 2005; 3(2): 151-6.

[184] Feltis BN, Sexton BA, Glenn FL, Best MJ, Wilkins M, Davis TJ. A hand-held surface plasmon resonance biosensor for the detection of ricin and other biological agents. Biosens Bioelectron 2008; 23(7): 1131-6.

[185] Balasubramanian S, Sorokulova IB, Vodyanoy VJ, Simonian AL. Lytic phage as a specific and selective probe for detection of Staphylococcus aureus-A surface plasmon resonance spectroscopic study. Biosens Bioelectron 2007; 22(6): 948.

[186] Endo T, Kerman K, Nagatani N, *et al*. Multiple Label-Free Detection of Antigen-Antibody reaction using localized surface plasmon resonance-based core-shell structured nanoparticle layer nanochip. Anal Chem 2006; 78(18): 6465-75.

[187] Pang L, Chen HM, Wang L, Beechem JM, Fainman Y. Controlled detection in composite nanoresonant array for surface plasmon resonance sensing. Opt Express 2009; 17(17): 14700-9.

[188] Ji J, O'Connell JG, Carter DJD, Larson DN. High-throughput nanohole array based system to monitor multiple binding events in real time. Anal Chem 2008; 80(7): 2491-8.

[189] Daaboul GG, Yurt A, Zhang X, Hwang GM, Goldberg BB, Ünlü. High-throughput detection and sizing of individual low-index nanoparticles and viruses for pathogen identification. Nano Letters 2010; 10(11): 4727-31.

[190] Özkumur E, Needham JW, Bergstein DA, *et al*. Label-free and dynamic detection of biomolecular interactions for high-throughput microarray applications. Proc Natl Acad Sci U S A 2008; 105(23): 7988-92.

[191] Lazcka O, Del Campo FJ, Munoz FX. Pathogen detection: A perspective of traditional methods and biosensors. Biosens Bioelectron 2007; 22: 1205-17.

[192] Gronewold TMA. Surface acoustic wave sensors in the bioanalytical field: recent trends and challenges. Anal Chim Acta 2007; 603(2): 119-28.

[193] Lange K, Rapp BE, Rapp M. Surface acoustic wave biosensors: a review. Anal Bioanal Chem 2008; 391(5): 1509-19.

[194] Tai DF, Lin CY, Wu TZ, Huang JH, Shu PY. Artificial receptors in serologic tests for the early diagnosis of dengue virus infection. Clin Chem 2006; 52(8): 1486-91.

[195] Campbell GA, Mutharasan R. Detection and quantification of proteins using self-excited PZT-glass millimeter-sized cantilever. Biosens Bioelectron 2005; 21(4): 597.

[196] Campbell GA, Mutharasan R. Detection of Bacillus anthracis spores and a model protein using PEMC sensors in a flow cell at 1 mL/min. Biosens Bioelectron 2006; 22(1): 78.

[197] Gaster RS, Hall DA, Nielsen CH, *et al*. Matrix-insensitive protein assays push the limits of biosensors in medicine. Nat Med 2009; 15(11): 1327 – 32.

[198] Goldschmidt MC. The use of biosensor and microarray techniques in the rapid detection and identification of salmonellae. J AOAC Int 2006; 89(2): 530-7.

[199] Aubree-Lecat A, Hervagault C, Delacour A, Beaude P, Bourdillon C, Remy MH. Direct electrochemical determination of glucose oxidase in biological samples. Anal Biochem 1989; 178(2): 427-30.

[200] Wolfson SK, Jr., Chan LT, Krupper MA, Yao SJ. Electrochemical glucose sensing at low potentials. Biomed Biochim Acta 1989; 48(11-12): 919-24.

[201] Boyaci IH, Aguilar ZP, Hossain M, Halsall HB, Seliskar CJ, Heineman WR. Amperometric determination of live Escherichia coli using antibody-coated paramagnetic beads. Anal Bioanal Chem 2005; 382(5): 1234-41.

[202] Mittelmann AS, Ron EZ, Rishpon J. Amperometric quantification of total coliforms and specific detection of Escherichia coli. Anal Chem 2002; 74(4): 903-7.

[203] Thomas JH, Kim SK, Hesketh PJ, Halsall HB, Heineman WR. Bead-based electrochemical immunoassay for bacteriophage MS2. Anal Chem 2004; 76(10): 2700-7.

[204] Hafeman D, Parce J, McConnell H. Light-addressable potentiometric sensor for biochemical systems. Science 1988; 240(4856): 1182-5.

[205] http://www.moleculardevices.com/pages/reagents/threshold.html. Accessed on 5/22/2010.

[206] Evans D, Johnson S, Laurenson S, Davies AG, Ko Ferrigno P, Walti C. Electrical protein detection in cell lysates using high-density peptide-aptamer microarrays. J Biol 2008; 7(1): 3.

[207] Qavi AJ, Washburn AL, Byeon J-Y, Bailey RC. Label-free technologies for quantitative multiparameter biological analysis. Anal Bioanal Chem 2009; 394(1): 121-35.

[208] Liedberg B, Nylander C, Lunström I. Surface plasmon resonance for gas detection and biosensing. Sensors and Actuators 1983; 4: 299-304.

[209] Homola J. Present and future of surface plasmon resonance biosensors. Anal Bioanal Chem 2003; 377(3): 528-39.

[210] Mullett WM, Lai EPC, Yeung JM. Surface plasmon resonance-based immunoassays. Methods 2000; 22: 77-91.

[211] Homola J, Yee SS, Gauglitz G. Surface plasmon resonance sensors: review. Sensors Actuators B 1999; 54(1-2): 3-15.

[212] http://www.biacore.com/lifesciences/index.html. Accessed 5/20/2010.

[213] Genet C, Ebbesen TW. Light in tiny holes. Nature 2007; 445(7123): 39-46.

[214] Slutsky B, Pang L, Ptasinski J, Fainman Y. Optofluidics fundamentals, devices, and applications. In: Fainman Y, Luke LP, Psaltis D, Yang CH, editors. Biophotonics. New York: McGraw-Hill; 2010. p. 313-48.

[215] Brolo AG, Gordon R, Leathem B, Kavanagh KL. Surface plasmon sensor based on the enhanced light transmission through arrays of nanoholes in gold films. Langmuir 2004; 20(12): 4813-5.

[216] Ebbesen TW, Lezec HJ, Ghaemi HF, Thio T, Wolff PA. Extraordinary optical transmission through sub-wavelength hole arrays. Nature 1998; 391: 667-9.

[217] Leebeeck AD, Swaroop Kumar LK, de Lange V, Sinton D, Gordon R, Brolo AG. On-chip surface-based detection with nanohole arrays. Anal Chem 2007; 79(11): 4094-100.

[218] Hwang GM, Pang L, Mullen EH, Fainman Y. Plasmonic sensing of biological analytes through nanoholes. IEEE Sensors Journal 2008; 8(11-12): 2074-9.

[219] Pang L, Hwang GM, Slutsky B, Fainman Y. Spectral sensitivity of two-dimensional nanohole array surface plasmon polariton resonance sensor. App Phys Lett 2007; 91(12).

[220] Steiner G. Surface plasmon resonance imaging. Anal Bioanal Chem 2004; 379(3): 328-31.

[221] Stewart ME, Mack NH, Malyarchuk V, *et al.* Quantitative multispectral biosensing and 1D imaging using quasi-3D plasmonic crystals. Proc Natl Acad Sci U S A 2006; 103(46): 17143-8.

[222] http://gwctechnologies.com/gwcPublications.htm. Accessed 5/21/2010.

[223] http://www.discoversensiq.com/. Accessed on 5/21/2010.

[224] http://www.ibis-spr.nl/. Accessed on 5/20/2010.

[225] http://www.genoptics-spr.com/. Accessed on 5/21/2010.

[226] Fan XD, White IM, Shopoua SI, Zhu HY, Suter JD, Sun YZ. Sensitive optical biosensors for unlabeled targets: A review. Anal Chim Acta 2008; 620(1-2): 8-26.

[227] Daaboul GG, Vedula RS, Reddington A, *et al.* LED-based spectral reflectance imaging biosensor for label-free high-throughput multi-analyte and single-pathogen detection. SPIE Photonics West San Francisco, California: USA 2010.

[228] Daaboul GG, Lopez C, Connor JH, Hwang G, Ünlü MS. LED-based spectral reflectance imaging biosensor for label-free high-throughput multi-analyte and single-pathogen detection. New England Regional Center of Excellence Biodefense and Emerging Infectious Disease Research; Newport, RI: USA 2009.

[229] Özkumur E, Ahn S, Yalcin A, *et al.* Label-free microarray imaging for direct detection of DNA hybridization and single-nucleotide mismatches. Biosens Bioelectron 2010; 25(7): 1789-95.

[230] Özkumur E, Lopez CA, Yalçın A, *et al.* Spectral reflectance imaging for a multiplexed, high-throughput, label-free, and dynamic biosensing platform. IEEE J Sel Top Quant Electron 2010; 16(3): 635-46.

[231] http://www.zoiray.com/Technology.html. Accessed on 5/22/2010.

[232] Principi N, Esposito S. Antigen-Based Assays for the Identification of Influenza Virus and Respiratory Syncytial Virus: Why and How to Use Them in Pediatric Practice. Clin Lab Med 2009; 29(4): 649-60.

[233] http://www.who.int/csr/disease/avian_influenza/guidelin es/RapidTestInfluenza_web.pdf. Accessed 04/04/2010.

[234] Sambol AR, Abdalhamid B, Lyden ER, Aden TA, Noel RK, Hinrichs SH. Use of rapid influenza diagnostic tests under field conditions as a screening tool during an outbreak of the 2009 novel influenza virus: practical considerations. J Clin Virol 2010; 47(3): 229-33.

[235] Hurt AC, Alexander R, Hibbert J, Deed N, Barr IG. Performance of six influenza rapid tests in detecting human influenza in clinical specimens. J Clin Virology 2007; 39(2): 132-5.

[236] Smit M, Beynon KA, Murdoch DR, Jennings LC. Comparison of the NOW Influenza A & B, NOW Flu A, NOW Flu B, and directigen Flu A+B assays, and immunofluorescence with viral culture for the detection of Influenza A and B viruses. Diagn Microbiol Infect Dis 2007; 57(1): 67-70.

[237] Welch DF, Ginocchio CC. Role of Rapid Immunochromatographic antigen testing in diagnosis of Influenza A virus 2009 H1N1 infection. J Clin Microbiol 2010; 48(1): 22-5.

[238] Hatchette TF, Pilpn. The limitations of point of care testing for pandemic influenza: what clinicians and public health professionals need to know. Can J of Public Health 2009; 100(3): 204-7.

[239] http://www.binaxnow.com/influenza_a__b.aspx. Accessed on 5/23/2010.

[240] http://www.bd.com/ds/productCenter/256010.asp Accessed on 5/23/2010.

[241] Landry ML, Ferguson D. SimulFluor respiratory screen for rapid detection of multiple respiratory viruses in clinical specimens by immunofluorescence staining. J Clin Microbiol 2000; 38(2): 708-11.

[242] Sabetta J, Smardin J, Burns L, *et al.* Performance of rapid influenza diagnostic tests during two school outbreaks of 2009 pandemic influenza A (H1N1) virus infection - Connecticut, 2009. MMWR Morb Mortal Wkly Rep 2009; 58(37): 1029-32.

[243] Barenfanger J, Drake C, Mueller T, Troutt T, O'Brien J, Guttman K. R-Mix cells are faster, at least as sensitive and marginally more costly than conventional cell lines for the detection of respiratory virus.J Clin Virol 2001; 22(1): 101-10.

[244] http://www.luminexcorp.com/rvp/. Accessed on 5/23/2010.

[245] Ginocchio CC, Zhang F, Manji R, *et al.* Evaluation of multiple test methods for the detection of the novel 2009 influenza A (H1N1) during the New York City outbreak. J Clin Virol 2009; 45(3): 191-5.

[246] Paulson J. 3M Rapid Detection Flu A + B Test: a new diagnostic test for rapid detection of influenza A and influenza B. Mol Diagn Ther 2009; 13(1): 15-8.

[247] Ginocchio CC, Lotlikar M, Falk L, *et al.* Clinical performance of the 3M Rapid Detection Flu A plus B Test compared to R-Mix culture, DFA and BinaxNOW Influenza A&B Test. Journal of Clinical Virology 2009 Jun; 45(2): 146-9.

[248] Dale SE, Mayer C, Mayer MC, Menegus MA. Analytical and clinical sensitivity of the 3M rapid detection influenza A+B assay. J Clin Microbiol 2008; 46(11): 3804-7.

[249] Valley JK, Neale S, Hsu HY, Ohta AT, Jamshidi A, Wu MC. Parallel single-cell light-induced electroporation and dielectrophoretic manipulation. Lab on a Chip 2009; 9(12): 1714-20.

[250] Choi YJ, Kim HJ, Park JS, *et al.* Evaluation of new rapid antigen test for the detection of pandemic influenza A/H1N1 2009 virus. J Clin Microbiol 2010; 48(6): 2260-2.

[251] Diederen B, Veenendaal D, Jansen R, Herpers B, Ligtvoet E, IJzerman E. Rapid antigen test for pandemic (H1N1) 2009 virus. Emerg Infect Dis 2010; 16(5): 897-8

[252] Drexler JF, Helmer A, Kirberg H, *et al.* Poor clinical sensitivity of rapid antigen test for influenza A pandemic (H1N1) 2009 virus. Emerg Infect Dis 2009; 15(10): 1662-4.

[253] http://www.fujirebio.co.jp/english/product/other.html. Accessed on 5/23/2010.

[254] http://rockeby.com/pdf/AIV_Brochure.pdf. Accessed on 5/23/2010.

[255] http://www.quidel.com/products/product_detail.php? prod=101&group=1. Accessed on 5/23/2010.

[256] Karre T, Maguire HF, Butcher D, Graepler A, Weed D, Wilson ML. Comparison of Becton Dickinson Directigen EZ Flu A+B Test against the CDC real-time PCR assay for detection of 2009 pandemic Influenza A/H1N1 virus. J Clin Microbiol 2010; 48(1): 343-4.

[257] Kok J, Blyth CC, Foo H, *et al.* Comparison of a rapid antigen test with nucleic acid testing during cocirculation of pandemic Influenza A/H1N1 2009 and seasonal Influenza A/H3N2. J Clin Microbiol 2010; 48(1): 290-1.

[258] Louie JK, Guevara H, Boston E, *et al.* Rapid Influenza antigen test for diagnosis of pandemic (H1N1) 2009. Emerg Infect Dis 2010; 16(5): 824-6.

[259] Mehlmann M, Bonner AB, Williams JV, *et al.* Comparison of the MChip to viral culture, reverse transcription-PCR, and the QuickVue influenza A plus B test for rapid diagnosis of influenza. J Clin Microbiol 2007; 45(4): 1234-7.

[260] Noyola DE, Clark B, O'Donnell FT, Atmar RL, Greer J, Demmler GJ. Comparison of a new neuraminidase detection assay with an enzyme immunoassay, immunofluorescence, and culture for rapid detection of influenza A and B viruses in nasal wash specimens. J Clin Microbiol 2000; 38(3): 1161-5.

[261] http: //www.alaskascientific.net/products/biostar_flu_oia _rapid_diagnostic.htm. Accessed on 5/23/2010.

[262] Rodriguez WJ, Schwartz RH, Thorne MM. Evaluation of diagnostic tests for influenza in a pediatric practice. Pediatr Infect Dis J 2002; 21(3): 193-6.

[263] Ruest A, Michaud S, Deslandes S, Frost EH. Comparison of the directigen Flu A+B test, the QuickVue influenza test, and clinical case definition to viral culture and reverse transcription-PCR for rapid diagnosis of influenza virus infection. J Clin Microbiol 2003; 41(8): 3487-93.

[264] http: //www.oxoid.com/UK/blue/prod_detail/prod_detail. asp ?pr=R24600&c=UK&lang =EN. Accessed on 5/23/2010.

[265] Vasoo S, Stevens J, Singh K. Rapid antigen tests for diagnosis of pandemic (Swine) influenza A/H1N1. Clin Infect Dis 2009; 49(7): 1090-3.

[266] Weinberg A, Walker ML. Evaluation of three immunoassay kits for rapid detection of influenza virus A and B. Clin Diagn Lab Immunol 2005; 12(3): 367-70.

[267] Uyeki TM, Prasad R, Vukotich C, *et al.* Low S\sensitivity of rapid diagnostic test for Influenza. Clin Infect Dis 2009; 48(9): E89-E92.

[268] Tholen DW, Linnet K, Kondratovich M, *et al.* Protocols for determination of limits of detection and limits of quantitation; approved guideline. International Federation of Clinical Chemistry and Laboratory Medicine; 2004.

[269] Metzker ML. Sequencing technologies - the next generation. Nat Rev Genet 2010; 11(1): 31-46.

[270] Ngundi MM, Kulagina NV, Anderson GP, Taitt CR. Nonantibody-based recognition: alternative molecules for detection of pathogens. Expert Rev Proteomics 2006; 3(5): 511-24.

[271] Bunka DHJ, Stockley PG. Aptamers come of age - at last. Nat Rev Microbiol 2006; 4(8): 588-96.

[272] Soleymani L, Fang ZC, Sargent EH, Kelley SO. Programming the detection limits of biosensors through controlled nanostructuring. Nat Nanotechnol 2009; 4(12): 844-8.

[273] Ray S, Mehta G, Srivastava S. Label-free detection techniques for protein microarrays: prospects, merits and challenges. Proteomics 2010; 10(4): 731-48.

[274] Zhang Z, Chen SF, Jiang SY. Dual-functional biomimetic materials: Nonfouling poly(carboxybetaine) with active functional groups for protein immobilization. Biomacromolecules 2006; 7(12): 3311-5.

[275] Zhang Z, Vaisocherova H, Cheng G, Yang W, Xue H, Jiang SY. Nonfouling behavior of polycarboxybetaine-grafted surfaces: structural and environmental effects. Biomacromolecules 2008; 9(10): 2686-92.

[276] Zhang Z, Zhang M, Chen SF, Horbetta TA, Ratner BD, Jiang SY. Blood compatibility of surfaces with superlow protein adsorption. Biomaterials 2008; 29(32): 4285-91.

[277] Braunschweig AB, Huo FW, Mirkin CA. Molecular printing. Nat Chem 2009; 1(5): 353-8.

[278] Giljohann DA, Mirkin CA. Drivers of biodiagnostic development. Nature 2009; 462(7272): 461-4.

[279] Huo F, Zheng Z, Zheng G, Giam LR, Zhang H, Mirkin CA. Polymer Pen Lithography. Science 2008; 321(5896): 1658-60.

[280] Zheng ZJ, Daniel WL, Giam LR, *et al.* Multiplexed protein arrays enabled by polymer pen lithography: addressing the inking challenge. Angew Chem Int Ed 2009; 48(41): 7626-9.

CHAPTER 3

MALDI-TOF MS for Identification of Microorganisms: A New Era in Clinical Microbiological Research and Diagnosis

M. Welker[*]

BioMérieux – R&D Microbiology, 3 route de Port Michaud, La Balme les Grottes, 38390, France

Abstract: In medical microbiology, the identification of microorganisms in clinical specimens is a key step for successful therapy. In the last few years, new technologies have emerged for routine identification, among which matrix assisted laser desorption/ionization time of flight mass spectrometry (MALDI-TOF MS), a technology that appears very promising as it is currently becoming established in microbiological laboratories worldwide. MALDI-TOF MS allows the identification of microorganisms – bacteria as well as fungi – by so called intact-cell mass spectrometry, and the comparison of a sample's mass spectrum to reference mass spectra in a database. The key factors to the success of this technology are: i) the fact that a uniform sample preparation procedure is utilized for many different types of microorganisms, ii) the short time to a result, and 3) the comparatively low cost per analysis. Additionally, mass spectrometry based identification can be readily expanded to different microbiological fields, including food, industrial and veterinary microbiology.

In this chapter, the basic principles of MALDI-TOF MS are briefly described, followed by an introduction to intact-cell mass spectrometry of microorganisms and mass based identification. Further, limits of the technology are reviewed in the light of expected future developments. Finally, possible consequences of the broad introduction of MALDI-TOF MS based on microbial identification systems for practical and theoretical issues of medical microbiology are discussed.

Keywords: Mass Spectrometry, MALDI-TOF MS, Mass Spectra, Diagnostic Microbiology, Microbial Taxonomy, Spectral comparison.

1. THE IDENTIFICATION OF MICROORGANISMS IN CLINICAL SAMPLES

The identification of microorganisms is a crucial step in the diagnosis and therapy of human, animal, and plant diseases. Since the recognition of bacteria and fungi as etiologic agents of illnesses more than a century ago, elaborate methods have been developed for the selective isolation and identification of pathogens from all kinds of clinical and veterinary specimens. Most of the procedures used for the identification of microorganisms until recently depended on the isolation of a clonal sample and its culture on an array of multiple media containing particular substrates. The metabolisation of these substrates is then signalled by a colour change of an indicator, resulting in a pattern of positive and negative reactions. The metabolic pattern obtained is then used to identify the organism by comparing it to a database of reaction patterns of reference strains. Commercially available systems for the routine identification of clinical isolates have been automated to a high degree, allowing high throughput identification. However, despite the success and wide application of such systems, a number of disadvantages are becoming increasingly evident, including technical as well as conceptual problems. One category of disadvantages involves identification issues relating to isolates that are not able to metabolise most of the tested substrates and hence commonly are called "non-fermenting" bacteria. Further, automated identification using these systems requires the preparation of an ideally homogenous suspension, which is not always possible for particular bacteria, and practically impossible for filamentous fungi. Consequently, the latter organisms are not routinely identified using current commercially available identification systems.

The principle of biochemical identification has been developed in accordance to a species concept which in

---

*Address correspondence to M. Welker: BioMérieux – R&D Microbiology, 3 route de Port Michaud, La Balme les Grottes, 38390, France; Email: martin.welker@biomerieux.com

John P. Hays and W. B. van Leeuwen (Eds)

turn has been largely based on metabolic patterns. Hence, this biochemical identification procedure is prone to circular reasoning and is considered problematic in the light of new available data and techniques. Since the advent of the genomic era, a number of species concepts for prokaryotes have been postulated, discussed, and rejected, but without agreement on a broadly acceptable concept [1-3]. Consequently, bacterial species are still defined by conventions and parameters that are considered as objective phylogenetic markers, *i.e.*, the nucleotide sequence of the 16S rRNA gene and DNA-DNA-hybridisation values between clones [4, 5]. However, both of these markers possess flaws as they are either not discriminative enough, or are impractical in times when the sequencing of a complete bacterial genome can be performed relatively rapidly. Further, the concept of a "tree of life" (comprising a bifurcating phylogeny) has been challenged by the analyses of complete genomes of large numbers of bacterial strains [6], with genomic studies revealing that the number of shared genes between clones of the same species (as defined by taxonomists) - can be as low as 40% [7]. In this light, the identification of bacterial species by metabolic patterns is prone to errors, especially if non-typical clones are analysed. These non-typical clones may lack or may have acquired genes coding for fermentative enzymes that generate a deviation from the "conventional" metabolic pattern observed in typical clones of the same species. Therefore, classical clinical microbiology will likely face various paradigm shifts in the near future that will also profoundly affect the way in which routine microbiological diagnosis is performed. These shifts will require the development and application of new technologies, such as Matrix Assisted Laser Desorption/Ionization Time-of-Flight Mass Spectrometry (MALDI-TOF MS, Figs. **1** and **2**).

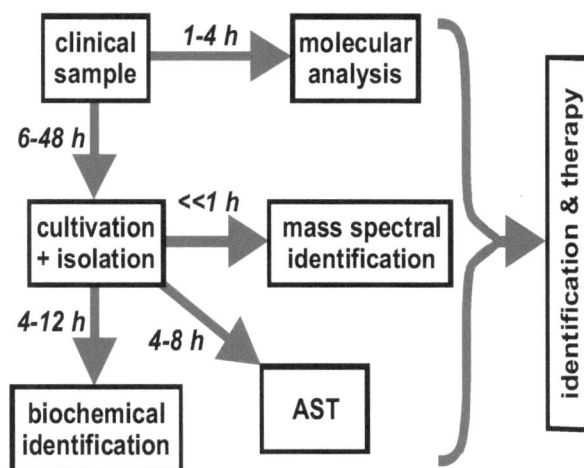

Fig. (1). Principle work-flow in clinical microbial diagnostics, indicating the advantages of IC-MS (MALDI-TOF MS)-based identification systems in terms of time-to-result. AST: antibiotic susceptibility testing.

2. PRINCIPLES OF MALDI-TOF MS

MALDI-TOF MS is a recently developed technology, with the first fundamental studies being published in the mid-1980s [8]. The key publications which eventually lead to a commercially available instrument were published in 1988 independently by two groups, and were later honoured by a Nobel prize bestowed on one of the authors [9,10]. Essentially, two main features of MALDI-TOF MS have triggered the rapid and profound success of this new technique. Firstly, it became possible to detect molecules as non-fragmented ions with molecular masses exceeding 100,000 Da for the first time. Secondly, biological samples could be analysed after a very simple sample preparation without the need for a preceding separation step, for example, chromatography. Both of these features were exploited in what was soon called 'intact cell mass spectrometry' (IC-MS), the analysis of whole microbial cells. In fact however, the analysed bacterial cells cannot be considered as intact, as the sample preparation procedure causes substantial cell wall disintegration, meaning that the term 'whole cell mass spectrometry' would be more appropriate. However, because the term IC-MS has been used in many previously published studies, this term will be used in this chapter.

Initial studies using IC-MS of bacteria showed that the mass spectral pattern of different species differ substantially [11,12]. Further, in these early studies, the potential of the use of IC-MS for bacterial identification was discussed but it required a number of further studies in the following years to prove that this could indeed be achieved. Unfortunately, a detailed description of MALDI-TOF MS cannot be given here, and the reader is advised to consult analytical chemistry textbooks for further information. Nonetheless, the basic principles required to understand the concept of mass-based microbial identification are outlined in this chapter (Fig. **2**).

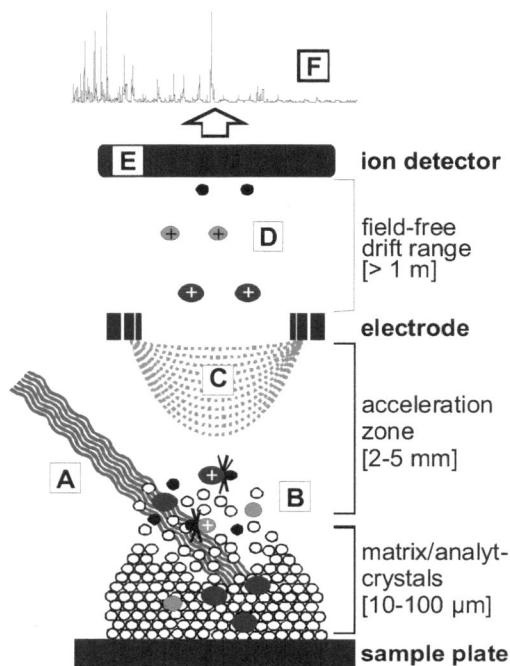

Fig. (2). Schematic illustration of principles of matrix assisted laser desorption/ionisation time-of-flight mass spectrometry (MALDI-TOF MS). Letters refer to individual steps of a single laser pulse cycle. **A:** laser pulse; **B:** desorption and ionisation of matrix and analyte molecules; **C:** build-up of electromagnetic field in which ions are accelerated; **D:** separation of ions *via* their mass-dependent velocities; **E:** detection of ions; **F:** recording and accumulation of time-resolved spectra.

During mass spectrometry-based analysis, the molecules to be detected (the analytes) are embedded in crystals of a matrix compound. The matrix compound is required for two reasons. Firstly, the matrix is able to absorb photonic energy from a laser beam. Secondly, the matrix facilitates the transfer of electrical charge from matrix molecules to analyte molecules. The matrix compound should ideally be a small molecular weight compound in order to avoid interference with analyte molecules, which usually possess a much higher molecular mass. Commonly used matrix compounds include primarily small aromatic organic acids, as these possess high energy absorbance coefficients at the wavelengths of commonly used lasers, and can act as both proton donors and proton acceptors. The most common matrix compounds used are 2,5-dihydroxybenzoic acid, α-cyanohydroxy cinnamic acid, and sinapic acid, with the co-crystallisation of matrix and analyte molecules being generally achieved by simple room-temperature evaporation of a matrix solvent/analyte mix directly on the sample plate. For analysis, a laser beam is focused at the matrix/analyte crystals and fired in pulses of a few hundred nanoseconds. The absorbed photonic energy causes the desorption of matrix and analyte molecules (under the high-vacuum conditions present within the instrument ($<10^{-6}$ mbar)), into the gas phase, whereupon charge transfer occurs between the photonically excited matrix and the analyte molecules [13]. All ions produced are then accelerated in an electromagnetic field that is built up between the sample plate and a grid or ring electrode placed a distance of a few millimetres apart. In modern instruments, the electromagnetic field is engaged with a short delay of 0.1-1 microseconds after the laser pulse has hit the sample so that either positively or negatively charged ions are accelerated depending on the polarity, *i.e.*, whether a positive or negative ion "extraction mode" is chosen. This delayed extraction procedure has proven crucial in improving the precision and resolution of mass spectral analysis [14]. After passing the electrode, the accelerated ions are directed into a "flight tube" at the end of which is an ion detector. In the flight tube, no further acceleration of ions takes place (hence the term "field-free drift range"), and the energy that the ions have gained when passing through the grid or ring electrode is related to the velocity of travel through the flight tube. This velocity is inversely proportional to the mass of the ion, as heavier molecules require a greater momentum. Consequently, the heavier a molecule, the longer the time-of-flight required to reach the ion detector at the end of the flight tube. The time of ion impact is then recorded and amplified with a high degree accuracy. Because matrix molecules are also charged by the laser energy, matrix ions are also accelerated and reach the detector. In fact, the number of matrix molecules reaching the detector generally far exceeds that of analyte molecules when a full mass range is recorded. For this reason, mass spectral analysis below m/z 500 is generally not performed, and ions in the lower mass range are diverted from the detector by a so- called "ion gate" (the term m/z refers to the mass of the molecule divided by the charge). In fact, in MALDI-TOF MS, proteins are detected primarily as singly charged ions, so that the term m/z generally equals the molecular mass of the analyte, *i.e.*, $M+H^+$ (in positive ion extraction mode) [13]. Finally, so-called "deconvolution" procedures have been developed in order to further reduce the number of peaks observed in an intact-cell mass spectrum, *via* the identification of multiple charge states of individual proteins, [15].

A full MALDI-TOF MS measurement consists of many cycles of laser pulse-mediated desorption, ionisation, acceleration, separation, and detection, repeated at a few to hundreds of Hertz. Single laser pulse mass spectra are accumulated into a resulting mass spectrum. In principle, each single laser pulse cycle yields an individual mass spectrum and no two such individual mass spectra are completely identical [16]. The major reason for this inhomogeneity is the fact that matrix and analyte molecules are not distributed homogeneously in the sample. Therefore, each laser pulse effectively hits a different microsample. Even when the laser focus remains unchanged, at each laser pulse material is desorbed, generating craters on the crystal surface [17]. Consequently, the laser never hits the same matrix/analyte crystal twice. This results in an uncertainty intrinsic to the technique itself that needs to be taken into account for mass-based identification techniques (discussed below).

The sample preparation procedures for IC-MS for microbial identification are generally simple and rapid. Fresh cells are transferred from a culture medium (solid or liquid) in small amounts to the sample plate and extracted immediately using an aqueous mixture of organic solvents containing the matrix compound [18]. For some samples, the optimisation of preparation procedures and matrix compounds may considerably improve the quality of mass spectra and hence the analytical outcome [19, 20], or alternatively allow the safe handling of highly pathogenic microorganisms [21].

The minimum amount of cells for an analysis depends largely on the preparation technique used, with a manual preparation technique requiring at least approximately 10^5 to 10^6 cells per sample. In the near future, miniaturisation and automation will possibly allow the preparation of smaller amounts of cells [22], based on the very low quantities of microorganism actually required for detection [23].

3. CELLULAR COMPOUNDS THAT ARE DETECTED BY WHOLE-CELL MASS SPECTROMETRY

When comparing the mass spectra obtained from different microbial species, the differences are immediately evident in most cases, as is the similarity of mass spectra of different isolates of a single species. However, this statement is especially applicable to spectra obtained in the mass range from 3000 to 20000 Da, as mass spectral patterns in the lower mass range (1000-3000 Da) are less consistent with current microbial taxonomy. The observation that proteins are mainly detected by IC-MS raises questions as to whether the taxonomic identification of microorganisms should actually be based on the detection of proteins, the presence of which in microbial cells is largely influenced by the metabolic regulation of gene expression. As a consequence, different culture conditions could conceivably generate variable protein expression profiles and hence variable mass spectroscopy patterns for identical isolates. However, even without detailed knowledge of the proteins actually detected by mass spectroscopy, early studies concluded that – at least for bacteria and yeasts – the mass spectroscopy patterns obtained from identical isolates remain generally stable.

Studies on cellular fractions (and later using *in silico* whole cell microbial genomics), showed that a major share of the proteins detected in whole cell mass spectra are actually ribosomal proteins [24-27], though the number of ribosomal proteins, in the mass range generally used, is lower than the total number of proteins generally detected. In bacteria, for example, some 40 ribosomal proteins can potentially be detected, though in most mass spectra, more than 100 further distinct peaks are recorded, though the correct annotation of these 100 peaks to their corresponding proteins is not yet possible for most microbial taxa [28-30]. This problem will however be overcome *via* the increasing number of microbial whole genome sequences available and the subsequent performance of *in silico* / IC-MS studies [31].

More importantly perhaps, a comparison of mass spectral patterns from related species reveals that individual peaks are specific at different taxonomic levels. In Fig. **3**, for example, a number of individual mass signals arare present in the spectra of either all, or most, of the species of Enterobacteriaceae shown. Further, genus and species-specific peaks are observed, together with peaks that are variable at the species level, potentially facilitating the development of sub-species typing.

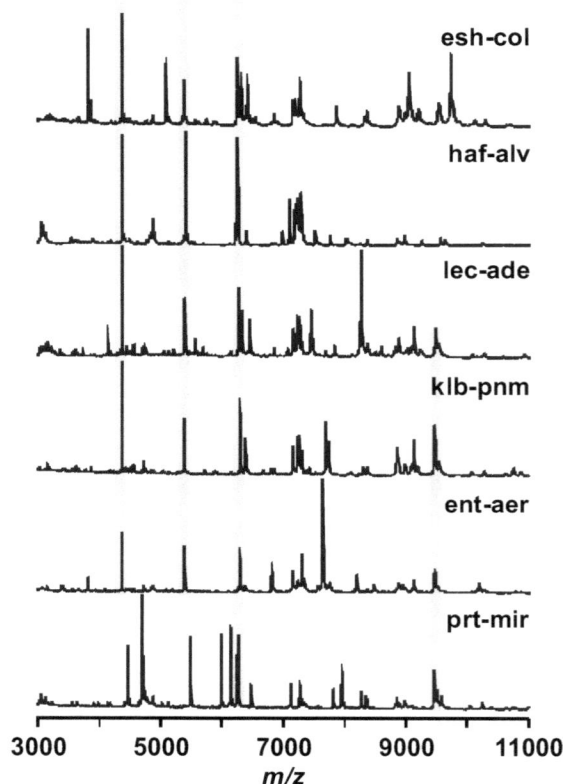

Fig. (3). Examples of mass spectra of Enterobacteriaceae isolates. esh-col: *Escherichia coli*; haf-alv: *Hafnia alvei*; lec-ade: *Leclercia adecarboxylata*; klb-pnm: *Klebsiella pneumonia*; ent-aer: *Enterobacter aerogenes*; prt-mir: *Proteus mirabilis*. Mass spectra were acquired using a Voyager DE Pro instrument (Applied Biosystems) with DHB as matrix. Grey shades indicate some prominent mass signals that were recorded for multiple species.

Detailed comparisons of mass spectra often reveal that mass shifts of particular protein peaks are explained by single amino acid exchanges [32, 33]. However, as previously mentioned, even without an absolute identification for all of the sample proteins detected by IC-MS, several studies have still shown that mass spectroscopy patterns obtained from an individual bacterial isolate is generally stable, irrespective of culture conditions, instrumentation, and sample preparation procedures [34-37]. However, for filamentous fungi such as dermatophytes and *Aspergillus* spp., the situation is somewhat different as mass spectral patterns and mass signal intensities may change considerably in response to different culture conditions [38].

In conclusion, for all microorganisms, it can be stated that culture conditions may substantially contribute to the variability in mass spectral patterns obtained from an identical isolate cultured under different conditions. This can result in individual spectra with similarities as low as 60 % shared mass signals obtained from a single isolate (author's own data, unpublished). Further, physico-chemical and technical factors such as laser power, sample preparation procedure or matrix to analyte ratios, may also contribute to this dissimilarity. Nevertheless, this 'background-uncertainty' observed when analysing microorganisms by IC-MS does not impede MALDI-TOF MS-based microbial identification, as the dissimilarity observed among spectral patterns of isolates belonging to different species is usually very much greater than that obtained from identical isolates grown under different conditions.

4. THE IDENTIFICATION OF MICRO-ORGANISMS BY MALDI-TOF MS-BASED SPECTRAL COMPARISON

Numerous studies have been published describing the mass spectrometric differentiation of more or less closely related microbial species (for a recent overview see reference [26]). The possibility of differentiating between species is an essential, but insufficient, prerequisite for the identification of microorganisms present within clinical samples using MALDI-TOF MS, as the identification of an unknown sample can only be performed by comparing the clinical isolate's mass spectrum to an independently acquired database of reference mass spectra. Therefore the most important part of an mass-based identification system is an extensive database containing reference spectra of all relevant microbial species, together with spectra of closely related species. Further, to cover intra-species variability, multiple reference spectra are required for the same microbial species [39]. Consequently, a database for clinical routine diagnostics must contain approximately 600 bacterial and 150 fungal species, based on current estimates of clinically relevant microorganisms, together with about the same number of related non-pathogenic species. These numbers are, however, far lower than the estimated number of microbial species that comprise the human microbiome (see next section). Moreover, for veterinary applications, the number of microbial species in the database has to be increased for each species of domestic and farm animal under consideration.

As well as a reference mass spectrum database of relevant species, mathematical algorithms need to be established that facilitate the comparison of mass spectrum patterns and which provide a measure of the significance of the similarity found between sample and reference spectra, eventually allowing the unambiguous identification of the sample microorganism. For this purpose, several mathematical approaches based on cluster analysis algorithms, or multivariate analysis approaches have been proposed:

- A cross-correlation analysis was proposed by Arnold and Reilly [40], which was applied to the mass spectra obtained from 25 *E. coli* strains by dividing the full spectrum in a varying number of intervals (bins), allowing the discrimination of individual strains whose mass spectra were very similar.

- Bright *et al.* [41] applied a pattern recognition algorithm to mass spectra in the range of *m/z* 500-10,000 by translating each quality-controlled mass spectrum into a single point vector in an n-dimensional space that was compared to a reference library containing 35 bacterial strains from 20 species.

- An algorithm for the extraction of fingerprints from the mass spectra (*m/z* 1,000-10,000) of bacteria developed by Jarman *et al.* [42] considered variability in replicate analyses of an individual strain. The resulting mass spectral 'fingerprints' were used for the comparison of blinded samples against a reference library of fingerprints by assessing similarities between sample and reference fingerprints based on the absence and presence of mass signals.

- A hierarchical clustering algorithm in combination with analysis of variance (ANOVA) to extract biomarkers from multiple isolates belonging to 6 human pathogens was applied by Hsieh *et al.* [43]. This set of specific markers was then reduced to 2-4, which was sufficient to identify isolates of the same species correctly (within a limited dataset).

Notably, a comparison of different algorithms revealed that they all generate very similar results [44], underlining the robustness of IC-MS based identification procedures.

Currently, two commercially available systems are running in clinical diagnostic laboratories, namely the MALDI biotyper by Bruker [45] and the AXIMA@SARAMIS by Shimadzu and AnagnosTec [26, 46]. These systems utilize relatively simple procedures for the comparison of mass spectra to identify unknown microorganisms. In both systems a sample's mass spectral pattern is compared to reference data in a database by assessing similarities based on matching peaks whilst taking into consideration an error range calculated from the respective instrument's analytical accuracy. The MALDI biotyper uses so-called "MainSpectra" for reference data that represent the spectral patterns obtained from single strains, usually obtained from public strain collections [47]. Peak height is also taken into account for the calculation of a score (as a measure of similarity). SARAMIS uses so-called "SuperSpectra" that consist of consensus spectra of multiple isolates of a species obtained from public collections, as well as from clinical laboratories, the individual peaks of which are weighted by their specificity [26]. To calculate the confidence value of the probable identification the sum of peak weights of matching masses is computed. This "specificity weighting" reduces background similarity, *i.e.*, between species of the same genus, allowing stronger discrimination between closely related species or even subspecies. A similar weighting has been successfully used to discriminate subspecies of the plant pathogen *Erwinia* sp. [48]. Despite the relative simplicity of their algorithms, both systems perform well in routine diagnostics [49], underlining the fact that the quality and quantity of reference data is of greater importance than the mathematical procedures utilized to compare spectra.

5. MALDI-TOF MS AND MODERN MICROBIAL TAXONOMY

In the "pre-genomic" era species have been distinguished often based on a single or a few metabolic reactions, without taking into consideration their over-all genomic similarity (due to technological limitations). With the advent in recent years of new technologies, bacterial and fungal taxonomy has come under continuous revision, mainly due to the increasing availability of genomic sequence data. Indeed, several 'classical' clinical species have now been renamed or further divided into multiple species. As examples, *Enterobacter sakazakii* has changed to *Cronobacter sakazakii* [50], and *Peptostreptococcus micros* was first changed to *Micromonas micros* and then to *Parvimonas micra* [51]. The clinical relevance of these taxonomic revisions may however not be easy to interpret by clinical microbiologists or general practitioners. Nevertheless, because IC-MS and subsequent pattern analysis of microbial strains is generally consistent with molecular phylogenetic analyses, it is obvious that IC-MS-based identification procedures should utilize the more recent taxonomies as a reference [52] for naming microbial species in a database.

A further major challenge for the clinical microbiologist is the rapidly increasing number of bacterial species associated with humans that are of potential medical significance. Although estimates of the total taxonomic diversity of the human microbiome vary considerably (approximately 1000 [53] to more than 40,000 [54] bacterial species estimated for the human gut microbiome alone), there is no doubt that the number of validly described species is only a very minor fraction of the number of actually existing microbial species. Advances in modern technology mean that the number of potentially pathogenic species of bacteria and fungi will increase considerably in the near future. In this light, it is evident, that a modern system for the routine identification of microorganisms must be highly flexible in order to be able to handle the increasing number of new and emerging pathogens that need to be identified in clinical specimens. Therefore, IC-MS reference databases should be regularly updated in order to include the most recent microbial taxonomic revisions. In this respect, one major advantage of MALDI-TOF MS based identification systems, compared to classical biochemical identification systems, is the fact that such systems are easily updated and expanded. New reference spectra obtained from new microbial species may be directly added to MALDI-TOF MS reference databases and easily compared to mass spectra of related species [55]. New species can be added to a database as soon as a single well characterized strain is available. This has been shown, for example, for species of the *Burkholderia cepacia* complex that have recently been transformed from the status of genomovars to validly described bacterial species [44]. Further, the comparison of mass spectra can rapidly reveal potentially new microbial species and consequently MALDI-TOF MS is increasingly applied in systematic microbiology [56, 57]. The generally observed high level of congruency of cluster analyses observed for microbial mass spectral patterns, compared to cluster analyses based on nucleotide sequences of housekeeping genes [33, 58], allows the rapid classification of bacterial strains and the recognition of subspecies, or even putative new species, at first hand [59]. Even without a formal species description, MALDI-TOF MS-based taxonomic units can be included in an IC-MS reference database to detect the re-occurrence and spread of a particular microbial pathogen. This may by itself provide valuable information with respect to therapeutic options and epidemiological data.

6. SOME POSSIBLE LIMITATIONS ASSOCIATED WITH THE MASS SPECTROMETRY-BASED ANALYSIS OF MICRO-ORGANISMS

A large number of studies, using mass spectral analysis of diverse taxa of microorganisms, emphasizes that IC-MS is applicable in principle for the species identification of all taxa of archeae, bacteria, yeasts, and moulds [26]. In some cases, it may be necessary to slightly modify the sample preparation procedure, for example, for yeasts, by introducing an additional extraction step with formic acid [60]. Otherwise, no principle restrictions on IC-MS-based microbial identification have been encountered so far. Indeed, the application of IC-MS technology has been extended for use in the discrimination of higher animals such as nematodes and insects [61, 62]. However, though this extension of IC-MS to larger organisms has been successful, the mass spectral analysis of viruses appears to be a limit for this technology due to the need for a sample comprising more or less of pure virus particles, which is generally not the case for clinical samples. Further, the protein patterns obtained from virus particles may not be complex enough to allow the distinction of important types of viruses and only MS-MS approaches may yield enough spectral information for this purpose. For diagnostic purposes, virus identification by MALDI-TOF MS can therefore probably only be achieved *via* a preceding PCR based sample preparation [63]. Nevertheless, a few studies have been published indicating that the direct MALDI-TOF MS of virus particles is a promising technology for fundamental virology [64, 65].

One aspect of IC-MS for clinical applications that is often considered as a major disadvantage compared to DNA-based methods, is the need to first obtain a clonal culture (which can be a small colony on an agar plate) prior to analysis. This is indeed a major time-consuming part of the entire IC-MS process, largely due to the fact that the growth rate of individual microorganisms has intrinsic limits that cannot be substantially increased, even when using new culturing methods. In practice, this need for selective culture is dependant on: 1), the absolute amount of microbial cellular material needed for analysis, and 2) the purity of the sample, *i.e.*, a pure clonal isolate of a particular microorganism free of complex background matrices. The amount of cells required for IC-MS can likely be further substantially reduced using improved sample handling techniques, and new technologies are currently being developed for this, including single-cell analysis [66]. The need for clonal cultures for IC-MS-based identification is not an absolute and in this context, the nature of the analysis has to be considered. In contrast to PCR-based methods, no selectivity in the choice of amplification target is required in IC-MS. As a consequence, those molecules that have the highest abundance within the sample are generally preferentially detected with the highest peaks (though this is a gross simplification because many factors affect the detection of a molecule including stoichiometry, hydrophilicity, and amino acid composition etc [13, 67, 68]). Nevertheless, it is a general rule for the analysis of mixtures of bacteria,that mass signals of cellular compounds of the dominant bacterial species will be found to dominate the mass spectrum obtained (Fig. **4**). However, mass signals from 2 mixed bacteria can be recorded only within a relatively narrow range of bacterial density ratios (approximately 1:4 to 4:1), a range that leads to an overlay of 2 spectra from which a sufficient number of specific mass signals can be recognized to allow the identification of both species. Beyond this range of density ratios, the majority of mass signals of the minority population are lost within the background noise. However, particular mass signals of a bacterium can occasionally be recorded despite a low representation, for example *m/z* 4410 of *Enterococcus faecalis* at a ratio of 1:10 to *Stapylococcus aureus* (Fig. **4**). Detailed analysis of this spectrum could reveal *E. faecalis* contamination of an *S. aureus* sample at 1:4 and 1:10 ratio, though this is not possible at the opposite 10:1 ratio due to the mass spectrum signal intensities of *S. aureus* being generally more evenly distributed and hence more easily lost.

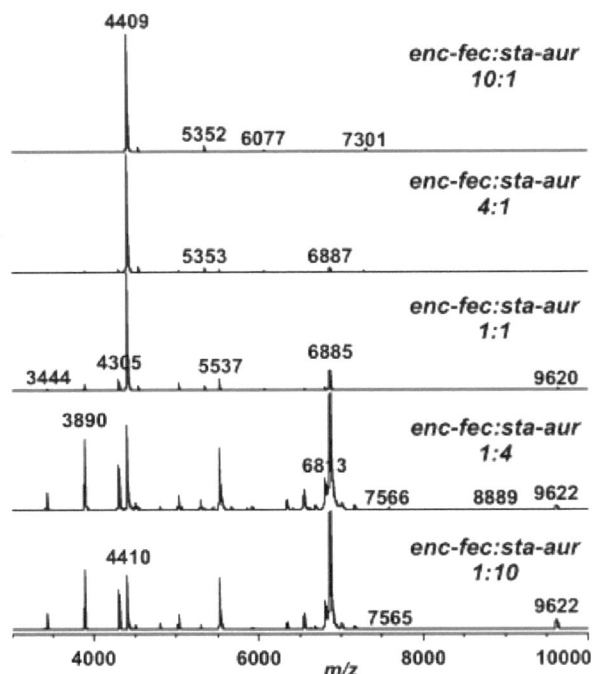

Fig. (4). Mass spectra of mixtures of *Enterococcus faecalis* (enc-fec) and *Staphylococcus aureus* (sta-aur). Cell numbers were estimated from optical density measurements of suspensions from which cells were harvested and mixed in ratios as indicated. Mass spectra were acquired using an AXIMA CFR+ instrument (Shimadzu) using DHB as the matrix.

The same effect of signal suppression is observed in samples of bacteria present within complex biological matrices such as urine, blood, and spinal fluid. Indeed, even in the presence of clonal or nearly clonal microbial infections, IC-MS and subsequent microbial species identification can generally only be achieved after a separation of bacterial cells from any other sample constituents. In fact, cellular separation actually allows the application of MALDI-TOF MS to positive blood culture samples, using such specimen preparation protocols as gel filtration, detergents, and centrifugation [69-71]. In all of these (and other) positive blood culture studies, the critical issues were found to be the absolute quantity of microbial cells available for analysis, and the relative purity of the bacterial pellet. In general however, the direct detection of microorganisms in clinical specimens is not feasible due to the low number of microbial cells present in the primary sample (especially problematic with important specimens such as spinal fluids). Encouraging results have, however, been reported for the direct identification of bacteria and yeasts in urine samples [72], facilitated by the relatively large number of microbes present within the primary urine sample (*e.g.* 10^5 cells per mL [73]).

The identification of antibiotic resistance types by IC-MS has been proposed for some microbial species in several publications [74-77], but has not yet become established in routine diagnostics. The major reason for this is the fact that IC-MS generally allows a discrimination of isolates in accordance to their phylogenetic distance, whilst the distribution of antibiotic resistance genes is most often the result of lateral gene transfer and rapid evolution [78, 79]. Therefore, the direct discrimination of resistant and susceptible isolates by IC-MS will likely not be achievable in the near future. One possibility to obviate this limitation could be to sub-type isolates of a given species and to then correlate resistance patterns to individual mass pattern types. This could allow the discrimination of different phylogenetic lineages associated with each antimicrobial resistance pattern, and eventually facilitate the comparison of reference (resistant sub-type) mass spectra against mass spectra obtained from clinical samples in order to predict resistance [33]. At the moment, a combination of taxonomic identification and classical antibiotic susceptibility testing is required (Fig. **1**).

Other possible limitations of IC-MS could be of a more technical nature. No microbial taxon has yet been recognized that is in principle inaccessible to IC-MS, meaning that the number of microbial species present in an IC-MS reference database is not limited by the methodology itself. Rather, limitations could be due to a gradual reduction in taxonomic resolution associated with an increasing number of reference species present within a database. Therefore, there is no guarantee that MALDI-TOF MS-based identification systems will still perform reliably if the current number of species (or taxonomic units) increases by orders of magnitude. On the other hand, no evidence for such a fundamental limitation has yet been produced. A further constraint could paradoxically be the continuing improvement of IC-MS instrumentation, which is leading to mass spectra containing an increasingly higher number of peaks due to an enhancement in sensitivity and resolution. Hence, technological advances could hamper the comparison of previously archived mass spectral patterns to those recently acquired using more sensitive instruments. Because, MALDI-TOF MS is essentially a chemical analytical method, the absence of a peak in a spectrum is not equivalent to the absence of a particular protein, but strictly speaking, its possible presence below the detection limit. A change in detection limits, for example through an increase in detector sensitivity of new instruments, can consequently lead to an altered peak pattern for an isolate. This is a major difference compared to nucleic acid sequence analyses, where old and new technologies, such as Sanger- and pyro-sequencing, yield essentially the same result, namely a sequence consisting of four distinct bases.

7. CONSEQUENCES OF MALDI-TOF MS IDENTIFICATION FOR THE ROUTINE CLINICAL MICROBIOLOGY DIAGNOSTIC LABORATORY

The rapid increase in acceptance of IC-MS in clinical diagnostic laboratories indicates that this technology has the potential to revolutionize clinical microbiology [80, 81]. Integration into a laboratory's work-flow scheme is facilitated by the fact that a single system may serve for the analysis of all types of clinical samples using high-throughput formats [82]. The time from specimen reception to identification and result depends primarily on the time that is required to cultivate microorganisms to visible colonies, a range of 8-48 h for most microbial species. Sample preparation for IC-MS and the measurement itself is accomplished on average in a few minutes per sample when batches of samples are analysed, meaning that the total time required from clinical specimen receipt to release of a result can be reduced by several hours compared to conventional microbiological identification techniques. For clinical diagnostics, a switch from biochemical to mass-based identification procedures will bring a number of changes:

- Automation of the entire work-flow from clinical specimen to final result.

- Shift of expenses from low investment & high consumables to high investment & low consumables.

- More samples can be analysed with higher accuracy at lower costs compared to classical biochemical methods.

- Identification and species assignment of isolates in accordance with recent taxonomy.

- New or cryptic microbial species may be recognized with a high probability.

One major prerequisite for the successful application of MALDI-TOF MS as an identification tool is a strong concordance of the detected proteome to the genomic sequence of microorganisms. Mass spectrum fingerprints could then be considered as an indirect genotyping tool (*e.g.* multi-locus sequence analysis), so that differences and similarities in mass spectral patterns would, to a large extent, represent phylogenetic relationships However, results obtained using an IC-MS approach to microbial identification are generally in accordance to a taxonomy strictly based on phylogenetic evidence. As a consequence, categories or groups of bacteria that have been established prior to the genomic era, and in use for decades, cannot be expected to be identified within the results of mass spetrum-based identification. For example, the direct discrimination of Gram-positive and Gram-negative bacteria by IC-MS is not possible and this information has to be obtained retrospectively, after species or genus identification. The same applies for coagulase-negative staphylococci [83], viridans streptococci [84], non-fermenting bacteria [85] *etc.* This means that laboratory reports will have to be adapted to include a number of 'new' microbial species and the medical staff will need to be prepared accordingly in order to understand how to interpret the information in the correct context.

Interestingly, the identification by IC-MS of several microbial taxa is far superior to any currently available biochemical systems. This is particularly true for non-fermenting and anaerobic bacteria, for which biochemical identification is often difficult and where any current difficulties in mass spectrometry-based identification are primarily due to the incompletely resolved taxonomy of these microbial groups [59, 86]. On the other hand, discrimination of clinically relevant species may be hampered, for example the correct identification of *Shigella* spp., and of pneumococci (*Streptococcus pneumoniae*). Both taxa are easily distinguishable from their closest relatives, *Escherichia coli* and *Streptococcus mitis*, respectively, using simple biochemical tests such as lactose fermentation or optochin resistance. In both cases however, it is not fully clear whether a negative test does indeed fully correlate to pathogenicity, as *Shigella* species, for example, are not clearly distinguishable from enteroinvasive *E. coli* [87], both of which cause similar illnesses. However, such constraints have not significantly affected the general acceptance of mass spectrometry-based identification in routine diagnostic microbiology laboratories.

The eventual development of high throughput systems will provide much more health-related value than economics alone, though economics may ultimately be the most substantial argument for replacing classical biochemistry with MALDI-TOF MS based systems. However, the effect of faster delivery and an increased number of results on medical microbiology laboratories remains to be seen. One emerging issue is the much higher diversity of microorganisms observed in clinical specimens, as well as the higher frequency of unexpected species, such as those commonly considered as 'environmental' microorganisms, but whose identification generates possible medical implications. Last but not least, the introduction of mass spectrometry-based identification systems coupled to advances in automation, may lead to a loss in microbiological knowledge of the personnel within microbiological diagnostic laboratories. The fact that no pre-selective sample preparation is required, together with the simplicity of sample preparation, renders microbiological expertise apparently superfluous. Indeed, the successful identification of microorganisms may be achieved by IC-MS-based systems even after minimal training of laboratory personnel, and could perhaps in the near future even be performed by a robot. How high-throughput automation can be achieved without losing the essential microbiological knowledge required to verify and check identification results is still an unresolved issue, especially in the light of an expected general shortage of trained laboratory staff.

8. CONCLUSIONS AND FUTURE PERSPECTIVES

It is not a vague prophecy for the author to predict that MALDI-TOF MS-based microbiological identification systems will be rapidly established within diagnostic laboratories in the very near future, certainly not if one considers the increasing number of participants at IC-MS related microbiological sessions at scientific meetings, and the increasing number of publications in this field.

As outlined in the previous section, the introduction of MALDI-TOF MS based identification systems into routine diagnostic laboratories will not only replace existing microbial identification technologies, but will also increase the number and accuracy of analyses available to the clinician, generating an impact on clinical therapeutic decision-making, helping decrease time-to-diagnosis for microbial pathogens, and expand further our understanding of infection and the disease process itself. Together with modern molecular techniques, MALDI-TOF MS will likely facilitate a new era in medical microbiology and generate a paradigm shift in our thinking, for example, by the recognition of the presence of a much greater diversity of clinically relevant pathogens than traditionally has been assumed. Despite the excellent performance and wide-spread acceptance of mass spectrometry-based identification, the full potential of MALDI-TOF MS in analytical microbiological diagnostics has not yet been fully exploited. For example, besides clinical microbiology, other fields such as environmental, veterinary, and industrial microbiology are already starting to adopt the technology. Further, beyond strictly clinical identification applications, MALDI-TOF MS is used in several other diverse fields of life-sciences, for example, for MALDI-imaging or Single-Nucleotide-Polymorphism detection [88, 89]. Although currently applied almost exclusively to microorganisms, intact-cell mass spectrometry-based analysis may be expanded to higher animals and plants, as well as to the quality control of food, histological samples, and the study of cell lines [90-93]. In fact, the principle of comparing the mass spectrum of a biological sample to reference mass spectra obtained from well-characterized biological samples can be applied globally. Within this global context, continued research and diagnostic applications will rapidly increase the availability and size of MALDI-TOF MS reference databases, which in turn will hasten the development of further clinical applications.

Finally, it is expected that MALDI-TOF MS will be introduced as a routine analytical technique not only in medical microbiology, but also in other microbiological and medical disciplines, so that a mass spectrometer will likely become a familiar piece of equipment within medical diagnostic laboratories of the future.

REFERENCES

[1]   Cohan FM. What are bacterial species? Annu Rev Microbiol 2002; 56: 457-87.

[2]   Rosello-Mora R, Amann RI. The species concept for prokaryotes. FEMS Microbiol Rev 2001; 25: 39-67.

[3]   Bapteste E, Boucher Y. Lateral gene transfer challenges principles of microbial systematics. Trends Microbiol 2008; 16: 200-7.

[4]   Stackebrandt E, Frederiksen W, Garrity GM, *et al.* Report of the *ad hoc* committee for the re-evaluation of the species definition in bacteriology. Int J Syst Evol Microbiol 2002; 52: 1043-7.

[5]   Goris J, Konstantinidis KT, Klappenbach JA, Coenye T, Vandamme P, Tiedje JM. DNA-DNA hybridization values and their relationship to whole-genome sequence similarities. Int J Syst Evol Microbiol 2007; 57: 81-91.

[6]   Dagan T, Artzy-Randrup Y, Martin W. Modular networks and cumulative impact of lateral transfer in prokaryote genome evolution. Proc Natl Acad Sci U S A 2008; 105: 10039-44.

[7]   Bapteste E, O'Malley MA, Beiko RG, *et al.* Prokaryotic evolution and the tree of life are two different things. Biol Direct 2009; 4: 34.

[8]   Karas M, Bachmann D, Hillenkamp F. Influence of the wavelength in high-irradiance ultraviolat laser desorption mass spectrometry of organic molecules. Anal Chem 1985; 57: 2935-9.

[9]   Karas M, Hillenkamp F. Laser desorption ionization of proteins with masses exceeding 10,000 Da. Anal Chem 1988; 60: 2299-303.

[10]   Tanaka K, Waki H, Ido Y, Akita S, Yoshida Y, Yoshida T. Protein and polymer analyses up to m/z 100 000 by laser ionization time-of-flight mass spectrometry. Rapid Comm Mass Spectrom 1988; 2: 151-3.

[11]   Krishnamurty T, Ross PL. Rapid Identification of Bacteria by Direct Matrix-assisted Laser Desorption/Ionization Mass Spectrometric Analysis of Whole Cells. Rapid Comm Mass Spectrom 1996; 10: 1992-6.

[12]   Holland RD, Wolkes JG, Rafii F, *et al.* Rapid identification of intact whole bacteria based on spectral patterns using Matrix-assisted Laser Desorption/Ionization with Time-of-flight Mass Spectrometry. Rapid Comm Mass Spectrom 1996; 10: 1227-32.

[13]   Karas M, Glückmann M, Schäfer J. Ionization in matrix-assisted laser desorption/ionization: singly charged molecular ions are the lucky survivors. J Mass Spectrom 2000; 35: 1-12.

[14]   Bahr U, Stahl-Zeng J, Gleitsmann E, Karas M. Delayed extraction time-of-flight MALDI mass spectrometry of proteins above 25000 Da. J Mass Spectrom 1997; 32: 1111-6.

[15]   Wilkes JG, Buzatu DA, Dare DJ, *et al.* Improved cell typing by charge-state deconvolution of matrix-assisted laser desorption/ionization mass spectra. Rapid Comm Mass Spectrom 2006; 20: 1595-603.

[16]   Feldman AB, Antoine M, Lin JS, Demirev PA. Covariance mapping in matrix-assisted laser desorption/ionization time-of-flight mass spectrometry. Rapid Comm Mass Spectrom 2003; 17: 991-5.

[17]   Dreisewerd K. The desorption process in MALDI. Chem Rev 2003; 103: 395-425.

[18]   Liu H, Du Z, Wang J, Yang R. Universal sample preparation method for characterization of bacteria by matrix-assisted laser desorption/ionization time-of-flight mass spectrometry. Appl Environ Microbiol 2007; 73: 1899-907.

[19]   Dong HJ, Kemptner J, Marchetti-Deschmann M, Kubicek CP, Allmaier G. Development of a MALDI two-layer volume sample preparation technique for analysis of colored conidia spores of *Fusarium* by MALDI linear TOF mass spectrometry. Anal Bioanal Chem 2009; 395: 1373-83.

[20]   Jaskolla TW, Lehmann WD, Karas M. 4-Chloro-a-cyanocinnamic acid is an advanced, rationally designed MALDI matrix. Proc Natl Acad Sci U S A 2009; 105: 12200-5.

[21]   Lasch P, Beyer W, Nattermann H, *et al.* Identification of *Bacillus anthracis* by using matrix-assisted laser desorption ionization-time of flight mass spectrometry and artificial neural networks. Appl Environ Microbiol 2009; 75: 7229-42.

[22]   van Wuijckhuijse AL, Stowers MA, Kleefsman WA, van Baar BLM, Kientz CE, Marijnissen JCM. Matrix-assisted laser desorption/ionisation aerosol time-of-flight mass spectrometry for the analysis of bioaerosols: development of a fast detector for airborne biological pathogens. Journal of Aerosol Science 2005; 36: 677-87.

[23]   Jespersen S, Niessen WMA, Tjaden UR, *et al.* Attomole detection of proteins by matrix-assisted laser desorption/ionization mass spectrometry with the use of picolitre vials. Rapid Comm Mass Spectrom 1994; 8: 581-4.

[24]   Teramoto K, Sato H, Sun L, *et al.* Phylogenetic classification of *Pseudomonas putida* strains by MALDI-MS using ribosomal subunit proteins as biomarkers. Anal Chem 2007; 79: 8712-9.

[25]   Demirev PA, Feldman AB, Kowalski P, Lin JS. Top-down proteomics for rapid identification of intact microorganisms. Anal Chem 2005; 77: 7455-61.

[26]   Kallow W, Erhard M, Shah HN, Raptakis E, Welker M. MALDI-TOF MS and microbial identification: years of experimental development to an established protocol. In: Shah HN, Gharbia SE, Encheva V, editors. Mass spectrometry for microbial proteomics.Chichester: Wiley; 2010. p. 255-76.

[27]   Dieckmann R, Strauch E, Alter T. Rapid identification and characterization of *Vibrio* species using whole-cell MALDI-TOF mass spectrometry. J Appl Microbiol 2010; 109: 199-211.

[28]   Holland RD, Duffy CR, Rafii F, *et al.* Identification of bacterial proteins observed in MALDI TOF mass spectra from whole cells. Anal Chem 1999; 71: 3226-30.

[29]   Karty JA, Lato S, Reilly JP. Detection of the bacteriological sex factor in *E. coli* by matrix-assisted laser desorption/ionization time-of-flight mass spectrometry. Rapid Comm Mass Spectrom 1998; 12: 625-9.

[30]   Fagerquist CK. Amino acid sequence determination of protein biomarkers of *Campylobacter upsaliensis* and *C. helveticus* by "composite" sequence proteomic analysis. J Proteome Res 2007; 6: 2539-49.

[31]   Wynne C, Fenselau C, Demirev PA, Edwards N. Top-down identification of protein biomarkers in bacteria with unsequenced genomes. Anal Chem 2009; 81: 9633-42.

[32]   Dieckmann R, Helmuth R, Erhard M, Malorny B. Rapid classification and identification of Salmonellae at the species and subspecies level by whole-cell matrix-assisted laser desorption ionization - time of flight mass spectrometry. Appl Environ Microbiol 2008; 74: 7767-78.

[33]   Rezzonico F, Vogel G, Duffy B, Tonolla M. Whole cell MALDI-TOF mass spectrometry application for rapid identification and clustering analysis of *Pantoea* species. Appl Environ Microbiol 2010.

[34]   Williams TL, Andrzejewski D, Lay JO, Musser SM. Experimental factors affecting the quality and reproducibility of MALDI TOF mass spectra obtained from whole bacteria cells. J Am Soc Mass Spectrom 2003; 14: 342-51.

[35]   Wunschel DS, Hill EA, McLean JS, *et al.* Effects of varied pH, growth rate and temperature using controlled fermentation and batch culture on Matrix Assisted Laser Desorption/Ionization whole cell protein fingerprints. J Microb Meth 2005; 62: 259-71.

[36]   Valentine NB, Wunschel SC, Wunschel DS, Petersen CE, Wahl KL. Effect of culture conditions on microorganism identification by matrix-assisted laser desorption ionization mass spectrometry. Appl Environ Microbiol 2005; 71: 58-64.

[37]   Burak S, Engels-Schwarzlose S, Erhard M, Welker M, Gehrt A. Official accreditation of a MALDI-TOF MS based identification system for diagnostic microbiology. Int J Med Microbiol 2010; 299: 9.

[38]   Erhard M, Hipler UC, Burmester A, Brakhage AA, Wöstemeyer J. Identification of dermatophyte species causing onychomycosis and tinea pedis by MALDI-TOF mass spectrometry. Exp Dermatol 2008; 17: 365-71.

[39]   Lartigue MF, Hery-Arnaud G, Haguenoer E, *et al.* Identification of *Streptococcus agalactiae* isolates from various phylogenetic lineages by matrix-assisted laser desorption ionization-time of flight mass spectrometry. J Clin Microbiol 2009; 47: 2284-7.

[40] Arnold RJ, Reilly JP. Fingerprint matching of *E. coli* strains with matrix-assisted laser desorption/ionization time-of-flight mass spectrometry of whole cells using a modified correlation approach. Rapid Comm Mass Spectrom 1998; 12: 630-6.

[41] Bright JJ, Claydon MA, Soufian M, Gordon DB. Rapid typing of bacteria using matrix-assisted laser desorption ionisation time-of-flight mass spectrometry and pattern recognition software. J Microbiol Methods 2002; 48: 127-38.

[42] Jarman KH, Daly DS, Peterson CE, Saenz AJ, Valentine NB, Wahl KL. Extracting and visualizing matrix-assisted laser desorption/ionization time-of-flight mass spectral fingerprints. Rapid Comm Mass Spectrom 1999; 13: 1586-94.

[43] Hsieh S-Y, Tseng C-L, Lee Y-S, *et al.* Highly efficient classification and identification of human pathogenic bacteria by MALDI-TOF MS. Mol Cell Proteom 2008; 7: 448-56.

[44] Vanlaere E, Sergeant K, Dawyndt P, *et al.* Matrix assisted laser desorption ionization-time of flight mass spectrometry of intact cells allows rapid identification of *Burkholderia cepacia* complex species. J Microb Meth 2008; 75: 279-86.

[45] Pusch W. Bruker Daltronics: leading the way from basic research to mass-spectrometry-based clinical applications. Pharmacogenomics 2007; 8: 663-8.

[46] Kallow W, Dieckmann R, Kleinkauf N, Erhard M, Neuhof T, inventors; Method of identifying microorganisms using MALDI-TOF-MS. European Patent patent EP 1 253 655 B1. 2000.

[47] Freiwald A, Sauer S. Phylogenetic classification and identification of bacteria by mass spectrometry. Nat Prot 2009; 4: 732-42.

[48] Sauer S, Freiwald A, Maier T, *et al.* Classification and identification of bacteria by mass spectrometry and computional analysis. PLoS One 2008; 3: e2843.

[49] Cherkaoui A, Hibbs J, Emonet S, *et al.* Comparison of two matrix-assisted laser desorption ionization-time of flight mass spectrometry methods with conventional phenotypic identification for routine identification of bacteria to the species level. J Clin Microbiol 2010; 48: 1169-75.

[50] Iversen C, Mullane N, McCardell B, *et al. Cronobacter* gen. nov., a new genus to accommodate the biogroups of *Enterobacter sakazakii,* and proposal of *Cronobacter sakazakii* gen. nov., comb. nov., *Cronobacter malonaticus* sp. nov., *Cronobacter turicensis* sp. nov., *Cronobacter muytjensii* sp. nov., *Cronobacter dublinensis* sp. nov., *Cronobacter* genomospecies 1, and of three subspecies, *Cronobacter dublinensis* subsp. *dublinensis* subsp. nov., *Cronobacter dublinensis* subsp. *lausannensis* subsp. nov. and *Cronobacter dublinensis* subsp. *lactaridi* subsp. nov. Int J Syst Evol Microbiol 2008; 58: 1442-7.

[51] Tindall BJ, Euzéby JP. Proposal of *Parvimonas* gen. nov. and *Quatrionicoccus* gen. nov. as replacements for the illegitimate, prokaryotic, generic names *Micromonas* Murdoch and Shah 2000 and *Quadricoccus* Maszenan *et al.* 2002, respectively. Int J Syst Evol Microbiol 2006; 56: 2711-3.

[52] Euzéby JP. List of Prokaryotic names with Standing in Nomenclature (http://www.bacterio.net). Int J Syst Bacteriol 1997; 47: 590-2.

[53] Qin J, Li R, Raes J, *et al.* A human gut microbial gene catalogue established by metagenomic sequencing. Nature 2010; 464: 59-65.

[54] Frank DN, Pace NR. Gastrointestinal microbiology enters the metagenomics era. Curr Opin Gastroenterol 2008; 24: 4-10.

[55] Kroppenstedt RM, Mayilraj S, Wink JM, *et al.* Eight new species of the genus *Micromonospora, Micromonospora citrea* sp. nov., *Micromonospora echinaurantiaca* sp. nov., *Micromonospora echinofusca* sp. nov., *Micromonospora fulviviridis* sp. nov., *Micromonospora inyonensis* sp. nov., *Micromonospora peucetia* sp. nov., *Micromonospora sagamiensis* sp. nov., and *Micromonospora viridifasciens* sp. nov. Syst Appl Microbiol 2005; 28: 328-39.

[56] Clermont D, Diard S, Motreff L, *et al.* Description of *Microbacterium binotii* sp. nov., isolated from human blood. Int J Syst Evol Microbiol 2009; 59: 1016-22.

[57] Ali Z, Cousin S, Fruhling A, *et al. Flavobacterium rivuli* sp nov., *Flavobacterium subsaxonicum* sp nov., *Flavobacterium swingsii* sp nov and *Flavobacterium reichenbachii* sp nov., isolated from a hard water rivulet. Int J Syst Evol Microbiol 2009; 59: 2610-7.

[58] Stackebrandt E, Päuker O, Erhard M. Grouping Myxococci (*Corallococcus*) strains by matrix-assisted laser desorption ionization time-of-flight (MALDI TOF) mass spectrometry: comparison with gene sequence phylogenies. Curr Microbiol 2005; 50: 71-7.

[59]   Wildeboer-Veloo ACM, Erhard M, Welker M, Welling GW, Degener JE. Identification of Gram-positive anaerobic cocci by AXIMA@SARAMIS MALDI-TOF Mass Spectrometry. Syst Appl Microbiol 2010; submitted.

[60]   Amiri-Eliasi B, Fenselau C. Characterization of protein biomarkers desorbed by MALDI from whole fungal cells. Anal Chem 2001; 73: 5228-31.

[61]   Perera MR, Vanstone VA, Jones MGK. A novel approach to identify plant parasitic nematodes using matrix-assisted laser desorption/ionization time-of-flight mass spectrometry. Rapid Comm Mass Spectrom 2005; 19: 1454-60.

[62]   Feltens R, Görner R, Kalkhof S, Gröger-Arndt H, von Bergen M. Discrimination of different species from the genus *Drosophila* by intact protein profiling using matrix-assisted laser desorption ionization mass spectrometry. BMC Evol Biol 2010; 10: 95.

[63]   Sjöholm MIL, Dillner J, Carlson J. Multiplex detection of human herpesviruses from archival specimens by using matrix-assisted laser desorption ionization–time of flight mass spectrometry. J Clin Microbiol 2008; 46: 540-5.

[64]   Yao ZP, Demirev PA, Fenselau C. Mass spectrometry-based proteolytic mapping for rapid virus identification. Anal Chem 2002; 74: 2529-34.

[65]   Swatkoski S, Russell S, Edwards N, Fenselau C. Analysis of a model virus using residue-specific chemical cleavage and MALDI-TOF mass spectrometry. Anal Chem 2007; 79: 654-8.

[66]   Russell SC. Microorganism characterization by single particle mass spectrometry. Mass Spectrom Rev 2009; 28: 376-87.

[67]   Krause E, Wenschuh H, Jungblut PR. The dominance of arginine-containing peptides in MALDI-derived tryptic mass fingerprints of proteins. Anal Chem 1999; 71: 4160-5.

[68]   Horneffer V, Forsman A, Strupat K, Hillenkamp F, Kubitscheck U. Localization of analyte molecules in MALDI preparations by confocal laser scanning microscopy. Anal Chem 2001; 73: 1016-22.

[69]   Ferreira L, Sanchez-Juanes F, Guerra IP, *et al.* Microorganisms direct identification from blood culture by MALDI-TOF mass spectrometry. Clin Microbiol Infect 2010; in press.

[70]   La Scola B, Raoult D. Direct identification of bacteria in positive blood culture bottles by matrix-assisted laser desorption ionisation time-of-flight mass spectrometry. PLoS One 2009; 4.

[71]   Stevenson LG, Drake SK, Murray PR. Rapid identification of bacteria in positive blood culture broths by matrix-assisted laser desorption ionization-time of flight mass spectrometry. J Clin Microbiol 2010; 48: 444-7.

[72]   Ferreira L, Sanchez-Juanes F, Gonzalez-Avila M, *et al.* Direct identification of urinary tract pathogens from urine samples by MALDI-TOF (Matrix-Assisted Laser Desorption Ionization Time-of-Flight) mass spectrometry. J Clin Microbiol 2010; 48: 2110-5.

[73]   Kass EH. Asymptomatic infections of the urinary tract. J Urol 2002; 167: 1016-9.

[74]   Edwards-Jones V, Claydon MA, Evason DJ, Walker J, Fox AJ, Gordon DB. Rapid discrimination between methicillin-sensitive and methicillin-resistant *Staphylococcus aureus* by intact cell mass spectrometry. J Med Microbiol 2000; 49: 295-300.

[75]   Du Z, Yang R, Guo Z, Song Y, Wang J. Identification of *Staphylococcus aureus* and determination of its methicillin resistance by matrix-assisted laser desorption/ionization time-of-flight mass spectrometry. Anal Chem 2002; 74: 5487-91.

[76]   Camara JE, Hays FA. Discrimination between wild-type and ampicillin-resistant *Escherichia coli* by matrix-assisted laser desorption/ionization time-of-flight mass spectrometry. Anal Bioanal Chem 2007; 389: 1633-8.

[77]   Xu CX, Lin XM, Ren HX, Zhang YL, Wang SY, Peng XX. Analysis of outer membrane proteome of *Escherichia coli* related to resistance to ampicillin and tetracycline. Proteomics 2006; 6: 462-73.

[78]   Enright MC, Robinson DA, Randle G, Feil EJ, Grundmann H, Spratt BG. The evolutionary history of methicillin-resistant Staphylococcus aureus (MRSA). Proc Natl Acad Sci U S A 2002; 99: 7687-92.

[79]   Holden MT, Feil EJ, Lindsay JA, *et al.* Complete genomes of two clinical *Staphylococcus aureus* strains: evidence for the rapid evolution of virulence and drug resistance. Proc Natl Acad Sci U S A 2004; 101: 9786-91.

[80]   Seng P, Drancourt M, Gouriet F, *et al.* Ongoing revolution in bacteriology: routine identification of bacteria by matrix-assisted laser desorption ionization time-of-flight mass spectrometry. Clinical Infectious Diseases 2009; 49: 543-51.

[81]   Sauer S, Kliem M. Mass spectrometry tools for the classification and identification of bacteria. Nat Rev Microbiol 2010; 8: 74-82.

[82]   van Veen SQ, Claas EC, Kuijper EJ. High-throughput identification of bacteria and yeast by matrix-assisted laser desorption ionization-time of flight mass spectrometry in conventional medical microbiology laboratories. J Clin Microbiol 2010; 48: 900-7.

[83]   Dupont C, Sivadon-Tardy V, Bille E, *et al.* Identification of clinical coagulase-negative staphylococci, isolated in microbiology laboratories, by matrix-assisted laser desorption/ionization time-of-flight mass spectrometry and two automated systems. Clin Microbiol Infect 2009.

[84]   Friedrichs C, Rodloff AC, Chhatwal GS, Schellenberger W, Eschrich K. Rapid identification of viridans streptococci by mass spectrometric discrimination. J Clin Microbiol 2007; 45: 2392-7.

[85]   Mellmann A, Cloud J, Maier T, *et al.* Evaluation of Matrix-Assisted Laser Desorption Ionization-Time-of-Flight mass spectrometry in comparison to 16S rRNA gene sequencing for species identification of nonfermenting bacteria. J Clin Microbiol 2008; 46: 1946-54.

[86]   Degand N, Carbonnelle E, Dauphin B, *et al.* Matrix-assisted laser desorption ionization-time of flight mass spectrometry for identification of nonfermenting gram-negative bacilli isolated from cystic fibrosis patients. J Clin Microbiol 2008; 46: 3361-7.

[87]   Lan R, Alles MC, Donohhoe K, Martinez MB, Reeves PR. Molecular evolutionary relationships of enteroinvasive *Escherichia coli* and *Shigella* ssp. Infect Immun 2004; 72: 5080-8.

[88]   Burnum KE, Frappier SL, Caprioli RM. Matrix-assisted laser desroption/ionization imaging mass spectrometry for the investigation of proteins and peptides. Annu Rev Anal Chem 2008; 1: 689-705.

[89]   Sauer S, Reinhardt R, Lehrach H, Gut IG. Single-nucleotide polymorphisms: analysis by mass spectrometry. Nat Prot 2006; 1: 1761-71.

[90]   Mazzeo MF, Giulio BD, Guerriero G, *et al.* Fish authentication by MALDI-TOF mass spectrometry. J Agric Food Chem 2008; 56: 11071-6.

[91]   Wang J, Kliks MM, Qu W, Jun S, Shi G, Li QX. Rapid determination of the geographical origin of honey based on protein fingerprinting and barcoding using MALDI TOF MS. J Agric Food Chem 2009; 57: 10081-8.

[92]   Schwamborn K, Caprioli RM. Molecular imaging by mass spectrometry - looking beyond classical histology. Nat Rev Cancer 2010; 10: 639-46.

[93]   Römpp A, Guenther S, Schober Y, *et al.* Histology by mass spectrometry: label-free tissue characterization obtained from high-accuracy bioanalytical imaging. Angew Chem Int Ed Engl 2010; 49: 3834-8.

CHAPTER 4

The Role of New (Meta-) Metabolomic Technologies in Medical Systems Microbiology

M.-E. Guazzaroni, L. Fernández-Arrojo, N. López-Cortés and M. Ferrer[*]

Department of Applied Biocatalysis, Institute of Catalysis, CSIC, Marie Curie 2, 28049 Madrid, Spain

Abstract: During the last few years, there have been enormous strides in the ability of microbiologists to analyse complete microbial genomes, the amount of information obtained from these sequences being quite astonishing, not least with respect to deciphering the role of microbial interactions within an environmental context. However, the measurement of metabolic changes could offer even deeper insights into biological mechanisms (as compared to simple DNA sequencing alone), by actually defining and interpreting the responses of microbial systems to environmental and/or genetic modifications. In this respect, (meta-) metabolomics is a recent discipline that attempts to study metabolites and their concentrations, interactions and dynamics at a global level within complex samples. It constitutes one of the tools of the post-genomic era, all of which are concerned with the study of the different functional levels of biological systems, *i.e.* the (meta-) transcriptome, the (meta-) proteome and the (meta-) metabolome.

The analysis of small metabolites is important because these molecules participate in the metabolic reactions necessary for the normal functioning, maintenance and growth of a cell. In this context, the primary goal of this chapter is to provide a general overview of the techniques, problems and prospects of microbial (meta-) metabolomics with respect to medical microbiological research and diagnosis. A key objective is to show how the fingerprinting analysis of intra- and extracellular metabolites can be used as a reflection of metabolic microbial activities that impact on microbial cell physiology, microbe-microbe interactions, microbe-host interactions, and on the analysis of whole microbial communities.

Keywords: Metabolomics, (Meta-) Metabolomics, Metabolomic Footprinting, Mass Spectroscopy, Nuclear Magnetic Resonance, Microbiome, Metabolite Extraction.

1. THE CONCEPT OF (META-) METABOLOMICS

Metabolomics is the analysis of the metabolite profile of cells from any origin. If the analysis is applied to a complex sample, such as whole microbial communities, then, the term (meta-) metabolomics is often used. The origin of the metabolic molecules that comprise the "metabolome" can be either endogenous *e.g.* the products of biosynthesis and catabolism, or exogenous *e.g.* nutrients, pharmaceutical compounds or degradation products. Therefore, the study of the chemical diversity and range of concentrations of both the intra- and extracellular (meta-) metabolomes are essential if a complete understanding of a biological system is to be obtained. Further, though analysis of cellular metabolites allows inferences to be made regarding the biochemical functioning of organisms [1], this information is by no means comprehensive unless it is complemented by accompanying studies investigating the different functional levels of a biological system, *i.e.* the (meta-) genome, the (meta-) transcriptome and the (meta-) proteome [2-5] (Fig. **1**). Additionally, when studying the diversity and range of concentrations of intra- and extracellular metabolic molecules, it should be remembered that (meta-) metabolomics only provides a blueprint of metabolic reactions (and the possible role of each reaction) based upon a particular environment [6-8], *i.e.* not every metabolite is produced under all environmental conditions. Indeed, the metabolic molecules obtained from microbial specimens and communities may be formed only under specific conditions, and usually in response to external environmental stimuli *e.g.* aerobic versus anaerobic culture, *etc.* [9,10]. Finally, slight variations in the techniques used for sample preparation, metabolite measurement/quantification and data analyses may be observed between

*Address correspondence to M. Ferrer:** Department of Applied Biocatalysis, Institute of Catalysis, CSIC, Marie Curie 2, 28049 Madrid, Spain; E-mail: mferrer@icp.csic.es

John P. Hays and W. B. van Leeuwen (Eds)

different laboratories [11]. However, metabolites (such as substrates, intermediates, products and cofactors) are essentially the "fingerprints" of combined enzyme and transporter system activity within cells [12, 13]. Therefore, the identification and quantification of metabolites within a biological system is especially interesting for biomedical research and diagnosis, as it facilitates the identification and fingerprinting of biochemical perturbations caused by, for example, disease, drugs and toxins [14,15].

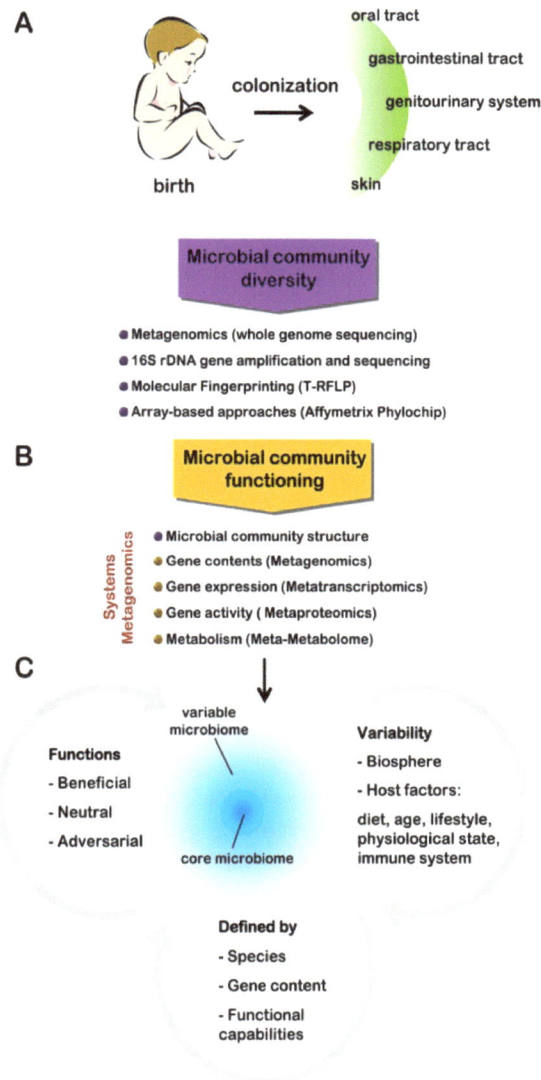

Fig. (1). Metagenomics applications and the study of the human microbiome. **(A)** The microbial colonization of skin, genitourinary system, oral- respiratory- and gastrointestinal- tracts begins immediately at birth. It is estimated that a human adult body contains approximately 100 trillion microbial cells that outnumber the host's own cells by approximately ten to one [101]. Currently, the study of host microbial diversity utilizes high-throughput technologies that aim to identify stable phylogenetic markers (metagenomic and rRNA-based techniques) rather than methods that rely in growing organisms in pure cultures. **(B)** In order to fully understand the functioning of the complete microbial community, a (meta-) genomic, transcriptomic, proteomic and metabolomics approach (systems metagenomics) is required. One of the main goals of human-microbial systems metagenomics is to determine whether a core microbiome (*i.e.* a set of microbial genes present in a given habitat in all or the vast majority of humans) exists, how variable this core microbiome is, and to understand if changes in the human microbiome can be correlated with human health (either beneficial, neutral or adversarial). Variation in the human microbiome could result from a combination of factors related to, i) the host (immune response, nutritional status etc), ii) the surrounding biosphere (nosocomial, rural, urban environments etc), and iii) features linked to the populations of microorganisms (gene content, number of species present, functional capabilities).

Before describing the state-of-the-art of medical microbial (meta-) metabolomics, a number of definitions need to be introduced [16]. "Metabolites" are the intrinsically complex small-to-medium sized molecules (Mr lower than 1000 Da) that direct cell differentiation and maintenance within the cell cycle. The complete set of metabolites in a biological system is named the "metabolome", while the actual measurement of metabolites may have different definitions, - "metabolomics" and "metabonomics" are used to define the static and dynamic identification and quantification of the metabolic space (*i.e.* the total population of metabolites), respectively. Further, if quantitative analysis is restricted to the analysis of a limited set of metabolites within a selected biochemical pathway, then, the most appropriate term to use is "metabolic profiling" [1,17]. In this context, the term "metabolic fingerprint" is used to classify and discriminate between the global intra- and extracellular metabolomic patterns generated by samples in response to specific external stimuli [18, 19]. If the analysis is restricted to excreted metabolites that are generated in a cell culture as a reflection of metabolite excretion or uptake, the term "metabolic footprinting" is used [20]. Also, at this stage, the study of the metabolome should be distinguished from the analysis of "metabolic capabilities" [21], which provides a complete analysis of all cell constituents including the genomic, proteomic and biochemical fingerprints of communities, and yields information regarding the taxonomy, functions, physiology, and abundance of community members. Further, the measurement of "metabolic activity" (*i.e.* total sample enzyme activity) may be combined with the analysis of metabolites, in order to determine the level of activity of specific microbial populations [12, 22, 23].

With respect to microbiological research and diagnosis, metabolomic profiling of biochemical reaction products, may be used to elucidate metabolic pathways and metabolic bottlenecks that may be useful for antimicrobial therapy, and in the context of microbial communities, may useful in tracking the complex metabolic interactions between microorganisms in response to, for example, quorum sensing signals. Further, metabolomics may be used to identify potential metabolic differences between microbial and mammalian cells [1], possibly useful in the development of novel diagnostic testing technologies.

2. THE HISTORY OF –OMICS AND (META-) METABOLOMICS

The first –omics term to be introduced was "genome" [2], followed in 1988 by the term "genomics" [2]. One year later, the concept of "meta-genomics" come into use, defined as the application of modern genomics techniques to the study of communities of microbial organisms directly in their natural environments, bypassing the need for isolation and lab cultivation of individual species [2]. This field actually had its roots in the culture-independent retrieval of 16S rRNA genes, pioneered by Pace and colleagues more than two decades ago [24]. Since then, (meta-) genomics has revolutionized microbiology by shifting the research focus away from single microbial isolates towards the estimated 99% of microbial species that cannot currently be cultivated [2]. While a genome represents the full genetic (DNA) complement of a single organism, (meta-) genomes represent the DNA of an entire community of organisms, and there are now thousands of genomes, including (meta-) genomes, available for study (see the Genomes Online Database at http://www.genomesonline.org) [25]. For example, in 2007, the Global Ocean Survey published scientific analyses of 41 (meta-) genomes [26], and as of October 2008, the submission of user-generated (meta-) genomes to the public MG-RAST annotation server surpassed 1300 [27]. We have now entered an era of so-called '(mega-) sequencing projects' that now include, as examples, the Genomic Encyclopedia of Bacteria and Archaea (GEBA) project [http://www.jgi.doe.gov/programs/GEBA/] and the Human Microbiome Project [http://nihroadmap.nih.gov/hmp/], with many more equally visionary projects on the horizon.

Proteomics (the study of whole cell protein production and function), followed genomics somewhat later in 1997, with proteomics research rapidly growing until the number of proteomics publications surpassed the number of genomics publications in 2009, now plateauing at approximately 3000 publications a year [2]. Although, protein isolation techniques have been traditionally applied to pure cultures of microorganisms, advances in "high-throughput" proteomics provided new tools for obtaining an integrated insight into the functioning of complex biological samples. In this context, the term (meta-) proteogenomics or (meta-) proteomics was introduced in 2004 to study the complex mixtures of proteins from an environmental sample [28-30]. Techniques such as 2-dimensional electrophoresis (2-DE) coupled to high-throughput mass spectrometry-based analytical platforms can now be used to separate and identify hundreds of proteins from a microbial community of more than 50 species, and it is even possible to identify proteins from a mixture of bacteria with unsequenced genomes [31, 32].

The term "transcriptomics" followed in 1999 and is used to define the monitoring of global changes in gene expression (RNA). However, in contrast to genomics and proteomics, transcriptomics research did not initially increase significantly in popularity due to the inherent technical problems associated with transcriptomic analysis, namely that microarrays (used to detect RNA transcripts) are organism-specific, and that the genome sequence of the organism being researched should be known [2]. However, at the moment, the number of papers is steadily increasing, with approximately 200 publications per year [33, 34], largely due to, the introduction of environmental microarrays that can measure the expression levels of hundreds to thousands of genes at the same time (the so-called (meta-) transcriptome), and perhaps more importantly, the introduction of whole transcriptome RNA sequencing within the last five years [for review see 35]. Whole transcriptome sequencing allows the analysis of community expression profiling *via* direct sequencing of reverse transcribed RNA, without prior knowledge of (meta-) genome sequences [36, 37].

In 1998, the term "metabolome" was introduced in a paper relating to the yeast genome by Oliver *et al.*, the term being based upon an analogy with the already introduced terms genome, proteome and transcriptome (see above). The term "metabolomics" came into use in the year 2000. In fact, the identification and quantification of metabolites was performed a long time before, using the techniques of thin layer and gas and liquid chromatography to study medicinal plant extracts and essential oils.

The number of publications relating to metabolomics (and metabonomics) shows a slower growth than genomics or proteomics publications, with approximately 600 publications in 2008 [2]. This slow growth may be attributed to the fact that metabolomics has no well defined method of analysis, unlike genomics and proteomics, issues that will be discussed further below. However, advances in metabolomic analysis, including: 1) advances in chromatographic techniques; such as the development of capillary columns for GC and small particle HPLC columns; 2) an increased resolution for mass spectrometry (MS)-Nuclear Magnetic Resonance (NMR); 3) the wider application of two-dimensional techniques; 4) advances in cyclotron resonance mass spectrometry and chemometrics; and 5) the direct identification of the metabolites in crude extracts or samples, may facilitate the wider use of metabolomics techniques, leading to an increase in metabolomics publications [16, 38-44].

Though the study of metabolomics has been extensively used for the analysis of single organisms, its use in complex samples (so-called (meta-) metabolomics), has been scarce, with most (meta-) metabolomic studies to date being limited to samples containing a low microbial complexity [28-30]. In the case of microbiology [8], such studies have mainly involved the investigation of metabolites in the digestive and urinary tracts (see examples in Table **1**). Unfortunately, the high amount of initial, intermediate, and dead-end, intra- and extracellular metabolites observed using (meta-) metabolomics is a major drawback, as these originate from thousands of metabolic flux networks involving thousands of enzymatic processes [13] (Fig. **2**). Further, some metabolites are prone to decomposition due to their inherent instability [45], meaning that certain metabolic fluxes may remain undetected and hence unknown. As an example of the complexity involved, it has been estimated that up to 20,000 different microbial species may be found in 1 gram of soil, comprising approximately 10^{12} genes. The majority of these genes will be contributing to the overall (meta-) metabolomic profile, with changes in metabolite level profiles continually changing over time [2]. This exceptional complexity means that the majority of (meta-) metabolomic studies have been centred around the analysis of the (meta-) metabolite profiles of body fluids or tissues during disease, or during response to specific disease therapies [1, 6, 46]. These complex samples tend to comprise homogenous cells that produce similar metabolites, and are thus technically less complex than microbial communities, such as those found in human gut.

Nevertheless, metabolomics is currently a young and vibrant (post-genomic) field of research entering its own exponential growth phase [16], having recently become more popular and accessible *via* a combination of new technologies and applications, including new faster sampling methods [*e.g.* 47], analytical tools [*e.g.* 48], isotope analysis [49] and molecular connectivity distribution [13] analyses. However, most of this growth has been related to the study of single organisms, and research involving metabolomic approaches in complex biological system is still rare, being mainly restricted to mammalian and clinically-related samples (biomedical research) [1, 50].

Table 1: List of human body samples in which (meta-) metabolomic analysis have been performed.

Organism	Microbiome	Major findings	Applied methodology	Ref.
Mouse (gut, liver, kidney, urine)	Gut	Metabotypes derived from different biological matrices from germ-free and conventional mice were characterized and it was shown that the metabolic impact of the microbiota extended beyond the intestinal tissue and biofluids to major organs such as the liver and kidney.	^{1}H NMR spectroscopic approach	[102]
Mouse (liver, plasma, urine and ileal Flushes)	Gut (humanized microbiome mouse model)	Authors compared germfree mice colonized by a human baby flora (HBF), or a normal flora, to conventional mice. Top-down multivariate analysis of metabolic profiles revealed a significant association between specific metabotypes and the resident microbiome. Data indicated that the microbiome modulates absorption, storage and energy harvest from the diet at the systems biology level.	^{1}H nuclear magnetic resonance, GC-FID[a]	[82]
Mouse (plasma, urine, fecal extracts, liver tissues and ileal flushes)	Gut (humanized microbiome mouse model)	Probiotic exposure generated microbiome modification and resulted in altered hepatic lipid metabolism coupled with lowered plasma lipoprotein levels and apparently stimulated glycolysis.	NMR spectroscopy, UPLC-MS	[103]
Human (urine samples)	Gut	Results confirmed that in humans the gut microflora metabolism is strongly linked to the obesity phenotype	NMR spectroscopy	[104]
Mouse (plasma and urine)	Gut	Authors demonstrated a close relationship between the metabolism of gut microbiota and the susceptibility of rodents to insulin resistance in high-fat diet studies.	^{1}H NMR spectroscopic approach	[105]
Human (fecal and urinary samples)	Gut	At the species level, the authors found structural differences between Chinese family gut microbiomes and those reported from American volunteers, a model consistent with population microbial co-metabolic differences reported in other epidemiological studies.	NMR spectroscopy	[106]
Rat (plasma and urine)	Gut	The authors showed that hydrazine toxicity was more severe in germfree rats compared with conventional rats for equivalent exposures, indicating that bacterial presence altered the nature or extent of response to hydrazine and that the toxic response can vary markedly in the absence of a functional microbiome.	^{1}H NMR spectroscopic approach	[107]

[a]Chromatography flame-ionization-detection (GC-FID).

3. TECHNICAL ISSUES IN THE FIELD OF (META-) METABOLOMICS

The development of robust and reliable experimental protocols for all steps in the analysis of metabolic profiles is a key issue in (meta-) metabolomics [47], with issues relating to the optimization of metabolite quenching and metabolite extraction procedures being particularly important [45]. Ideally, cell samples to be analyzed should be harvested under the same conditions as some metabolites are prone to decomposition because of their inherent instability, for example, ATP has a half-life of less than 0.1s [51]. Therefore, in order to obtain an accurate snapshot of actual metabolite levels at a particular moment in time, sampling procedures have to be significantly faster than the turn-over time of the metabolite pool, with any metabolic activity being halted instantaneously as cells are harvested. Ideally, the best protocol would combine specimen sampling, inactivation of metabolic activity, and extraction of intracellular metabolites, all in a single continuous process, which would minimize the number of handling operations required [47].

Current metabolite quenching methods include: 1) direct heating at 95°C [52, 53]; 2) dilution of the cell in cold (–48 or –45°C) methanol solution [54, 55]; 3) direct spraying of cell samples in perchloric acid [56, 57]; 4) fast filtration [58]; and 5) freezing in liquid nitrogen (N_2) [59]. Recently, integrated sampling and quenching protocols have also been developed, using either automated (*i.e.* stopped flow sampling systems) or manual devices [47, 52]. However, extensive evaluation of these and other novel methods is warranted for every sample type to be investigated.

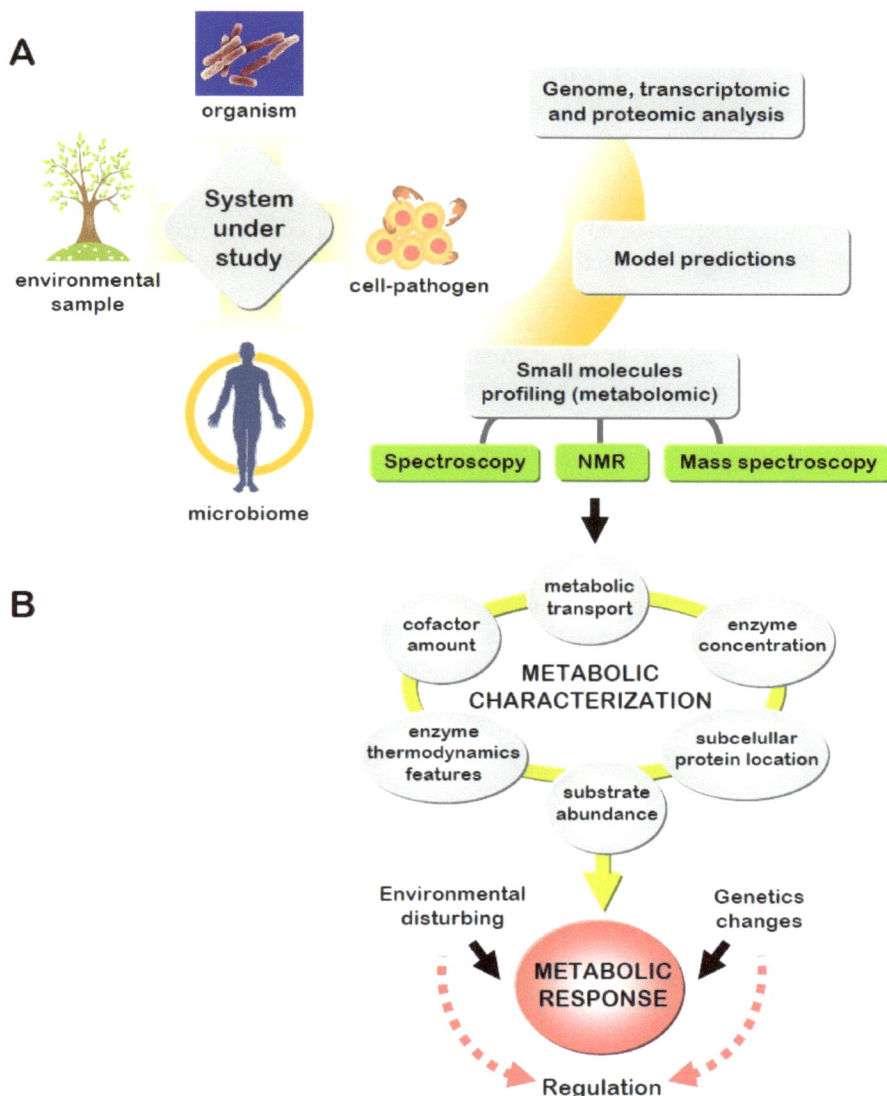

Fig. (2). Applications of metabolomic methods for understanding metabolite flux between and within species. Systems biology attempts to integrate global (holistic) approaches, in order to understand the functioning of whole systems (from individual organism, to cell-pathogen relationship, to microbiota-host interactions, and finally, microbiota inter-relationships within environments). Systems biology may therefore utilize a metabolomic profiling approach that is integrated with genome, transcription and proteome analysis, as well as *in silico* model prediction. Currently, several different technologies may be utilized to study small molecule (metabolite) profiles, including, Nuclear Magnetic Resonance (NMR) spectroscopy, Mass Spectroscopy (MS), and spectroscopy approaches (infrared [IR] or ultraviolet [UV]) often accompanied by Gas Chromatography [GC], Liquid Chromatography [LC], High-Performance Chromatography [HPLC], or Capillary Electrophoresis [CE] techniques. The functioning of microbial communities may be measured at several different levels. The ability to accurately characterize metabolic profiles is determined by interactions that occur at several different levels of regulation, including subcellular protein localization, enzyme, substrate/cofactor abundances, metabolic transport and features associated with enzyme thermodynamics. Genetic changes and environmental disturbances may affect these interplays and hence metabolic response and profile, which may then feed back into the system altering the regulation of gene expression, enzyme activity, and ultimately metabolite profile and metabolite changes (flux).

Advances in metabolite extraction methods constitute another of the key steps in metabolite analysis. Common approaches involve: 1) boiling the cell in ethanol-buffer solution; 2) diluting cells in perchloric acid; and 3) boiling the cell in hot water or cold chloroform [60, 61]. Of these methods, cold methanol / chloroform is most often preferred, because it is a mild protocol which seldom results in the loss of volatile metabolites [62, 63]. However, in the context of microbiology, both metabolite quenching and extraction procedures are heavily dependent on the type and range of microorganisms present in the sample, with samples containing a mixed microbial population being particularly problematic [47]. The difficulty in identifying and localizing metabolites and in determining the pool sizes of metabolic components are the major obstacle in applying a metabolomics approach to such complex samples.

As well as problems associated with metabolite quenching and extraction, a third problem is associated with the analysis of metabolomics itself. Metabolic fingerprinting can be performed using many diverse techniques, including: 1) UV and IR spectroscopy [64, 65]; 2) mass spectrometry; 3) nuclear and magnetic resonance; 4) GC or HPLC chromatography; and 5) a combination of techniques, such as GC-MS or LC-NMR. All of these techniques possess their own specific advantages and disadvantages [66, 67]. Further, though these methods may be applied to pure cultures of microorganisms, their low resolution may actually underestimate the number and nature of metabolites present [2]. Ultimately, the sensitivity and spatial resolution of the currently available methods still need to be improved.

All of the above issues should be taken into consideration when optimizing a (meta-) metabolome analysis since a biological sample may contain 10s, 100s, or 1000s of different metabolites, or even worse, an unknown number of unknown molecules. Further, a large variation in molecule abundance may exist, with some metabolites representing a high proportion of the total metabolome, and others only 0.001% or even less. Therefore, if the methods for sample preparation and analysis are not optimized, then a standard metabolome will capture: i) the entire amount of 'abundant' molecules; ii) most of the 'less abundant 'molecules; iii) a few of the 'low abundant' molecules; and iv) none of the 'rare' molecules. For example, bioactive molecules represent less than 10^{-6} % weight of some organisms, making their analysis technically very difficult.

4. EXPERIMENTAL CONSIDERATIONS ASSOCIATED WITH METABOLOMIC INVESTIGATIONS

(Meta-) metabolomics focuses on the complete analysis of all of the metabolites present within the sample to be investigated. However, it is virtually impossible to obtain a sample which permits the complete analysis of all of its constituent metabolites, not only because any insoluble or partly soluble compounds will be lost during the quenching and extraction reactions, but also because the further modification or derivatisation steps required for analysis may alter the molecular structure of the metabolite in such a way that the molecule become unstable. In this context, on-line tools have been developed to help in the preparation of micro-samples prior to analysis [68]. Further, quenching and extraction protocols need to take into account many chemical and physical aspects of metabolites, including:

- Metabolite diversity, *e.g.* acids, esters, amines, aliphatic compounds, peptides.

- Metabolite solubility, ranging from water soluble *e.g.* sugars, to oil soluble *e.g.* lipids.

- Metabolite concentration, which may range from very high *e.g.* sugars (can be up to 50% of a sample) and amino acids (0.5-10% of a sample), to minimal concentrations for intra-cellular signalling compounds, which often occur in the range of pg/ml to ng/ml quantities.

This means that metabolomics is very different in relation to other "-omics" technologies, requiring the analysis of thousands of different chemical compounds, often requiring multiple analyses. In fact, it is important to know how many metabolites are present within the sample under investigation in order to design appropriate methods for metabolite preparation and analysis. However, only rough estimates of the number of metabolic products within various sample types have been made. For example, in simple prokaryotes, there are expected to be approximately 1500-2000 chemical entities (both primary and secondary metabolites [2]), and this complexity increases between 2 to 5 times for *Arabidopsis* plants [69] and human cells [70]. Further, microbial (meta-) metabolomics of complex samples is much more complex than the metabolomics study of complex human samples (*e.g.* tissue or fluids), due to the enormous diversity of chemical entities (especially secondary metabolite diversity) within each microbial cell. Further, the quantities of both primary and secondary metabolites exhibit large variations and, in many cases, their concentrations lie much below the resolution of the current detection apparatus available. As one example of the problem, approximately 100,000,000,000 chemical entities are expected to be contained in 1 gram of soil [70], though only 200,000 natural compounds are known [71]. In this respect, chromatographic and NMR-based data collection and spectral processing techniques are very important in helping to ensure that, for example, replicate samples provide identical spectral fingerprints.

5. CURRENT 'GOLD STANDARD' TESTING METHODOLOGIES FOR SAMPLE PREPARATION AND METABOLITE EXTRACTION

Most laboratories use their own specific method of sample preparation for metabolomics research. It is particularly important that the reproducibility of the procedure is the best possible in order to minimize errors during sample selection [65], sample preparation, and during sample measurement [72]. Prior to sample collection, one should also consider the nature of the sample (soil, liquid, intestinal, *etc.*), and their exposure to external environmental factors that could potentially cause variation in metabolite profiles, such as storage at room temperature or frozen, the presence of artefacts that may arise due to interactions with solvents, or metabolic changes due to residual enzymatic activity.

A standard quenching procedure for metabolite measurement is outlined below (for further examples see references 20,47, 62). It should be noted that a single solvent will not be sufficient to analyse the metabolome as completely as reasonably possible [73], though a reasonable coverage of all metabolites may be obtained using two solvents, namely an organic solvent (*e.g.* chloroform) and a water-based solvent (*e.g.* water or water–methanol). However, both types of solvents have their disadvantages, for example the co-extraction of (non-metabolite) major cell components such as lipids, and sugars, by chloroform and water, respectively.

1. Microbial cultures (5 ml) grown to exponential growth phase are rapidly sprayed using an automatic pipette into pre-cooled centrifuge tubes and centrifuged at 14,000 x g for 20 seconds at 4°C.

2. The supernatants are then removed, and the cell pellets are re-suspended in 2 ml of cold wash solution (NaCl 0.9%).

3. The samples are subjected to a second quick centrifugation at 14,000 x g for 20 seconds at 4°C.

4. The supernatant is removed and cell pellets frozen by immersion in liquid N_2.

Human associated metabolites are by their nature generally labile species, chemically very diverse, and often present in a very wide dynamic range. In addition, when analyzing a living tissue or living cells, metabolic enzymes will still be active, and metabolite turnover will continue until quenched. Therefore, it is important to quench any metabolism as quickly as possible, or the system will equilibrate, and metabolite information will be compromised. With respect to unicellular organisms *e.g.* bacteria, metabolic activity can be stopped immediately, by spraying the sample into very cold (<-40°C) buffered methanol [74]. For plant or animal tissues, it is usual to "snap freeze" these samples in liquid nitrogen (N_2), after which mechanical disruption is employed to release the metabolites [75]. The above quenching methods are, however, realistic only in a laboratory setting. For the analysis of human biofluids (*e.g.* blood, urine, tears, breath, and saliva), it may not always be possible to spray these immediately into cold methanol. In this case, metabolism quenching of biofluids and organs, when applied to human or animal samples, may be performed as follows:

1. Biofluids - urinary samples are collected in a solution of 1% (wt/vol) sodium azide and centrifuged at 4°C to remove solid particles and kept at <-80°C until assayed. Blood (400 ml) should be collected into Li-heparin tubes, the plasma obtained by centrifugation, and the plasma frozen at <-70°C.

2. Organs - Organs are dissected and snap-frozen at <-70°C.

Alternatively, it may be useful to analyze the metabolites of the micro-flora associated with human organs. The most studied example is the gut. Below we summarize an example that illustrates the quenching method our laboratory uses with respect to the mouse gut (this methodology may also be applied to specimens originating in the human gut):

1. The intestinal tissue (*e.g.* from the stomach to the cecum) is removed.

2. The first 1 cm length after the stomach is considered to be duodenum and the rest is divided into three sections: the first 2/3 is designated as jejunum and the remaining 1/3 as ileum. Three-centimeter samples (3 cm) are excised from the middle of each section.

3. Ileal flush samples are obtained by rinsing the ileal lumen with 1ml of a phosphate buffer solution (0.2M Na_2HPO_4/0.04M NaH_2PO_4 (pH 7.4)) using a 1-ml sterile syringe.

4. Then, samples are retrieved in Eppendorf tubes and snap-frozen prior to appropriate analyses, *e.g.* NMR spectroscopy and UPLC–MS analyses.

5. Cecal content is collected upon animal autopsy, immediately snap-frozen and kept at <-80°C before analysis.

6. TECHNIQUES AVAILABLE FOR THE DETECTION AND ANALYSIS OF METABOLITES

Among the most widely used techniques in metabolomics analysis, currently mass spectrometry-based techniques / combinations and nuclear magnetic resonance are the most widely used. Mass spectrometry has a very high sensitivity and large dynamic range, and many different techniques can be distinguished within the field of mass spectrometry, varying by: 1) the method of introduction of the sample (direct, GC, LC); 2) in the method of ionisation (electron impact, MALDI, electrospray); and 3) in the method of detection (time-of-flight, FT-ICR). A recent review on MS techniques can be seen in ref. [11]. The most commonly used mass spectrometry platforms for metabolomics are described below:

GC-MS - Gas Chromatography – Mass Spectrometry. The high chromatographic resolving power of gas chromatography is combined with electron impact mass spectrometry. Electron impact ionisation (EI) provides a spectrum of masses for each sample tested, which *via* fragmentation, provides information regarding individual component identities. EI is the traditional method of sample ionisation, meaning that large databases of compounds already exist, making rapid identification possible. One major disadvantage of GC-MS is the fact that compounds need to be volatile to be analysed and that they should remain stable during analysis (high temperatures above 100°C are used). However, many non-volatile compounds can be converted into volatile adducts *e.g.* by silylation, acetylation or methylation, in a process called derivatisation [40]. Using this method, non-volatile sugars and amino acids may be analysed [40].

LC-MS - Liquid Chromatography - Mass Spectrometry. In this type of analysis, all types of compounds can be first separated by LC and subsequently analysed in-line using MS (usually electrospray-MS). High metabolite resolutions can be obtained using modern LC columns, *e.g.* UPLC. The electrospray mass spectra are, however, less informative then the EI mass spectra, and large reference databases are not (yet) available. Another problem with respect to electrospray mass spectrometry is the difficulty of ionisation of many compounds, though it is however possible to work in positive or negative ion mode. The advantage of being able to switch between modes is that certain substance ionize better dependant on the ion mode, *i.e.* sugars ionize better in the positive mode, whereas phenolic compounds and short fatty acids ionize better in the negative mode. An alternative approach to LC-MS profiling is to generate a representative metabolite fingerprint without using the chromatographic dimension, in which data variables are simply the detected mass values [76]. In such approaches [77 and references therein] the sample may be dissolved in an appropriate solvent and injected directly into the ion source (Direct Injection Mass Spectrometry, DIMS) or infused as a 'plug' flow using a HPLC system without a chromatography column (Flow Injection Electrospray Ionisation Mass Spectrometry, FIE-MS).

MALDI FT-ICR-MS - Fourier transform – ion cyclotron resonance – mass spectroscopy. This type of mass spectrometry has a very high resolution of up to 2,000 compounds, based on the exact masses [78]. However, isomers cannot be resolved. For metabolomics research, the chromatography step (which might actually prevent certain compounds arriving at the mass spectrometer) is often omitted. For these reasons, FT-ICR MS is an ideal technology for profiling metabolites in a high-throughput fashion. However, a preceding chromatographic separation step that sorts molecules into types is recommended for better MALDI FT-ICR-MS analytical performance.

CE-MS - Capillary electrophoresis – mass spectrometry. The coupling of CE to MS is rather new, but promising results have been obtained [79]. CE provides fast, highly efficient separations, without requiring rigorous sample pre-treatment, and with low running costs. The most attractive feature of CE though, is its small sample requirement (a few nanoliters at most), making it particularly well-suited for samples that are volume-limited. Poor concentration sensitivity, which is often cited as a disadvantage of CE alone (when fitted with absorbance-related detectors), does not pose a significant problem if using MS for detection. To date however, reports based on CE–MS constitute only a small fraction of publications, with most of these dealing with targeted metabolite analysis, and only a few dealing with comprehensive metabolomic analysis [79]. One major disadvantage of CE-MS however, is its low resolution in terms of the separation of a large number of molecules per sample.

In mass spectrometry, a single MH^+ signal indicates the presence of a compound with a specific molecular formula. However, no structural information is obtained and many isomers of a particular metabolite may exist. In this respect, the structural information content available using nuclear magnetic resonance (NMR), as well as the reproducibility and other quantitative aspects of metabolite detection, are superior to mass spectrometry, though the sensitivity of NMR is much lower. In ^1H NMR each signal corresponds to a specific hydrogen atom within a molecule, and within the spectrum, a signal is obtained for every hydrogen atom present within a molecule. Further, sample preparation is easier and the analysis more rapid. This makes NMR an ideal tool for the broad-range profiling of abundant metabolites and for metabolite fingerprinting of extensive sample collections [71, 80]. However, the number of compounds that can be detected by NMR in a single analysis is limited from one to several dozens [81, 82], largely because of the superimposition of signals when complex mixtures are analyzed. In contrast, the number of compounds that may be detected by mass spectrometry is much larger. A recent review on NMR techniques can be seen in ref. [83]. Nevertheless, the most commonly used two-dimensional NMR platforms [84] are currently the following:

1. 2D-COSY -indicates correlations between scalar coupled hydrogen atoms.

2. 2D-HSQC - indicates correlations between hydrogen atoms and the carbon atom to which they are attached.

3. 2D-HMBC - indicates correlations between hydrogen atoms and carbon atoms, generally two or three bonds away.

4. 2D-TOCSY - indicates correlations between all hydrogen atoms of a spin system.

5. J-resolved - chemical shift and coupling information are displayed in separate dimensions [79].

The tentative identification of most primary and secondary metabolites can be generally obtained using NMR techniques. However, in some cases it will be necessary to actually isolate compounds in order to correctly identify them. For the definitive identification of metabolite molecules a series of additional data (*i.e.* exact mass and MS/MS predicted structure) is generally necessary, which can be obtained with different techniques, mainly mass spectrometry coupled to different chromatographic tools (Fig. **3**).

Apart from the above most frequently used technologies, UV-visible and IF (infrared) spectroscopies are also used as non-invasive methods for metabolite analysis. These techniques are frequently used as metabolomic profiling methods in specific applications, *e.g.* in assessing an embryo's reproductive potential. Metabolomics by ultraviolet (UV) and near-infrared (NIR) spectroscopy, provide biological information by ascertaining the concentrations of key functional groups such as ROH, -SH, C=C, -CH, -OH and -NH groups. In the case of embryo selection, these methods allow detection of possible constituents of the culture media that could represent embryo viability changes, including albumin, lactate, pyruvate, glutamate and glucose. In an ongoing pilot study, the authors retrospectively investigated whether metabolomic profiling of spent culture media by NIR spectroscopy, correlated to ongoing pregnancy when transferred embryos were selected by conventional morphological selection criteria. The major disadvantage of these technologies is that they are restricted to certain molecules, and that many molecules (those of similar nature but differing in chemical structure) may have similar UV and IR patterns, which hinders their proper identification.

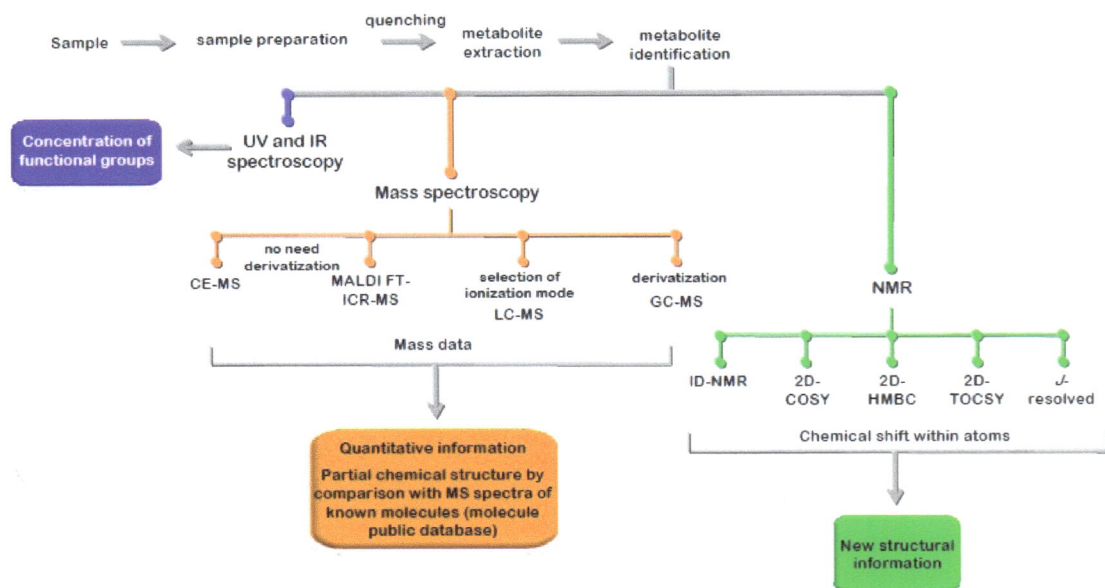

Fig. (3). Flow chart summarizing the different steps and techniques used to dissect the metabolome of biological samples.

7. TYPES OF LABORATORY EQUIPMENT REQUIRED FOR METABOLOMICS RESEARCH

A range of laboratory equipment may be required for metabolomics research in order to identify and measure metabolite levels:

1.   Centrifuge capable of > 16,000 g.

2.   Probe type sonicator.

3.   Rotor evaporator or similar (*i.e.* speed-vac).

4. High-performance liquid/GC/NMR chromatography (HPLC) vial with an insert and a pre-slit cap.

5. Flow-infection auto-sampler (*e.g.* from Gilson).

6. GC/TOF-MS - Agilent 6890N gas chromatograph interfaced to a Time-Of-Flight (TOF) Pegasus III mass spectrometer, Gas chromatograph 7890 (Agilent Technologies, Palo Alto, CA, USA) coupled to mass spectrometer 5975C (Agilent Technologies) and a DB-WAXetr column.

7. HILIC-LC/ESI-MS and LC-MS - Paradigm MS4 HPLC system coupled to an LTQ Orbitrap hybrid ion-trap/Fourier transform mass spectrometer. ZIC-pHILIC and Luna HILIC Diol columns are normally used.

8. ESI source of a LTQ Linear Ion Trap (LIT) mass spectrometer.

9. Fourier-Transform Ion Cyclotron Resonance MS (FT-ICR/MS) apparatus.

10. 1D ^{1}H NMR, 1D ^{13}C NMR, 2D ^{1}H, 1H TOCSY, 2D ^{1}H,13C HSQC, 2D JRES: i) Bruker Avance DRX600 NMR spectrometer (Bruker BioSpin, Rheinstetten, Germany), with a magnetic field strength of 14.1 T and resulting ^{1}H resonance frequency of 600 MHz, equipped with a 3 mm inverse flow probe; ii) Bruker DRX-600 spectrometer (for ^{1}H NMR TOCSY and SOFAST-HMQC), equipped with a TCI CryoProbe, 400 MHz Varian Unity equipped with a 5-mm-^{1}H (^{13}C / ^{29}Si / ^{15}N-31P) indirect detection PFG Probe; iii) ^{13}C- NMR and HSQC spectrometer (Bruker AVANCE 700) equipped with a ^{1}H inverse cryogenic probe with triple-axis gradients, operating at 700.15 MHz; iv) ^{1}H-^{13}C HSQC on an AVANCE-500 spectrometer (Bruker) equipped with a g-HR MAS 500 SB BL4 probe operating at 500.132 MHz for ^{1}H and 125.764 MHz for ^{13}C; v) Avance-700 NMR spectrometer equipped with an inverse triple-resonance CryoProbe with a z-axis gradient for 5 mm sample diameters operating at 700.153 MHz for ^{1}H and 176.061 MHz for ^{13}C, INOVA-600 MHz NMR spectrometer operating at 599.84 MHz.

Annotation of MS and MS/MS spectra can be performed using ad-hoc, commercial and publicly available databases *e.g.* NIST05/Wiley Registry, METLIN, Mass-Bank, Human Metabolome Database, Lipid Maps and BinBase [see 46 and references therein].

8. FUNCTION-DRIVEN (META-) METABOLOMICS: METABOLIC NETWORK TOPOLOGY AND METABOLIC FLUXES

Microbiological systems biology research treats microbial communities as a whole, integrating the fundamental biological knowledge gained using (meta-) metabolomics, as well as other "-omics" techniques, to create an integrated picture of how a microbial community communicates, operates and responds to environmental stimuli.

One approach toward reconstructing a metabolic network is through the analysis of all metabolite concentrations in a cell. If all intracellular and extracellular metabolites of a cell could be measured and perturbed, then the metabolic network topology (*i.e.* how each metabolic pathway interacts and communicates with each other) of that cell could be deduced. However, as has been previously mentioned, (chemo) systematic analysis and identification of metabolites is currently very difficult. For example, only 176 intracellular metabolites in *Escherichia coli* have been identified and quantified at different steady-state conditions, even using a total of 6 different analytical methods [60, 85, 86]. Since, identification and quantification of all metabolites in an organism (or a sample) is difficult, alternative methods dealing with targeted metabolic analysis (directly linked with molecule metabolism) are urgently needed in order to increase our ability to determine metabolic network topologies.

Flux analysis (*i.e.* the analysis of changes in metabolite concentrations associated with particular metabolic pathways over time), integrated with quantitative information obtained on cell, genome, mRNA and protein concentrations, contributes to a better understanding of how microbes deal with environmental perturbations both at the species [87], and at the community levels [5]. However, not all metabolites associated with a particular microbial network may contribute equally to ecosystem functioning, and the development of technologies that provide information on which metabolite groups are actually "flux-controlling" (*i.e.* metabolites whose concentrations provide information relating to key enzymatic processes that control particular metabolic pathways over time), may provide a first step in identifying "metabolic regulators" in complex microbial networks [5].

Metabolic flux networks (which are equivalent to changes in enzymatic reaction rates), cannot be measured directly, but are usually inferred, for example, from changes in metabolite levels over time. In this respect, metabolic flux analysis (MFA), using for example 13C-MFA, facilitates the dynamic quantification of intracellular fluxes by iteratively fitting the distribution of amino acid isotopomers that are present in cellular proteins to a stoichiometric model of central carbon metabolism [88]. This process allows quantitative predictions of the functional characteristics of metabolic networks to be made, without requiring prior knowledge of genomes or kinetic data [89]. For example, MFA analysis combined with sequence data results has been used to guide the metabolic engineering of at least one environmentally important species, *e.g. Geobacter sulfurreducens* [90]. Further, the flux solution space (*i.e.* the observed metabolic phenotype) can be further defined using transcriptomics and proteomics data to determine the active metabolic network, and exclude reactions that are thermodynamically unfeasible [91].

Another method used to gain an insight into metabolic flux is based on the paradigm that metabolic flux networks rely on enzyme catalysis. Enzymes in turn are encoded by genes, which allows the *in silico* reconstruction of metabolic network topologies using annotated genomic data [37]. However, the identification of all open reading frames (ORFs) present in an organism is a real challenge [92], and even in well-characterized model organisms, *e.g. E. coli* and *Saccharomyces cerevisiae*, only 940 out of 4472 (21%), and 1134 out of 5796 (20%) proteins encoded by genes have been characterized, respectively [93, 94]. The end result is that genome sequence-derived metabolic networks are typically characterized by missing reaction steps and dead-end metabolic pathways [95]. Ultimately therefore, versatile tools for the analysis of enzymatic activities (and therefore flux networks) at a given point in time, and under defined conditions, that do not require genome sequence information, are required. Some of the interesting methods in this direction are discussed below.

9. CURRENT ADVANCES IN THE FIELD OF ACTIVITY-DRIVEN (META-) METABOLOMIC FLUX ANALYSIS

Until recently, the functional assignment of metabolite pathways and metabolic network reconstruction has generally been dependant on both the genome sequence of the organism(s) in question, and the bioinformatic analysis of these sequences based on homology to known genes and proteins. Currently, however, many of the genes available in sequence databases have questionable annotations (many of them being hypothetical), or are not annotated at all, which hinders effective exploitation of the rapidly growing volume of genomic sequence data. Metabolomics provides new insights into the metabolic state of a cell under a given set of environmental parameters, or in response to changes in these parameters, independent of the knowledge of a genome sequence. However, problems of metabolite identification and quantification still exist. Further, functionally associating the metabolic profiles obtained to actual enzymes and pathways still depends heavily upon sequenced-based metabolic reconstructions. There is thus a need for new methods to causally link metabolites with cognate enzymes, which, in addition to delivering global descriptions of metabolic responses to given environmental conditions, will simultaneously provide annotation for the enzymes involved in the transformation or production of particular metabolites.

Following on from the above statement, methods in which the functional groups of enzymes are immobilized on mass spectrometry surfaces may be used to specifically target enzyme activity at high throughput scales and in complex biological mixtures. The Nanostructure-Initiator Mass Spectrometry

(NIMS) enzymatic (Nimzyme) assay is a recent development in this direction [96]. NIMS is more sensitive (sub-picogram level) than standard fluorescence- and colorimetric-based assays (500-fg and 50-pg level, respectively) and provides substrate stability at temperature as high as 100°C, thereby being potentially useful for screening enzymes that generate specific metabolites, even under harsh conditions. Here, the function, activity and chemistry of reactions are identified by mass spectrometry based on fluorous-tagged metabolites and using subsequent products as indicators. The technique has been successfully used for the detection of sialyltransferases and galactosidases in microbial community samples in a sequence independent manner.

Although, of potential interest for (meta-) metabolomics, these spectrometric approaches are not yet high-throughput systems, as it is difficult to prepare the required synthetic substrates at reasonable costs. However, the above study clearly demonstrates how future efforts in this field of research may be extremely useful for assigning functions to genetic sequences and to metabolites. These can then be further improved using software programs that allow graphical representation of the data, such as Cytoscape (http://www.cytoscape.org/) [97] the iPath web application (http://pathways.embl.de/) [98].

10. FUTURE PROSPECTS FOR (MICROBIAL) METABOLOMICS

Metabolomics has been frequently applied to compare perturbations in biological systems against unperturbed reference systems. Although, it is a relatively new field of research, its potential implications for (microbiological) diagnosis and research has catalyzed the development of metabolomics as a distinct and very active multi-disciplinary research field. The great diversity of metabolites in complex microbial communities makes it much more difficult to arrive at a routine procedure for sample preparation and analysis when compared to the metabolomic analysis of humans, plants or animals. This problem is currently one of the largest hurdles facing the use of metabolomics in microbiological diagnosis and research today. Finally, the integrative study of metabolic flux with meta-omics datasets (including metabolomics, transcriptomics, proteomics and genomics datasets), brings with it the demand for new computational approaches [99,100]. These new integrative approaches hold the promise of unparalleled insights into fundamental questions across a range of fields that include evolution, ecology, environmental biology, health and medicine. Finally, the development of high-throughput technologies that allow the detection of enzymatic activity and the identification of the products formed are urgently required. By doing so, the identification and activities of specific enzymes may be directly linked to the presence or absence of specific metabolite molecules, providing valuable data relating to microbial pathogenesis and identification.

ACKNOWLEDGEMENTS

This work is supported by BIO2006-11738, CSD2007-00005, GEN2006-27750-C-4-E, BFU2008-04398-E/BMC, KBBE-226977 (MAMBA), KBBE-245226 (MAGIC-PAH) and FEDER funds. M-*E.G.* thanks the CSIC for a JAE fellowship.

REFERENCES

[1] Wang J, Alexander P, Wu L, *et al.* Dependence of mouse embryonic stem cells on threonine catabolism. Science 2009; 325: 435-9.

[2] Vieites JM, Guazzaroni ME, Beloqui A, *et al.* Metagenomics approaches in systems microbiology. FEMS Microbiol Rev 2009; 33: 236-55.

[3] Snyder M, Gallagher JE. Systems biology from a yeast omics perspective. FEBS Lett 2009; 583: 3895-9.

[4] Barros E, Lezar S, Anttonen MJ, *et al.* Comparison of two GM maize varieties with a near-isogenic non-GM variety using transcriptomics, proteomics and metabolomics. Plant Biotechnol J 2010; 8: 436-451.

[5] Roling WF. Do microbial numbers count? Quantifying the regulation of biogeochemical fluxes by population size and cellular activity. FEMS Microbiol Ecol 2007; 62: 202-10.

[6] Young, SP, and Wallance, GR. Metabolomic analysis of human disease and its application to the eye. J Ocul Biol Dis Inform 2009; 2: 235-242.

[7]   Behrends V, Ryall B, Wang X, *et al.* Metabolic profiling of *Pseudomonas aeruginosa* demonstrates that the anti-sigma factor MucA modulates osmotic stress tolerance. Mol Biosyst 2010; 6: 562-9.

[8]   Kafsack BF, Llinas M. Eating at the table of another: metabolomics of host-parasite interactions. Cell Host Microbe 2010; 7: 90-9.

[9]   Seo JS, Keum YS, Li QX. Bacterial degradation of aromatic compounds. Int J Environ Res Public Health 2009; 6: 278-309.

[10] Yang S, Tschaplinski TJ, Engle NL, *et al.* Transcriptomic and metabolomic profiling of *Zymomonas mobilis* during aerobic and anaerobic fermentations. BMC Genomics 2009; 10: 34.

[11] Boccard J, Veuthey JL, Rudaz S. Knowledge discovery in metabolomics: an overview of MS data handling. J Sep Sci 2010; 33: 290-304.

[12] Fiehn O. Combining genomics, metabolome analysis, and biochemical modelling to understand metabolic networks. Comp Funct Genomics 2001; 2: 155-68.

[13] Dauner M. From fluxes and isotope labeling patterns towards *in silico* cells. Curr Opin Biotechnol 2010.

[14] Goodacre R. Metabolomics of a superorganism. J Nutr 2007; 137: 259S-66S.

[15] Davies H. A role for 'Omics' technologies in food safety assessment? Food Control 2009; doi: 10.1016/j.foodcont.2009.03.002 in press

[16] Nicholson JK, Lindon JC. Systems biology: Metabonomics. Nature 2008; 455: 1054-6.

[17] Lee JE, Hwang GS, Lee CH, Hong YS. Metabolomics reveals alterations in both primary and secondary metabolites by wine bacteria. J Agric Food Chem 2009; 57: 10772-83.

[18] Canelas AB, Ras C, ten Pierick A, van Dam JC, Heijnen JJ, van Gulik WM: Leakage-free rapid quenching technique for yeast metabolomics. Metabolomics 2008; 4:226-239.

[19] Pluskal T, Nakamura T, Villar-Briones A, Yanagida M. Metabolic profiling of the fission yeast S. pombe: quantification of compounds under different temperatures and genetic perturbation. Mol Biosyst 2010; 6: 172-88.

[20] Villas-Boas SG, Bruheim P. Cold glycerol-saline: the promising quenching solution for accurate intracellular metabolite analysis of microbial cells. Anal Biochem 2007; 370: 87-97.

[21] Salinero KK, Keller K, Feil WS, *et al.* Metabolic analysis of the soil microbe Dechloromonas aromatica str. RCB: indications of a surprisingly complex life-style and cryptic anaerobic pathways for aromatic degradation. BMC Genomics 2009; 10: 351.

[22] Arita M. What can metabolomics learn from genomics and proteomics? Curr Opin Biotechnol 2009; 20: 610-5.

[23] Hocquette JF, Cassar-Malek I, Scalbert A, Guillou F. Contribution of genomics to the understanding of physiological functions. J Physiol Pharmacol 2009; 60 Suppl 3: 5-16.

[24] Olsen GJ, Lane DJ, Giovannoni SJ, *et al.* Microbial ecology and evolution: a ribosomal RNA approach. Annu Rev Microbiol 1986; 40: 337-65.

[25] Liolios K, Mavromatis K, Tavernarakis N, Kyrpides NC. The Genomes On Line Database (GOLD) in 2007: status of genomic and metagenomic projects and their associated metadata. Nucleic Acids Res 2008; 36: D475-9.

[26] Rusch DB, Halpern AL, Sutton G, *et al.* The Sorcerer II Global Ocean Sampling expedition: northwest Atlantic through eastern tropical Pacific. PLoS Biol 2007; 5: e77.

[27] Meyer F, Paarmann D, D'Souza M, *et al.* The metagenomics RAST server - a public resource for the automatic phylogenetic and functional analysis of metagenomes. BMC Bioinformatics 2008; 9: 386.

[28] Wilmes P, Andersson AF, Lefsrud MG, *et al.* Community proteogenomics highlights microbial strain-variant protein expression within activated sludge performing enhanced biological phosphorus removal. Isme J 2008a, 2: 853-64.

[29] Wilmes P, Wexler M, Bond PL. Metaproteomics provides functional insight into activated sludge wastewater treatment. PLoS One 2008b, 3: e1778.

[30] Verberkmoes NC, Russell AL, Shah M, *et al.* Shotgun metaproteomics of the human distal gut microbiota. Isme J 2009; 3: 179-89.

[31] Beloqui A, Guazzaroni ME, Ferrer M. Procedures for protein isolation in pure culture and microbial communities. In: Handbook of Hydrocarbon and Lipid Microbiology. Springer Verlag Press, 2010; pp. 4813-4194.

[32] Tyson GW, Chapman J, Hugenholtz P, *et al.* Community structure and metabolism through reconstruction of microbial genomes from the environment. Nature 2004; 428: 37-43.

[33]   Parro V, Moreno-Paz M, Gonzalez-Toril E. Analysis of environmental transcriptomes by DNA microarrays. Environ Microbiol 2007; 9: 453-64.

[34]   Frias-Lopez J, Shi Y, Tyson GW, *et al.* Microbial community gene expression in ocean surface waters Proc Natl Acad Sci U S A 2008; 105: 3805-10.

[35]   Moran, M.A. Metatranscriptomics: eavesdropping on complex microbiol communities. Microbe 2009; 4: 329-335.

[36]   Bailly J, Fraissinet-Tachet L, Verner MC, *et al.* Soil eukaryotic functional diversity, a metatranscriptomic approach. Isme J 2007; 1: 632-42.

[37]   Feist AM, Herrgard MJ, Thiele I, *et al.* Reconstruction of biochemical networks in microorganisms. Nat Rev Microbiol 2009; 7: 129-43.

[38]   Schripsema J, Verpoorte R. Investigation of extracts of plant cell cultures by proton nuclear magnetic resonance spectroscopy. Phytochem Anal 1991; 2: 155–162.

[39]   Schripsema J, Erkelens C, Verpoorte R. Intra- and extracellular carbohydrates in plant cell cultures investigated by 1H-NMR. Plant Cell Rep 1991; 9: 527–530.

[40]   Fiehn O, Kopka J, Dormann P, *et al.* Metabolite profiling for plant functional genomics. Nat Biotechnol 2000; 18: 1157-61.

[41]   Chikayama E, Sekiyama Y, Okamoto M, *et al.* Statistical indices for simultaneous large-scale metabolite detections for a single. NMR spectrum Anal Chem 2010; 82: 1653-8.

[42]   Madsen R, Lundstedt T, Trygg J. Chemometrics in metabolomics--a review in human disease diagnosis. Anal Chim Acta 2010; 659: 23-33.

[43]   Ohta D, Kanaya S, Suzuki H. Application of Fourier-transform ion cyclotron resonance mass spectrometry to metabolic profiling and metabolite identification. Curr Opin Biotechnol 2010.

[44]   Sekiyama Y, Chikayama E, Kikuchi J. Profiling polar and semipolar plant metabolites throughout extraction processes using a combined solution-state and high-resolution magic angle spinning. NMR approach Anal Chem 2010; 82: 1643-52.

[45]   Tian J, Sang P, Gao P, *et al.* Optimization of a GC-MS metabolic fingerprint method and its application in characterizing engineered bacterial metabolic shift. J Sep Sci 2009; 32: 2281-8.

[46]   Urayama S, Zou W, Brooks K, Tolstikov V. Comprehensive mass spectrometry based metabolic profiling of blood plasma reveals potent discriminatory classifiers of pancreatic cancer. Rapid Commun Mass Spectrom 2010; 24: 613-20.

[47]   van Gulik WM. Fast sampling for quantitative microbial metabolomics. Curr Opin Biotechnol 2010;21(1):27-34.

[48]   Ramautar R, Somsen GW, de Jong GJ. CE-MS in metabolomics. Electrophoresis 2009; 30: 276-91.

[49]   Shaikh AS, Tang YJ, Mukhopadhyay A, Keasling JD. Isotopomer distributions in amino acids from a highly expressed protein as a proxy for those from total protein. Anal Chem 2008; 80: 886-90.

[50]   Ferrara CT, Wang P, Neto EC, *et al.* Genetic networks of liver metabolism revealed by integration of metabolic and transcriptional profiling. PLoS Genet 2008; 4: e1000034.

[51]   Walsh K, Koshland DE, Jr. Determination of flux through the branch point of two metabolic cycles. The tricarboxylic acid cycle and the glyoxylate shunt. J Biol Chem 1984; 259: 9646-54.

[52]   Schaub J, Schiesling C, Reuss M, Dauner M. Integrated sampling procedure for metabolome analysis. Biotechnol Prog 2006; 22: 1434-42.

[53]   Schaub J, Reuss M. *In vivo* dynamics of glycolysis in *Escherichia coli* shows need for growth-rate dependent metabolome analysis. Biotechnol Prog 2008; 24: 1402-7.

[54]   Winder CL, Dunn WB, Schuler S, *et al.* Global metabolic profiling of *Escherichia coli* cultures: an evaluation of methods for quenching and extraction of intracellular metabolites. Anal Chem 2008; 80: 2939-48.

[55]   Chassagnole C, Noisommit-Rizzi N, Schmid JW, *et al.* Dynamic modeling of the central carbon metabolism of *Escherichia coli.* Biotechnol Bioeng 2002; 79: 53-73.

[56]   Weuster-Botz D. Sampling tube device for monitoring intracellular metabolite dynamics. Anal Biochem 1997; 246: 225-33.

[57]   Larsson G, Tornkvist M. Rapid sampling, cell inactivation and evaluation of low extracellular glucose concentrations during fed-batch cultivation. J Biotechnol 1996; 49: 69-82.

[58]   Bolten CJ, Kiefer P, Letisse F, *et al.* Sampling for metabolome analysis of microorganisms. Anal Chem 2007; 79: 3843-9.

[59]   Mashego MR, van Gulik WM, Vinke JL, Heijnen JJ. Critical evaluation of sampling techniques for residual glucose determination in carbon-limited chemostat culture of *Saccharomyces cerevisiae.* Biotechnol Bioeng 2003; 83: 395-9.

[60] van der Werf MJ, Overkamp KM, Muilwijk B, *et al.* Microbial metabolomics: toward a platform with full metabolome coverage. Anal Biochem 2007; 370: 17-25.

[61] Bhattacharya M, Fuhrman L, Ingram A, *et al.* Single-run separation and detection of multiple metabolic intermediates by anion-exchange high-performance liquid chromatography and application to cell pool extracts prepared from Escherichia coli. Anal Biochem 1995; 232: 98-106.

[62] Faijes M, Mars AE, Smid EJ. Comparison of quenching and extraction methodologies for metabolome analysis of *Lactobacillus plantarum*. Microb Cell Fact 2007; 6: 27.

[63] Lange HC, Eman M, van Zuijlen G, *et al.* Improved rapid sampling for *in vivo* kinetics of intracellular metabolites in *Saccharomyces cerevisiae*. Biotechnol Bioeng 2001; 75: 406-15.

[64] Goodacre R. Making sense of the metabolome using evolutionary computation: seeing the wood with the trees. J Exp Bot 2005; 56: 245-54.

[65] Defernez M, Wilson RH. Infrared spectroscopy: instrumental factors affecting the long-term validity of chemometrics models. Anal Chem 1997; 69: 1288–94.

[66] Schauer N, Fernie AR. Plant metabolomics: towards biological function and mechanism. Trends Plant Sci 2006; 11: 508-16.

[67] Hall RD. Plant metabolomics: from holistic hope, to hype, to hot topic. New Phytol 2006; 169: 453-68.

[68] Priego Capote F, Luque de Castro MD. On-line preparation of microsamples prior to CE. Electrophoresis 2007; 28: 1214-20.

[69] Bino RJ, Hall RD, Fiehn O, *et al.* Potential of metabolomics as a functional genomics tool. Trends Plant Sci 2004; 9: 418-25.

[70] Guazzaroni ME, Ferrer M. (Meta-) genomics approaches in Systems Biology. In: Handbook for Molecular Microbial Ecology I: Metagenomics and Complementary Approaches, de Bruijn, F.J. 2010. Editor, Wiley - Blackwell Publisher. In press.

[71] Dixon RA, Gang DR, Charlton AJ, *et al.* Applications of metabolomics in agriculture. J Agric Food Chem 2006; 54: 8984-94.

[72] Maher AD, Zirah SF, Holmes E, Nicholson JK. Experimental and analytical variation in human urine in 1H NMR spectroscopy-based metabolic phenotyping studies. Anal Chem 2007; 79: 5204-11.

[73] Verpoorte R, Choi YH, Kim HK. NMR-based metabolomics at work in phytochemistry. Phytochem Rev 2007; 6: 3–14

[74] Tweeddale H, Notley-McRobb L, Ferenci T. Effect of slow growth on metabolism of *Escherichia coli*, as revealed by global metabolite pool ("metabolome") analysis. J Bacteriol 1998; 180: 5109-16.

[75] Viant MR, Lyeth BG, Miller MG, Berman RF. An NMR metabolomic investigation of early metabolic disturbances following traumatic brain injury in a mammalian model. NMR Biomed 2005; 18: 507-16.

[76] Beckmann M, Parker D, Enot DP, *et al.* High-throughput, non-targeted metabolite fingerprinting using nominal mass flow injection electrospray mass spectrometry. Nat Protoc 2008; 3: 486-504.

[77] Draper J, Enot DP, Parker D, *et al.* Metabolite signal identification in accurate mass metabolomics data with MZedDB, an interactive m/z annotation tool utilising predicted ionisation behaviour 'rules'. BMC Bioinformatics 2009; 10: 227.

[78] Murch SJ, Rupasinghe HP, Goodenowe D, Saxena PK. A metabolomic analysis of medicinal diversity in Huang-qin (*Scutellaria baicalensis* Georgi) genotypes: discovery of novel compounds. Plant Cell Rep 2004; 23: 419-25.

[79] Monton MR, Soga T. Metabolome analysis by capillary electrophoresis-mass spectrometry. J Chromatogr A 2007; 1168: 237-46, discussion 36.

[80] Lommen A, Weseman JM, Smith GO, Noteborn HPJM. On the detection of environmental effects on complex matrices combining off -line liquid chromatography and 1H-NMR. Biodegradation 1998; 9: 513–525.

[81] Krishnan P, Kruger NJ, Ratcliffe RG. Metabolite fingerprinting and profiling in plants using NMR. J Exp Bot 2005; 56: 255-65.

[82] Martin FP, Dumas ME, Wang Y, *et al.* A top-down systems biology view of microbiome-mammalian metabolic interactions in a mouse model. Mol Syst Biol 2007; 3: 112.

[83] Ludwig C, Viant MR. Two-dimensional J-resolved NMR spectroscopy: review of a key methodology in the metabolomics toolbox. Phytochem Anal 2010; 21: 22-32.

[84] Motta A, Paris D, Melck D. Monitoring real-time metabolism of living cells by fast two-dimensional NMR spectroscopy. Anal Chem 2010; 82: 2405-11.

[85] Rabinowitz JD. Cellular metabolomics of Escherichia coli. Expert Rev Proteomics 2007; 4:187-198.

[86] Cakir T, Hendriks MM, Westerhuis JA, Smilde AK. Metabolic network discovery through reverse engineering of metabolome data. Metabolomics 2009; 5: 318-29.

[87]   Daran-Lapujade P, Rossell S, van Gulik WM, *et al.* The fluxes through glycolytic enzymes in *Saccharomyces cerevisiae* are predominantly regulated at posttranscriptional levels. Proc Natl Acad Sci U S A 2007; 104: 15753-8.

[88]   Sauer U. Metabolic networks in motion: 13C-based flux analysis. Mol Syst Biol 2006; 2: 62.

[89]   Edwards JS, Palsson BO. Robustness analysis of the *Escherichia coli* metabolic network. Biotechnol Prog 2000; 16: 927-39.

[90]   Izallalen M, Mahadevan R, Burgard A, *et al. Geobacter sulfurreducens* strain engineered for increased rates of respiration. Metab Eng 2008; 10: 267-75.

[91]   Henry T, Fonseca R. Genomics and proteomics in multiple myeloma and Waldenstrom macroglobulinemia. Curr Opin Hematol 2007; 14: 369-74.

[92]   Li QR, Carvunis AR, Yu H, *et al.* Revisiting the *Saccharomyces cerevisiae* predicted ORFeome. Genome Res 2008a, 18: 1294-303.

[93]   Keseler IM, Bonavides-Martinez C, Collado-Vides J, *et al.* EcoCyc: a comprehensive view of Escherichia coli biology. Nucleic Acids Res 2009; 37: D464-70.

[94]   Christie KR, Hong EL, Cherry JM. Functional annotations for the *Saccharomyces cerevisiae* genome: the knowns and the known unknowns. Trends Microbiol 2009; 17: 286-94.

[95]   Satish Kumar V, Dasika MS, Maranas CD. Optimization based automated curation of metabolic reconstructions. BMC Bioinformatics 2007; 8: 212.

[96]   Northen TR, Lee JC, Hoang L, Raymond J, Hwang DR, Yannone SM, Wong CH, Siuzdak G. A nanostructure-initiator mass spectrometry-based enzyme activity assay. Proc Natl Acad Sci USA 2008; 105: 3678-3683.

[97]   Shannon P, Markiel A, Ozier O, *et al.* Cytoscape: a software environment for integrated models of biomolecular interaction networks. Genome Res 2003; 13: 2498-504.

[98]   Letunic I, Yamada T, Kanehisa M, Bork P. iPath: interactive exploration of biochemical pathways and networks. Trends Biochem Sci 2008; 33: 101-3.

[99]   Frolkis A, Knox C, Lim E, *et al.* SMPDB: The Small Molecule Pathway Database. Nucleic Acids Res 2010; 38: D480-7.

[100]   Wishart DS. Computational approaches to metabolomics. Methods Mol Biol 2010; 593: 283-313.

[101]   Savage DC. Microbial ecology of the gastrointestinal tract. Annu Rev Microbiol 1977; 31: 107-33.

[102]   Claus SP, Tsang TM, Wang Y, *et al.* Systemic multicompartmental effects of the gut microbiome on mouse metabolic phenotypes. Mol Syst Biol 2008; 4: 219.

[103]   Martin FP, Wang Y, Sprenger N, *et al.* Top-down systems biology integration of conditional prebiotic modulated transgenomic interactions in a humanized microbiome mouse model. Mol Syst Biol 2008; 4: 205.

[104]   Calvani R, Miccheli A, Capuani G, *et al.* Gut microbiome-derived metabolites characterize a peculiar obese urinary metabotype. Int J Obes (Lond) 2010.

[105]   Dumas ME, Barton RH, Toye A, *et al.* Metabolic profiling reveals a contribution of gut microbiota to fatty liver phenotype in insulin-resistant mice. Proc Natl Acad Sci U S A 2006; 103: 12511-6.

[106]   Li M, Wang B, Zhang M, *et al.* Symbiotic gut microbes modulate human metabolic phenotypes. Proc Natl Acad Sci U S A 2008b, 105: 2117-22.

[107]   Swann J, Wang Y, Abecia L, *et al.* Gut microbiome modulates the toxicity of hydrazine: a metabonomic study. Mol Biosyst 2009; 5: 351-5.

CHAPTER 5

The Use of Electronic Nose Devices in Clinical Microbiology

M. Bruins[1,2*], A. van Belkum[1] and A. Bos[2]

[1]*Erasmus Medical Center Rotterdam, Department of Medical Microbiology and Infectious Diseases, 's - Gravendijkwal 230, 3015 CE Rotterdam, The Netherlands and* [2]*C-it BV, Marspoortstraat 2, 7201 JB Zutphen, The Netherlands*

Abstract: This chapter describes the use of electronic noses in the field of clinical microbiology. These devices can be used to detect volatile organic compounds directly from clinical materials and can also be applied to monitor the production of volatiles during the process of microbiological culture. Various electronic nose appliances have been developed, but most need rigorous normalization and standardization each and every time that the sensors are renewed. In this chapter, the authors focus on a recently developed, patented micro-technology that does not require regular normalization. Using metal oxide sensors and electronic nose technology allows the dynamic analysis of volatile molecule production during bacterial fermentation to be performed, which will facilitate the real-time detection and identification of live bacteria present within clinical specimens.

Keywords: Electronic Nose, Smell, Quartz Microbalance, Conducting Polymers, Semi-conducting Metal Oxides, MonoNose, Pattern Fingerprints.

1. INTRODUCTION

Everyone who has ever cultured microorganisms knows that certain bacterial species produce odours during growth, some of which are species-specific, and belong to several clinically important bacteria. This odour may be a characteristic sign of the presence of a particular bacterial species, a fact that can be important in the field of bacterial diagnostics. An experienced person may be able to determine which microorganism is present within a specimen, just by carefully sniffing a specimen that has been cultured. A few examples of these bacterial species and the type of smell they produce are shown in Table **1**, and the relationship between disease and aroma producing microorganisms can be found in reference [1].

The use of smell as a diagnostic aid in the detection of infectious diseases has been known since ancient times. For example, Hippocrates mentioned the diagnostic value of smell in his work called "Aphorisms" written in 400 BC [2], and wrote: in Section IV:81.

Table 1: A list of bacterial species and their characteristic odours that are distinguishable using the human nose.

Bacterial species	Odour
Clostridium difficile	Horse-like
Haemophilus	Burnt Caramel
Streptococcus milleri	Butterscotch
Pseudomonas aeruginosa	Almond
Streptomyces spp	Earth
Eikenella corrodens	Bleach
Streptococcus constellatus	Caramel

*" If a patient passes blood, pus, and scales, in the urine, and if it has a heavy **smell**, ulceration of the bladder is indicated"; and in Section V: 11. "In persons affected with phthisis, if the sputa which they cough up have a heavy **smell** when poured upon coals, and if the hairs of the head fall off, the case will prove fatal."*

*****Address correspondence to M. Bruins:** C-it BV, Marspoortstraat 2, 7201 JB Zutphen, The Netherlands; Email: Marcel.Bruins@c-it.nl

John P. Hays and W. B. van Leeuwen (Eds)

These quotes show that the olfactory diagnosis of infectious diseases has a longstanding history, though the possibility of using odour to identify a particular bacterial species was only re-discovered in 1922, when Omelianski described the aroma producing capacities of several species of microorganisms [3]. In the current age of modern immunological and molecular diagnostics, the art of olfactory diagnosis is slowly disappearing. However, given the simplicity and ease of olfactory diagnostics, this field may still provide an attractive means for the laboratory-based identification of infections in real time. Ultimately, this will require the development of specific instrumentation that is not vulnerable to bias or to inter-individual quality variation. This is where modern electronics and software play an important role.

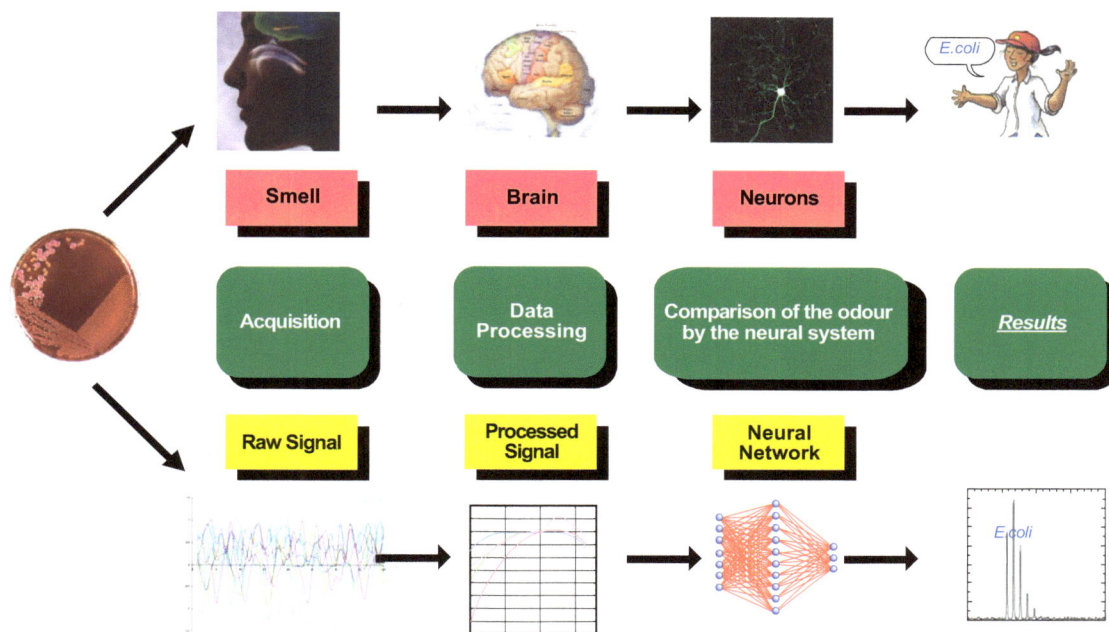

Fig. (1). Comparison of the steps required to detect an odour using either a biological or an electronic nose.

The concept of an electronic nose originated in the 70s of the previous century. Up to then, analytical chemistry had been pre-occupied with developing highly specific sensors and methods aimed at identifying unique substances. However the availability of personal computing made it possible to apply pattern recognition techniques to complex data measurements, including analytical chemistry measurements. The general idea was to develop a broadly responsive sensor system and use pattern recognition systems to match "unknown response" patterns to previously "observed response" patterns, thereby identifying the specific odours present within (complex) mixtures. In fact, this is analogous to how we humans smell complex mixtures of unknown substances that contain a characteristic odour, hence the name "electronic nose". The principles underlying this approach are illustrated in Fig. **1**.

An important consequence of this electronic nose concept is that a substance, or mixtures of substances, can only be recognized after a calibration phase. That is, in order to match a complex pattern of odours, it is first necessary to possess a database that defines one or more of the odour patterns. This means that all electronic noses currently available are reliant on the use of a searchable (digital) database where characteristic odour signal patterns obtained from previous measurements are stored. In this way novel odour signal patterns can be matched with an existing odour pattern result *via* comparative pattern recognition analysis, ultimately leading to pattern (and hence odour) identification.

At this moment in time, the electronic nose is most often commercially used in the food industry and in environmental monitoring. These are relatively simple applications as their main purpose is the detection of "abnormal" situations *i.e.* the electronic nose continuously monitors a process line or environment and detects anything deviating from the normal situation. This deviation then acts as a trigger to start looking for the reason of the deviation in odour. These kinds of applications are very useful in situations where every deviation from a normal situation is cause for action, especially when the "abnormal" situation rarely occurs.

Currently, there is no known device or application that utilizes electronic nose technology present within medical microbiology laboratories, though there has been research into the possible medical diagnostic applications of electronic nose technology, with in general, promising results [4-7]. In this chapter, the authors explain why these devices are not currently in use and how we think these problems can be solved.

2. CURRENT ELECTRONIC NOSE TECHNOLOGIES

Every sample preparation method that produces volatiles is usable in theory for "electronic nose detection", including methods that involve the heating, burning or chemical treatment of a sample, though these methods will of course destroy the actual sample. Also, in the literature, GC-MS (gas chromatography-mass spectrometry) systems are sometimes described as electronic nose devices. However, though gas chromatography and mass spectrometry can be used to separate, quantify and identify volatile chemicals, they do not indicate whether the compound is associated with an odour or not. In fact, an odour is mostly a "blend" of compounds that combine to create a specific odour. This blend is actually separated by GC-MS systems analysis, thereby destroying the specific odour itself and are therefore "technically speaking" not genuine electronic noses.

In effect the basic sensor technologies most commonly incorporated into modern electronic nose (e-nose) technologies are:

1. Quartz Microbalance (QMB)

2. Conducting polymers (CPs)

3. Semi-conducting metal oxides (MOS)

4. Miscellaneous

1. **Quartz Microbalance** (QMB) is a quartz crystal with a chemically active surface, usually a polymer. When gas molecules adsorb to the surface, the mass changes and the resonance frequency of the crystal shifts. These minute shifts are then measured using high frequency electronics (which are complex and expensive). However, small temperature variations in the environment may also generate similar frequency shifts requiring the maintenance of strict environmentally controlled temperature conditions. A variation of a QMB sensor is a SAW (surface acoustic wave) sensor, which is based upon changes in an acoustic wave applied to the surface. Changes in surface composition change the path of the wave and hence the wave's characteristics.

2. **Conducting Polymers** (CPs) are polymers which have been 'loaded' with graphite. The graphite provides an electrical resistance path that can be easily measured. When gas molecules associate with the polymer, it swells, breaking contact points between the graphite particles and thus changing the resistance. Similar to QMB sensors, temperature and/or humidity changes will result in expansion/contraction of the sensor and lead to changes in resistance profiles, again requiring the use of strictly controlled environmental temperature conditions. Although the number of possible polymer variants is enormous (and thus the number of sensor array variants), polymers tend to be rather unstable. Strong oxidizers such as chlorine and ozone can fairly easily disrupt these polymers and thereby destroy the sensor.

3. **Metal-Oxide** (MOS) are sensors based on the principle that certain metal-oxides behave as semiconductors at high temperatures. Sensors based on this principle are designed to bring together a heating element and a sensor element (usually a sintered metal-oxide with or without catalyst). Both elements are separated by a very thin isolating membrane. Redox-reactions occurring at the sensor surface

at elevated temperatures result in changes in resistance that can be measured using appropriate electronic hardware and software. These types of redox-reactions are dependent on the nature of the metal-oxide/catalyst, the reacting gas(ses), and the temperature. As a "rule-of-thumb", a minimum of 0.1% of ambient oxygen is required for normal operation. Dependant on sensor type and temperature, a very broad range of substances will exhibit redox reactions, though notable exceptions are CO_2 (which will not oxidize further) and the noble gases. At lower oxygen concentrations the resistance of the metal oxides decreases very drastically as can be seen in Fig. **2**.

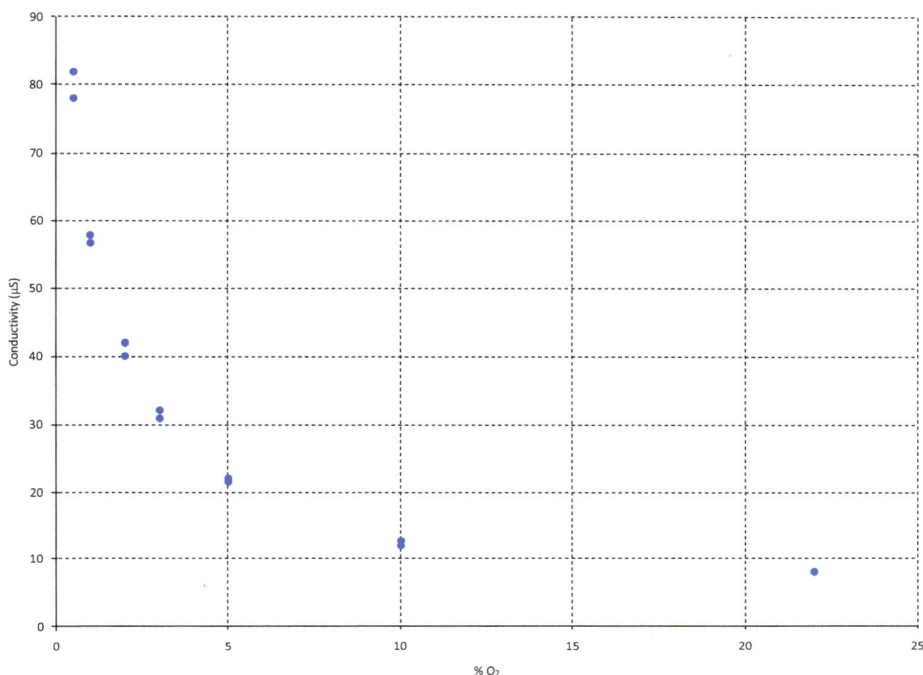

Fig. (2). The influence of oxygen concentration on the conductivity of a Metal Oxide Sensor (MOS).

4. As well as the 3 above mentioned techniques, there are several **Miscellaneous** sensor techniques that may be currently used within electronic nose devices. These techniques include: 1) Electrochemical sensors are based on the flow of electrons between an electrode surface and molecules in the surrounding air. The sensor mainly comprises 2 different electrodes with electron flow between the electrodes being measured as an indication of the presence of chemicals within the surrounding environment. These sensors can be made fairly specific for a range of chemical compounds, though a major drawback is the depletion of the chemical being detected which is actually consumed during the detection process; 2) Surface acoustic wave (SAW) sensors are largely based on the same principal as QMB sensors mentioned above. However, instead of measuring a change in weight, the SAW sensor measures a change in the length of the path that a high frequency wave has to travel. Similar to QMB sensors, SAW sensors require highly specific and very delicate high frequency equipment; 3) Optical sensors are based on changes in the scattering of light from a laser beam. The presence of particular chemical compounds cause light from a laser beam to scatter in a specific manner, which is detected by the sensor. This technique may also be incorporated into fire alarms, which are triggered by a major disturbance in the light signal or by total blocking of the light signal by particles created by the fire.

Nowadays, there is a definite commercial market for electronic nose devices, with the market leader for decades being the French company Alpha M.O.S. However, Smiths Detection (which acquired the Cyranose from Cyrano Sciences in 2004), and Scensive Ltd (which acquired the Bloodhound assets of Bloodhound Sensors Limited in 2005), are also well known. The e-nose devices of Smiths Detection and Scensive Ltd are based on conducting polymer arrays, whilst those of Alpha M.O.S use combinations of both QMB and arrays of conducting polymers. All of these devices are bulky, power-hungry and are intended to be used as laboratory instruments, requiring regular normalization, and cost in the region of $9,000-$150,000 per machine.

In contrast, the Consultatie-Implementatie technisch beheer (C-it) *MonoNose* technology described further in this chapter is based on metal oxide sensors and uses intelligent sensor modules for detection purposes. These intelligent modules contain everything needed to operate the sensor and make it easy to construct a measuring device containing a varied number of sensors, without adding additional complexity. Indeed, the electronics required for a device containing a single module does not differ from that of a device containing for example 12 modules, with the configuration of the device determining whether the modules operate in parallel on the same sample, or operate on a different sample per module. In essence, the philosophy of C-it is not to compete with the existing market, but to address a different niche *i.e.* the currently unoccupied niche of very cheap, low power, mass-producible and mass-employable electronic noses [2-4].

3. CURRENT MICROBIOLOGICAL DIAGNOSIS

The "gold standard" for microbiological diagnosis in the majority of diagnostic microbiological laboratories is the culture and identification of unknown microorganisms within a clinical sample using selective culture methods coupled to differential biochemical reactions (leading to variation in coloration, precipitation, gas production etc). For bulk analysis this process can now be achieved *via* automation using devices such as the Phoenix™ (Becton Dickinson) or the VITEK® (bioMérieux) apparatus. In essence, a sample is collected from a patient, inoculated into a suitable medium, and allowed to grow overnight (or longer dependent on the initial sample and amount and type of microorganisms). Identification of the organism begins after a positive result (*i.e.* microbial growth), is observed, meaning that the average time to identification of an organism lies between 12-24 hours after specimen inoculation. Further, the total time between arrival of the clinical specimen and definitive result can lie between 48 hours for "high microbiological-load" samples such as urine and faeces, and up to 168 hours for "low microbiological-load" samples such as blood. In fact, most of the samples that are processed in an average hospital are negative for pathogens and no further processing is required.

At the present moment in time, much effort is being focused towards the development of (molecular) techniques that can reduce the "time-to-diagnosis" for clinical specimens, such as Raman spectroscopy, MALDI-TOF etc [8-10]. However, most of these techniques require a certain amount of microbial biomass that has been obtained by culturing the clinical specimen on a solid medium. Further, these techniques are relatively expensive and complex. With respect to nucleic acid amplification technologies *e.g.* the Cepheid, GenExpert system, these types of systems are generally very specific, targeting a particular microbial species and therefore requiring separate primer and thermocycling combinations for each pathogen to be detected.

4. THE C-IT ELECTRONIC NOSE

Microorganisms have the ability to use a very broad range of compounds to create the components needed for their growth and development.

To process these compounds, microorganisms have developed a variety of metabolic pathways, with the activation of particular metabolic pathways being determined by both the (genetically determined) capabilities of the microorganism, and the compounds available for integration into the growing cell.

Additionally, if the mixture of available compounds changes over time *e.g.* by being depleted from the growth medium, then microorganisms are capable of adapting their metabolic pathways in response to these changes. Finally, the activity of particular metabolic pathways over time may be characteristic of particular microbial genera (or even species), and measurement of these pathways (*via* for example the measurement of resultant Volatile Organic Compounds (VOCs)), could lead to the development of a rapid, pan-specific, microbial identification system. It is with this concept in mind, that the C-it electronic nose is being developed.

C-it uses a small electronic nose device (patent pending) called the *MonoNose*, which continuously monitors the headspace gases above a broth in a culture flask of approximately 100 ml (Fig. **3**). The pattern of volatiles generated during culture is measured as a function of time *via* a sensor module (Fig. **4**), and is used to classify bacteria in real-time during growth. The pattern recognition techniques utilised to detect and identify volatile patterns employ dynamic time warping algorithms to match features as they develop in time during the growth process. Dynamic changes in the metabolic pathways used during microbial culture result in a dynamic change in the composition of volatile compounds in the headspace of the *MonoNose* device [11], providing information on the active metabolic pathways, thereby allowing robust identification of microbial genera or species. It is the head space that is the key factor in *MonoNose* technology. Interestingly though, the concept involved in *MonoNose* technology can also be used to perform exhaled breath analysis, where exhaled air is collected in a sample bag attached to the electronic nose for analysis purposes. One benefit of this approach is that the exhaled air is allowed to cool, thus removing excess water, and preventing condensation in the electronic nose device. This approach also eliminates the handling of contaminated patient materials containing infectious microbial agents, as the air can be filtered during collection. However, currently there is very little data available regarding the use of the *MonoNose* for exhaled breath analysis. Therefore, this chapter will only focus on *MonoNose* technology and the headspace analysis of cultivated microbiological samples, and on exhaled breath analysis.

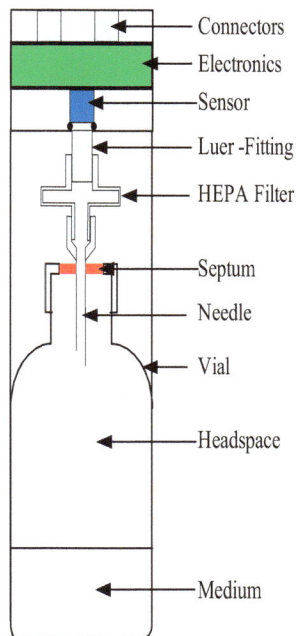

Fig. (3). Schematic representation of the C-it electronic nose. Measurements relating to the production of volatile compounds (an indication of variation in metabolic pathway use) are measured over time in the head space.

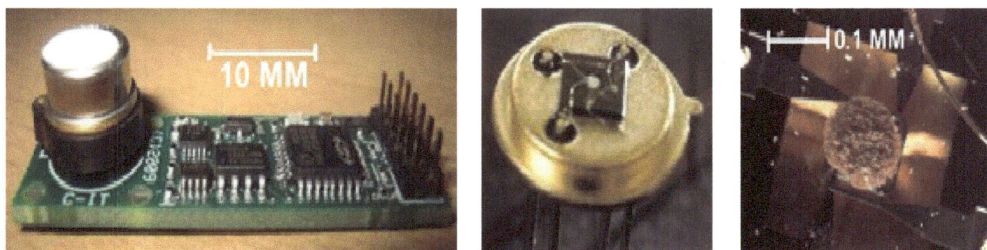

Fig. (4). The sensor module utilised in the e-nose technology described in this chapter. **Left:** A sensor module containing the sensor in a metal cap with a white teflon membrane on top, temperature controlling electronics and microprocessor. **Middle:** The sensor with cap removed (the white dot is the actual sensor material seen at 100 micron diameter). **Right:** A close-up of the sensor material with its attached electronics.

The *MonoNose* device uses a single Metal Oxide (MO) sensor instead of the multitude of sensors used in other electronic nose technologies [11]. The Fox2000 from Alpha M.O.S uses 6 metal oxide sensors [12], the NC State electronic nose uses 15 sensors [13], the Cyranose 32 uses 32 polymer sensors [14], whilst the Bloodhound BH114 uses 14 polymer sensors [15,16]. Though, the use of a single sensor within the *MonoNose* device tends to limit the specificity of volatile organic compound detection, the addition of a thermal cycle heating program to the sensor compensates for this lack of chemical specificity, facilitating the creation of a "virtual array" of sensors [17]. This is possible because the complex system of physical and chemical reduction/oxidation (RedOx) rates at the sensor surface is temperature dependent. The sensor thermal cycle used in the *MonoNose* varies from 240-320°C, following a sinusoid shaped profile to facilitate a smooth transition between the temperatures. For connected sets of *MonoNose* devices (when multiple samples are to be processed at the same time), the individual sensor heaters within each *MonoNose* device is calibrated using a proprietary electronics/software system (patent pending) that ensures a difference of less than 4°C in programmed temperature between individual devices over the full working temperature range. This strict temperature control minimizes shape distortion in the temperature curve analysis between individual *MonoNose* devices, which could arise due to differences in the working temperature of the individual devices. This procedure allows the reproducible comparison of the temperature/RedOx reaction curves of devices and the sharing of calibration models between different laboratories.

Progress in *MonoNose* development now allows the direct comparison of VOC pattern data between different *MonoNose* devices, a development aided by the maintenance of strict temperature control between different devices. The production process of these sensors, deposition of metal oxide vapour, will result in a different amount of active surface available for the RedOx reactions as the exact amount deposited cannot be controlled. A larger sensor surface area will have a higher initial resistance, meaning that changes in the VOCs present in the headspace generate larger changes in sensor signal as the sensor surface increases. In fact, it has been shown that these effects can be compensated for by using the shape of the pattern obtained during VOC sensor measurement, rather than using the amplitude of the signal obtained. The practicality of this methodology has been demonstrated with a set of 30 independently produced *MonoNose*s by M.Bruins *et al.* [11]. Ultimately, using this procedure means that any differences observed in VOC pattern data between different *MonoNose* devices is due only to the biological differences present in different clinical specimens.

5. THE C-IT ELECTRONIC NOSE IN MICROBIOLOGICAL DIAGNOSIS

Using headspace analysis allows a range of clinical specimen material to be tested. Specimens may vary from sputum [15, 18] and urine [12, 16, 19, 20], to wound swabs/dressings [21- 23] and blood [24, 25]. Most examples of electronic nose devices and microbiological diagnosis in the literature describe devices that are suited for identifying the presence and/or identification of micro-organisms, and require overnight culture in order to reduce the influence of the initial sample matrix and to increase the amount of microorganisms present within the culture (which increases device sensitivity). Further, the majority of electronic nose device experiments have reported results using a single "snapshot" of the VOC content at a specific point in time (for example after an overnight period of growth) [13, 26]. This may provide sufficient analytical information for that particular experiment, but the information gained may not be suitable for use as a comparative reference. This is because the headspace composition is dependent on several different factors, including, but not limited to, the initial inoculated amount of microorganisms, variations in the incubation temperature, and exact medium formulation. Therefore, defining an end-point at a specific moment in time assumes that all of these factors are identical between different experiments and also between different laboratories, which is almost impossible to regulate. In fact, a better standard for end-point measurement would be to define a particular headspace VOC pattern, or to define a specific sequence of headspace changes that occur using real-time measurement. The advantage of using multiple headspace VOC pattern measurements in real-time (compared to a single headspace VOC pattern measurement), is that different headspace VOC patterns may occur over time, but that they may ultimately all generate identical headspace VOC patterns sometime in the future. Moreover, real-time VOC pattern changes could be diagnostic for a particular microbial species, information that may be lost if only a single headspace VOC pattern measurement is taken. Some of the factors crucial in influencing headspace VOC patterns are described in more detail below. The resultant Figs. **5**, **6** and **7** are taken from experiments conducted with *Escherichia coli* strain ATCC 35218.

i) Initial Microbial Inoculation Concentration

The available resources available for microbial growth within a defined medium will be depleted faster as the initial microbial inoculation concentration is increased, and the timing of the headspace VOC pattern dynamics will also change accordingly. Fig. **5**, illustrates this effect. It can be clearly seen that an increase in the initial inoculation concentration causes characteristic changes in headspace VOC pattern dynamics (measured as changes in the conductivity of the sensor). The greater the initial microbial inoculation concentration, the sooner the time at which a distinctive signal change is achieved.

ii) Medium Composition

Changes in headspace VOC patterns occur as a result of the metabolic processes occurring during microbial growth. The number and type of metabolic pathways actually used by the microorganism is dependent on the availability of compounds within the growth medium being used, which in turn causes headspace composition to change over time.

Fig. **6** shows the influence of medium salt and amino acid concentration on the resultant sensor signal, with the X and Y axes indicating the concentration of salt and amino acid, respectively. A series of experiments have been conducted using a single sensor and *E. coli* strain ATCC 35218 grown with different media compositions. In order to compensate for any sensor drift, *i.e.* changes in sensor signals independent of any effects associated with the salt and amino acid concentration (for example differences in sensor ageing between different experiments), the signal is shown as the percentage change between the minimal and maximum sensor response values once the maximum value in the experiment has been reached. This is because the influence of sensor drift will be the same for both the minimum and the maximum values. In effect, the influence of the difference in initial microbial inoculation concentration is compensated by using the maximum value observed in the experiment instead of the value after a pre-defined period of time.

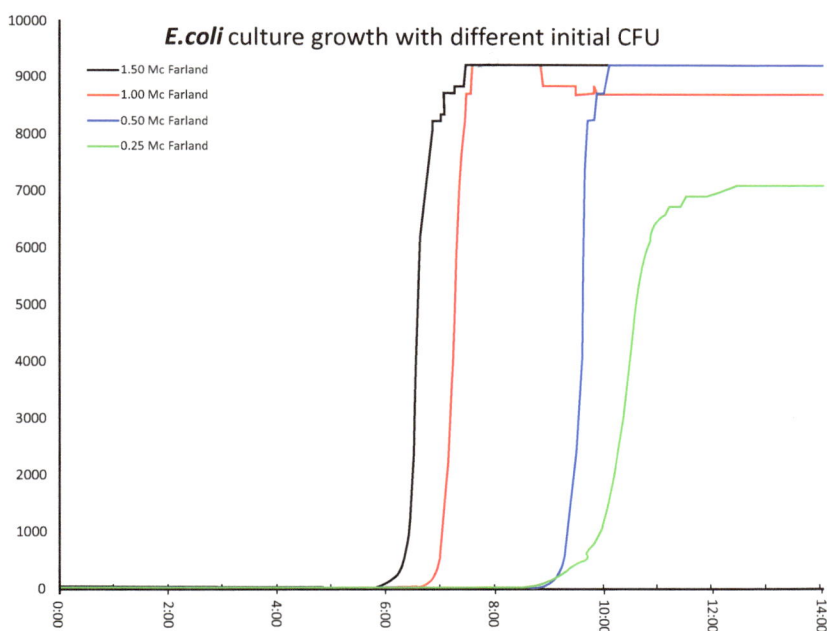

Fig. (5). The influence of initial microbial inoculation size on VOC headspace pattern dynamics. The x-axis shows the amount of time passed since inoculation (in hours) and the y-axis shows the conductivity of the sensor in μS. A McFarland unit is a measurement of turbidity where 0.25 McFarland unit corresponds to approximately 0.75×10^8 cells/ml, and 1.5 McFarland units 4.5×10^8 cells/ml (http://en.wikipedia.org/wiki/ McFarland_standard).

In Fig. **6** it is obvious that the salt and amino acid concentration greatly influencing the resultant headspace composition. *Escherichia coli* cultured on a medium containing a salt concentration of 8½ g/l and an amino acid concentration of 3½ g/l will generate different headspace VOC pattern than *Escherichia coli* cultured on media containing a salt concentration of for example 3½ g/l and an amino acid concentration of 6½ g/l.

6. *MONONOSE* PATTERN FINGERPRINTS

The *MonoNose* generates VOC RedOx reaction patterns in real-time, which means that looking at the entire 'odor-movie' during microbial growth may provide some specific "scenes" (specific changes in VOC patterns over time), that characterize a particular microbial genus or species present within the clinical specimen being tested. Moreover, this process may be aided by searching for specific combinations of patterns obtained at different time periods. These unique patterns may be useful in determining the "fingerprint" of a particular microorganism present within a clinical sample. Further, once these unique patterns have been identified, there is no need to continue with extended headspace monitoring.

The actual dynamic part of odour detection occurs over a relatively small period of time as can be seen in Fig. **5**. This dynamic period can emerge at any time throughout the measurement process, because the initial microbial inoculation concentration within the clinical specimen being tested is not known. The identification of a microorganism may however be based on specific fingerprint patterns so that the electronic nose monitoring device can be set up to continually scan for the emergence of relevant fingerprint patterns to ensure the shortest possible time-to-diagnosis identification time.

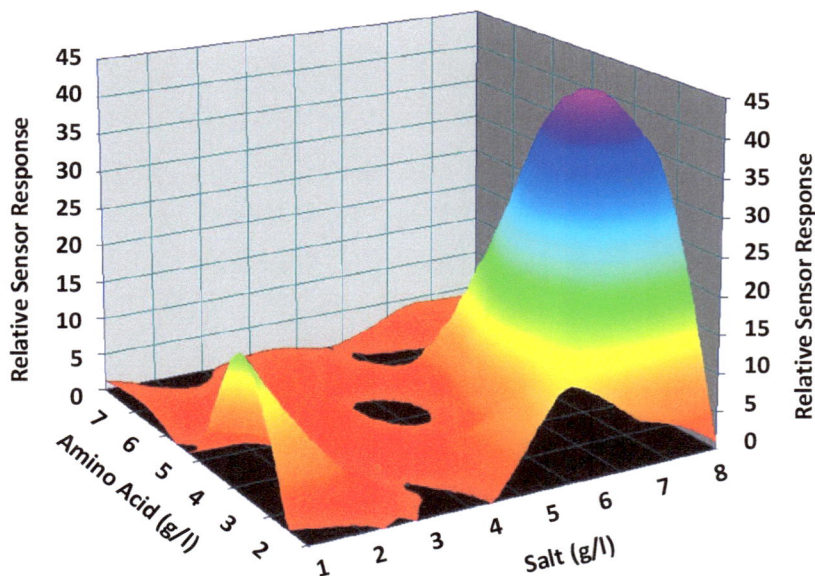

Fig. (6). The influence of medium composition on VOC headspace pattern dynamics. The x-axis indicates the amount of salt present in the media, the y-axis indicates the amount of amino acid present in the medium , and the z-axis is the compensated sensor signal. The compensated sensor signal is the percentage change between the minimal and maximum sensor response values .

The matching of a predetermined fingerprint for *Escherichia coli* in a full experiment is shown in Fig. **7**. The insert shows the predetermined fingerprint. The experiment was continually scanned for the emergence of a specific fingerprint using dynamic time warping algorithm software. In fact, such algorithms are designed to scan for fingerprint similarities instead of exact matches. This is because even a small change in temperature will generate a small change in the signal obtained, though the overall fingerprint pattern similarity will be maintained. This is clearly shown in Fig. **7**, where the inset shows a predetermined *E. coli* fingerprint, and the main figure shows a test specimen culture. The fingerprints look similar (and can be identified using dynamic time warping algorithm software), but are not identical.

This fingerprint profile is composed of 3 different descriptors derived from the signal recorded after applying a thermal heating profile. The descriptors used are the slope of the signal, the surface area of the signal and the difference between the maximum and minimum value in a thermal cycle. All of these values are normalized to 1. Ultimately, the development of microbial fingerprint pattern recognition such as presented in Fig. **7**, will allow electronic nose technology to become a rapid diagnostic tool for microbiological diagnosis of the future.

7. DISCUSSION

Despite all of the promising research performed using various electronic nose technologies over the past 10 years, the current status of electronic nose technology in the medical laboratory can be best summarised as:

... *may* be available in a few years.

... *may* find its way into the medical laboratory.

... *may* be commonplace in the future.

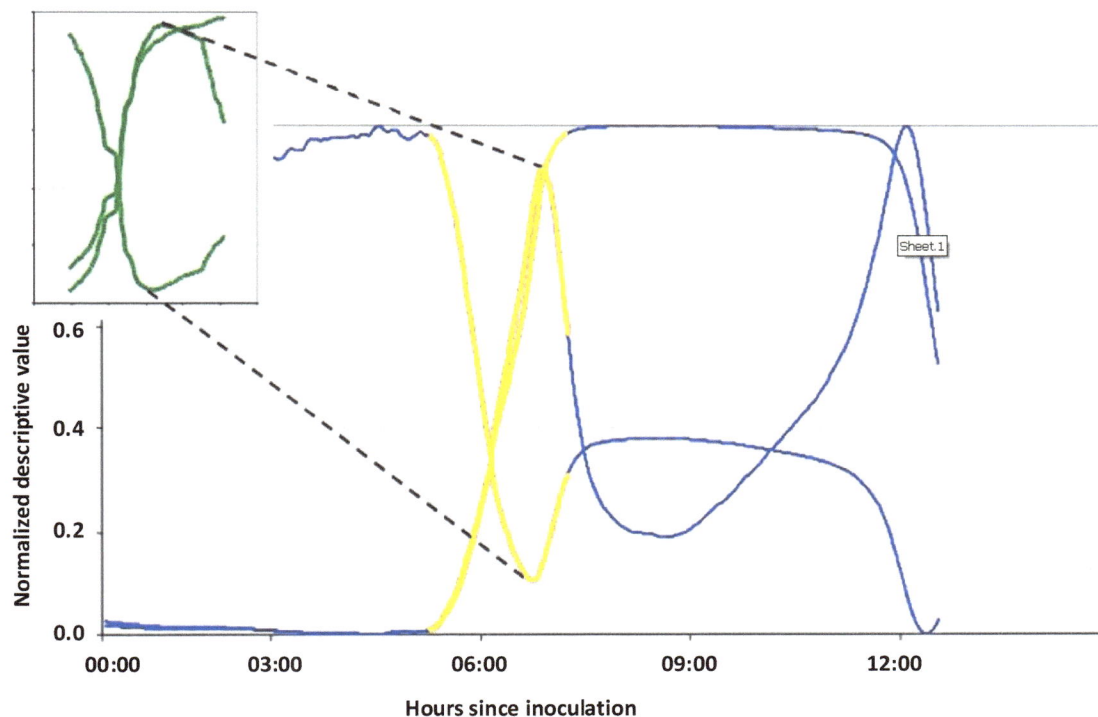

Fig. (7). A *MonoNose* real-time pattern obtained using *Escherichia coli* ATCC35218 grown in Todd Hewitt Broth medium for 12 hours. The position of the predetermined fingerprint pattern for *Escherichia coli* (shown in the inset) is marked in the experiment. The X-axis shows the time passed since inoculation and the y-axis shows the normalized descriptor values. The normalized descriptor value represents 3 different descriptors derived from the signal recorded after applying a thermal heating profile. The descriptors used are the slope of the signal, the surface area of the signal and the difference between the maximum and minimum value in a thermal cycle. All of these values are normalized to 1.

In fact, there are still no electronic noses currently in use in day to day medical diagnostics (including in medical microbiological diagnosis).

There are 3 fundamental factors keeping electronic noses from being introduced into the routine laboratory environment. These are:

1. **Calibration** – Reference VOC patterns are device dependent and not interchangeable between different electronic nose devices or between different electronic nose technologies. The necessity of calibrating every individual electronic nose device and the need to recalibrate regularly due to "sensor drift" creates a logistical nightmare and makes current real-time applications of electronic nose technology unfeasible.

2. **Timing** – Previous research tended to use measurements using a fixed arbitrary end-point in time, meaning that it was not certain whether any differences observed in the final results were a mere artefact of the arbitrary point-in-time chosen for measurement.

3. **Sample Matrix** – The majority of previous electronic nose experiments relating to medical microbiological diagnosis only measured the properties of pure isolates after selective culture, rather than clinical specimens consisting of a real life matrix. This required an initial culture step in order to obtain the pure microbial strain, even before electronic nose identification could take place. If the electronic nose could be utilized for the identification of microbes within clinical specimens immediately after inoculation into growth media, then detection could occur in real-time, possibly providing the microbial diagnostician with a more rapid test for the identification of microbial pathogens. With respect to these problems, strict temperature control in combination with the continuous monitoring of the inoculated headspace allows calibration models to be shared between different *MonoNose*s and eliminates the need to find a suitable end-point in time. Further, the *MonoNose* measurement principal of dynamic headspace development allows for samples from different matrices to be measured during the period normally needed to culture a pure microbial isolate.

An understanding of the above mentioned factors (which are unique to this field), is critical for the development of the electronic nose as a diagnostic tool in the field of medical microbiological diagnostics. *MonoNose* technology is developed with these factors in mind, it's approach being different from that of 'classical' electronic nose devices, meaning that and it stands an excellent chance of becoming a useful addition to the field of medical microbiological diagnostics and research.

REFERENCES

[1]   Pavlou AK, Turner APF. Sniffing out the truth : Clinical Diagnosis Using the Electronic Nose. Clin Chem Lab Med 2000; 38(2):99-112.

[2]   Adams F. Hippocratic writings: Aphorisms Sections IV and V http://classics.mit.edu/Hippocrates/aphorisms.html.

[3]   Omelianski VL. Aroma producing Microorganisms. J Bacteriol. 1923; July; 8(4): 393–419.

[4]   Pavlou AK, Magan N, Sharp D, Brown J, Barr H, Turner APF. An intelligent rapid odour recognition model in discrimination of Helicobacter pylori and other gastroesophageal isolates *in vitro*. Biosensors & Bioelectronics 2000; 15, 333-342.

[5]   Gibson TD, Prosser O, Hulbert JN, *et al.* Detection and simultaneous identification of microorganisms from headspace samples using an electronic nose Sensors and Actuators 1997; B 44, 413-422.

[6]   Moens M, Smet A, Naudts B, *et al.* Fast identification of ten clinically important micro-organisms using an electronic nose. Letters in Applied Microbiology 2006; 42: 121-126.

[7]   Rossi V, Talon R, Berdagué J. Rapid Discrimination of *Micrococcaceae* species using semiconductor gas sensors. Journal of Microbiological Methods 1995; 24 183-190.

[8]   Willemse-Erix DFM, Scholtes-Timmerman MJ, Jachtenberg J, *et al.* Optical Fingerprinting in Bacterial Epidemiology: Raman Spectroscopy as a Real-Time Typing Method. J Clin Microbiol., March 2009; 47, No. 3: 652-659,

[9]   Buijtels PCAM, Willemse-Erix HFM, Petit PLC, *et al.* Rapid Identification of Mycobacteria by Raman Spectroscopy. J Clin Microbiol, Mar.2008; 46,No.3:961–965.

[10]   O.Lay Jr J. MALDI-TOF Mass Spectrometry Of Bacteria. Mass Spectrometry Reviews, 2001; 20, 172-194.

[11]   Bruins M, Bos A, Petit PL, *et al.* Device-independent,real-time identification of bacterial pathogens with a metaloxide-based olfactory sensor Eur. J. Clin. Microbiol. Infect. Dis. 2009; 28:775–780.

[12] Kodogiannis V, Wadge E. The use of gas-sensor arrays to diagnose urinary tract infections. Int J Neural Syst. 2005; Oct;15(5):363-76.

[13] Schiffman SS, Wyrick DW, Gutierrez-Osuna R, Nagle HT. Effectiveness of an Electronic Nose for Monitoring Bacterial and Fungal Growth. 7th International Symp. On Olfaction and Electronic Nose, Brighton UK. 20-24 July 2000.

[14] Dutta R, Hines EL, Gardner JW, Boilot P. Bacteria classification using Cyranose 320 electronic nose. BioMedical Engineering OnLine, Vol.1 (No.4). ISSN 1475-925X.

[15] Fend R, Kolk AH, Bessant C, Buijtels P, Klatser PR, Woodman AC. Prospects for clinical application of electronic-nose technology to early detection of *Mycobacterium tuberculosis* in culture and sputum. J Clin Microbiol. 2006; Jun;44(6):2039-45.

[16] Pavlou AK, Magan N, McNulty C, *et al.* Use of an electronic nose system for diagnoses of urinary tract infections. Biosensors and Bioelectronics 2002;17:893-899.

[17] Pearce TC, Schiffman SS, Nagle HT, Gardner JW. Handbook of Machine Olfaction WILEY-VCH, 2003.

[18] Pavlou AK, Magan N, Jones JM, Brown J, Klatser P, Turner AP. Detection of *Mycobacterium tuberculosis* (TB) *in vitro* and in situ using an electronic nose in combination with a neural network system. Biosens Bioelectron. 2004;Oct 15;20(3):538-44.

[19] Aathithan S, Plant JC, Chaudry AN, French GL. Diagnosis of Bacteriuriaby Detection Of Volatile Organic Compounds in Urine Using an Automated Headspace Analyzer with Multiple Conducting Polymer Sensors. Journal of Clinical Microbiology July 2001;2590-2593.

[20] Kodogiannis VS, Lygouras JN, Tarczynski A, Chowdrey HS. Artificial odor discrimination system using electronic nose and neural networks for the identification of urinary tract infection. IEEE Trans Inf Technol Biomed. 2008;12(6):707-13.

[21] Bailey ALPS, Pisanelli AM, Persaud KC. Development of conducting polymer sensor arrays for wound monitoring. Sensors and Actuators B 2008;131:5-9.

[22] Pisanelli AM, Persaud KC, Bailey A, Stuczen M, Duncan R, Dunn K. Development of a diagnostic aid for bacterial infection in wounds. 13th International symposium on Olfaction and Electronic Nose. AIP Conference Proceedings, 2009;1137:133-135.

[23] Ritaban D, Ritabrata D. Intelligent Bayes Classifier (IBC) for ENT infection classification in hospital environment. BioMedical Engineering OnLine 2006;5:65.

[24] Yates JW, Chappell MJ, Gardner JW *et al.* Data reduction in headspace analysis of blood and urine samples for robust bacterial identification. Comput Methods Programs Biomed. 2005;79(3):259-71.

[25] Trincavelli M, Coradeschi S, Loutfi A, Soderquist B, Thunberg P. Direct Identification of Bacteria in Blood Culture Samples using an Electronic Nose. IEEE Trans Biomed Eng. 2010; May 10.

[26] Lechner M, Fille M, Hausdorfer J, Dierich MP, Rieder J. Diagnosis of bacteria *in vitro* by mass spectrometric fingerprinting: A pilot study. Current Microbiology 2005;51:267-269.

CHAPTER 6

Nanoparticles in Medical Microbiological Research and Diagnosis

J. Ikonomopoulos[1*], E. Liandris[1], I. Tachtsidis[2] and M. Gazouli[3]

[1]Faculty of Animal Science, Laboratory of Anatomy-Physiology, Agricultural University of Athens, 75, Iera Odos st., 11855 Athens, Greece; [2]Department of Medical Physics and Bioengineering, Malet Place Engineering Building, University College, London, Gower st., WC1E 6BT, London, UK and [3]Laboratory of Biology, School of Medicine, University of Athens, 11527, Athens, Greece[3]

Abstract: The social and financial impact of infectious diseases are unfortunately still very relevant today, and the development of new diagnostic tests with improved detection characteristics continues to be an important research priority. Currently, there is a demand for accurate and specific diagnostic tests that can be performed at the point-of-care without the need for dedicated equipment or highly trained personnel. In this respect, advances in the field of nanotechnology are already being utilized by several research groups around the world, and with very encouraging results. In fact, nanoparticles can now be conjugated to oligonucleotides, antibodies, and peptides, facilitating multi-labeling and hence multi-target detection, which (in the context of diagnostic applications) allows the genetic or immunogenic "footprint" of a microbial pathogen to be determined. Further, there exists a range of metal or polymer nanoparticle materials to choose from, and their choice is dependant on the properties of the material required. Here, we provide a concise description of the applications of 2 such materials, colloidal gold and quantum dots, which have already been utilized in several different applications that target pathogen detection. Emphasis is placed on the principles behind these novel applications, and the way in which the properties of nanoparticles are being used in the development of future microbiological applications.

Keywords: Nanoparticles, Quantum Dots, Functionalization, Quartz Crystal Microbalance, Dipstick, Biobarcode Assay.

1. INTRODUCTION

Despite the progress recorded to date, infectious diseases are still considered major causes of disability and death [1]. The problem is most intense in those countries that cannot afford to allocate the financial resources required for the application of effective control measures. Further, this situation applies not only to humans, but also to animals, which are often the source of transmission of pathogens to humans either directly or *via* the food chain. The accompanying social and financial impact of these infectious diseases has led to a focus on the development of new diagnostic tests with improved characteristics. These new diagnostics tests may vary in their methodology, dependant on the target application, but in general demonstrate high reproducibility, sensitivity and specificity, and a more rapid 'time-to-diagnosis'. Further, since the 1980s, molecular biology research has led to some successes in meeting the demands for such tests. PCR, PCR-RFLP, Real Time PCR, DNA sequencing, and DNA strip (dipstick) technologies have considerably improved the speed and accuracy of microbial detection, having facilitated the development of applications that are impossible using traditional means of diagnosis. However, the reliable application of these new methodologies requires highly-specialised personnel, dedicated equipment and distinct laboratory specimen preparation areas. This latter requirement is a consequence of avoiding "carry-over" (*i.e.* the accidental contamination of test samples by amplicons generated during previous PCR reactions), a consequence of the large numbers of amplicons generated during PCR thermocycling. Carry-over can easily lead to false positive results even in the presence of minute quantities of contaminating DNA. These disadvantages do not however apply to the use of "nanodiagnsotsics".

Recent advances in nanotechnology mean that nanoparticles can now be applied to the study of biological

*Address correspondence to J. Ikonomopoulos: Faculty of Animal Science, Laboratory of Anatomy-Physiology, Agricultural University of Athens, 75, Iera Odos st., 11855 Athens, Greece; Tel: 00302105294383; E-mail: ikonomop@aua.gr

processes at dimensions comparable to that of the atom. Further, nanoparticles permit a more efficient interaction between biological molecules due to the one-on-one interactions between the target molecule and the signal generating moieties. Nanotechnologies are becoming available with the ability to detect increasingly smaller amounts of biological materials, without the need for target amplification. Indeed, due to their unique chemical, optical and electronic properties, nanoscale probes are suitable for the detailed analysis of molecule-size receptors, pores, and other components of living cells. Further, nanoparticles can be conjugated to oligonucleotides, antibodies, and peptides, allowing multi-labeling (and multi-target) diagnostic applications to be designed that identify specific genetic and/or immunological pathogen "footprints". Most importantly, nanotechnology currently offers the means for the creation of novel technology platforms that are specifically designed for the diagnostic investigation of infectious diseases, including point-of-care applications with no reliance on specialized personnel or expensive equipment.

2. PROPERTIES OF NANO-PARTICLES

As previously mentioned, advances in the field of molecular biology have gradually become a major cornerstone of research in the "Life Sciences", all within a period of less than 20 years. The intra-disciplinary collaboration that this integration required was supported by a foundation of basic biology that was commonly available to all the interacting scientists. Unfortunately however, this common background does not apply to nanotechnology. In the case of nanotechnology, interacting scientists from the fields of physics, chemistry, molecular biology and microbiology all have to understand the many divergent concepts that are derived from these distinct fields. With this in mind, in this chapter, the authors aim to provide a concise description of the basic characteristics of nanoparticles in a rather simplistic manner in order to facilitate the understanding of their potential use in pathogen detection. Currently, biological imaging techniques in many applications rely heavily on the use of fluorescent proteins and organic dyes as markers. However, these markers suffer from several major disadvantages, such as low probe brightness, poor photostability, and oxygen sensitivity [2]. This means that there is often a need for signal amplification, which limits their usefulness in many *in vitro* and *in vivo* applications. Nanoparticles offer an exciting technological advancement that can eliminate and overcome the above problems, offering state of the art detection solutions for both *in vitro* and *in vivo* applications.

The term nanoparticle is commonly used to describe particles with dimensions less than 100 nm, as opposed to 'bulk material', which is expected to demonstrate a specific physical behavior regardless of size. In fact, nanoparticles may actually exhibit different properties dependant on their size and on the percentage of atoms located at their surface (the surface area of nanoparticles being significantly larger than that of bulk materials). Consequently, nanoparticles demonstrate an unexpected behavior, otherwise referred to as the 'quantum effect', which influences their optical, electrical, chemical and physical characteristics. For example, their high surface area to volume ratio gives them unique properties when used in dispersants, as they possess a very strong tendency to diffuse, avoiding deposition, or floating. In terms of their optical characteristics, an interesting feature of semiconductor nanoparticles is that the minimum amount of energy required for the release of an outer electron from its nucleus (bandgap) is size-dependent, which translates into a color shift from red to blue as the size of the particles decrease [3]. Further, the variable optical characteristics of these nanoparticles (compared to bulk materials) also extends to their electrical properties, allowing the construction of semiconductors whose conductivity can be accurately calibrated within a range of energies by using particles of specific sizes. Finally, colloidal particles can act as robust, broadly tunable nano-emitters that can be excited by a single light source, providing distinct advantages over current fluorescent markers (including organic dyes and fluorescent proteins).

There are a number of metal or polymer nanoparticle materials currently available, whose use is dependant on the properties required in a particular application. In the last few years, nanodiagnostic applications have tended to focus on colloidal gold and cadmium selenide quantum dots, which seem to be very promising materials in terms of pathogen detection.

Colloidal gold nanoparticles (AuNPs) range in size from 3-100 nm, they are stable, uniform and monodispersed particles that can be easily produced by various chemical processes, among which the reduction of chloroauric acid by citrate. Metal nanoparticles (or NPs) exhibit strong size-dependent optical resonance, tunable for emission in the near-infrared (NIR) part of the spectrum, which is generally known as Surface Plasmon Resonance (SPR) [4]. This resonance is pronounced in noble metal NPs because of the collective oscillations of conduction band electrons. SPR is especially interesting with reference to Au (and also silver (Ag)) NPs. When metal NPs are photo-activated, the plasmon couples with the excitation light to produce a large enhancement of the electromagnetic (EM) field. Interactions between the incident light and the oscillating electric fields result in the scattering and absorption of light. The enormous enhancement of the local EM field make metal NPs attractive in applications from optical devices to bioanalyses and bioimaging, and can be exploited to generate a color change (visual detection), or heat (for the construction of biosensors) [5].

AuNPs are negatively charged and are very sensitive to changes in the "dielectric constant" of a solution [6]. This sensitive change is significant in terms of their potential application in diagnostics, since (for typical citrate stabilized particles) the addition of NaCl neutralizes the surface charge and can cause a decrease in inter-particle distance. This decrease can be utilized to selectively deposit the AuNPs eventually resulting in a change of color detectable by visual observation [6]. The same result can be achieved by linkage of two or more functionalized (*i.e.* chemically modified for conjugation) AuNPs to a target molecule of DNA, which results in particle aggregation as the distance between the particles is decreased.

The properties of AuNPs have been utilized to construct several different types of detection mechanisms, including visual observation of a color change or measurement of optical absorption. In all cases, the basic idea is that in solution, monodispersed AuNPs appear red and exhibit a relatively narrow surface plasmon absorption band centered at around 520 nm in the UV-visible spectrum. In contrast, a solution containing aggregated AuNPs appears purple in color corresponding to a characteristic red shift in the surface plasmon resonance of the particles from 520 nm to 574 nm. Further, colloidal silver and gold particles offer some other unique features, they do not undergo any photodecomposition, which is a common problem encountered when using fluorescent dyes. Secondly, they are not toxic, in sharp contrast to the potential toxicity of semiconductor QDs (see later). Thirdly, they are reasonably stable and can be stored in a dry state. Lastly, there exists a capability to shift their 'Surface Plasmon Resonance' (SPR), in a controlled fashion, to the spectral region best suited for optical bioimaging and biosensing applications. Therefore the use of these materials as nanoparticle biosensors relies on signalling *via* a shift in the absorption of different wavelengths of light that can be measured mechanically, or be detected visually by a resulting change in color.

Nanometer-scale semiconductor crystallites, better known as Quantum Dots (QDs), are semiconductor crystals with physical dimensions smaller than the exciton Bohr radius [7]. A typical exciton Bohr radius for QDs is of a few nanometers, though this property does depend on the material used to construct the nanoparticles. Indeed, those metal and semiconductor nanoparticles in the size range of 2-6 nm are currently of considerable interest due to their dimensional similarities with biological macromolecules *i.e.* nucleic acids and proteins. Colloidal semiconductor nanocrystals can be produced using various semiconductors including Cadmium Selenide (CdSe), Cadmium Sulfide (CdS), indium arsenide (InAs), indium phosphide (InP).and lead sulfide (PbS). These materials exhibit size-dependent fluorescence-emission wavelengths (a defining feature of QDs), a very significant property in terms of their potential use as biosensors. When a photon of visible light hits such a semiconductor, some of their electrons are excited into higher energy states. When these electrons return to their ground state, a photon is emitted with a frequency that is characteristic of the semiconductor material. The ability of QDs to release photons (in effect their photoluminescence), can actually be improved using specific types of "inorganic shells". In more detail, the surface of QDs contain non-radiative recombination sites. When an electron returns to its valence state from the conduction band, it usually emits the excess energy in the form of heat instead of photons. In other words the presence of search sites causes a loss of optical signal, a process that can be avoided by blocking the relevant sites using inorganic shells (sites are "passivated") [8]. When blocked, the excited electrons will release photons upon their return to their valence band. In effect, the shell makes QDs brighter and more sensitive to change as the QDs then require less energy to be excited (*e.g.* adding a ZnS shell around a CdSe core [9]). Another very widely used coating material for QDs is silica [10]. This high-band-gap, oxidation-resistant, shell material has been widely investigated because it is less toxic and it imparts 'wettability' and biocompatibility to QDs. Further, silica surfaces can be easily modified to link to bioconjugators (such as avidin), meaning that silica coated nanoparticles are applicable to diagnostic methodologies utilizing biological interactions.

Once prepared, inorganic core-shell semiconductor nanoparticles are only soluble in hydrophobic solvents, yet to be used in biological applications, nanoparticles must be soluble in aqueous solutions, which requires an additional hydrophilic coating after quantum dot core/shell synthesis. There are two alternatives used to generate this coating: 1) surface ligand exchange; and 2) coating with an amphiphilic polymer, and a wide range of molecules serve as surface coatings, including thiolate ligands and silica.

In summary, a shell is a very important component of a QD, as it will protect the core from oxidation, minimize or eliminate core-derived toxicity and increase its water solubility. Importantly, these adaptations mean that QDs can be used as biosensors in hydrophilic solutions, for example with DNA solutions derived from clinical samples.

The bandgap energy of different QD materials determines the color of the light emitted so that QDs are ideal for the development of easy-to-read diagnostic assays that rely on color detection. As mentioned above the larger the dot the redder (lower energy) its fluorescence peak; thus the energy spectrum of a QD can be engineered by controlling its size [8]. In this respect, CdSe may be size-tuned to emit in the 450–650 nm range, CdTe (cadmium telluride) in the 500–750 nm range, and InAs or PbSe (lead selenide) above 800 nm [2]. The simultaneous detection of multiple targets (QDs of different sizes conjugated to biomolecules that hybridize to complimentary oligonucleotides or peptides), using a single excitation wavelength of light, is therefore feasible. In conclusion, these nanoparticles are proving superior biosensors when compared to traditional organic dyes as they are much brighter and more stable (being much less prone to photobleaching). It has been estimated that QDs are 20 times brighter and 100 times more stable than traditional fluorescent reporters [11]. In addition to their extremely high brightness, QDs also offer: i) a wide excitation window (which makes the use of a single excitation filter possible) [12]; ii) narrow and tuneable emission spectra (which reduces spectral overlap making the simultaneous use of multiple colours possible); iii) a large separation between the excitation and emission (which increases the detection sensitivity); and iv) resistance to photobleaching.

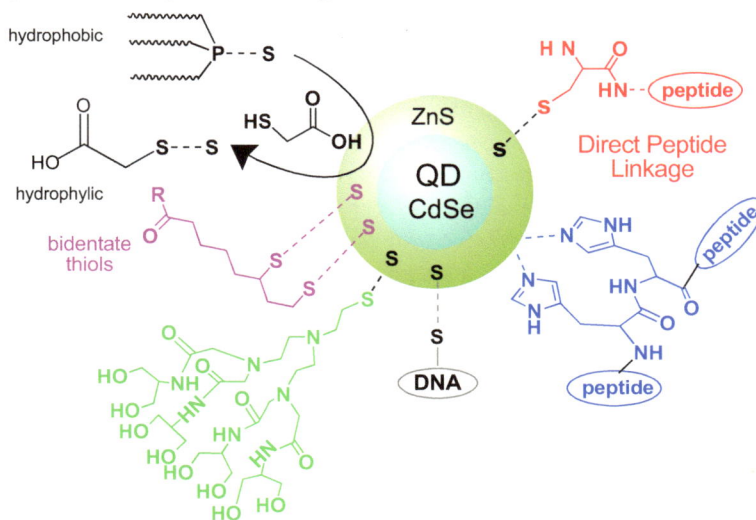

Fig (1). Chemical groups on the surface of nanoparticles that can be used for functionalization with biomolecules.

3. FUNCTIONALIZATION OF NANOPARTICLES

Nanoparticles first have to be "functionalized" if they are to be used as biosensors. This means that the nanoparticles and relevant probe biomolecules (*e.g.* specific oligonucleotides or monoclonal antibodies) first have to be modified in order to facilitate binding of the probe to the nanoparticle surface. Suitable chemical groups for this are nucleophiles or sulfhydryls (Fig. **1**), and the nanoparticle-biomolecule conjugate can be designed to carry functionally reactive groups *e.g.* biotin and avidin or streptavidin (the strongest interaction known between a ligand and a protein known[13]. Various functionalization methods have been developed [14], with the process being considerably improved by Brust *et al.*, [15], who utilized the reduction of metal salts in the presence of thiols as capping ligands. This allowed a range of noble metal cores (eg, Au, Ag, Pd, Pt) to be synthesized possessing specific functionalities. The initial ligand layer can be further developed *via* the Murray place-displacement reaction [16], facilitating the efficient binding of several biomolecules, and providing control over the final nanoparticle structure and function. In general, antibodies and proteins are usually functionalized with thiols and biotin [17], whilst DNA is functionalized at the 5′- or the 3′-end (or inbetween), by amino modification, thiol modification, phosphorylation or biotinylation. Genomic DNA is an ideal stabilizer/coating for QDs, allowing experimentation using DNA or RNA oligos and other biological macromolecules. In fact, a coating composed of biological macromolecules can streamline the subsequent functionalization of QDs by facilitating the conjugation of probes, aptamers or proteins to the nanoparticle surface.

4. DETECTION OF AUNPS

The detection of functionalized gold nanoparticles is possible by exploiting the basic properties of AuNPs (described in the previous section). These methods are categorized into two groups dependant on the phase of the medium utilized (liquid or solid).

4.1 Liquid Phase Detection

a. Cross-linking Method: A milestone in the use of gold nanoparticles was the discovery in 1996 by Mirkin *et al.* [18], that AuNPs can be effectively conjugated to oligonucleotides that can then hybridize to complementary DNA sequences. Hybridization decreases the distance between the particles causing a shift in the optical absorption of the solution, ultimately resulting in a visual color change. This change in color occurs when target is present, while negative samples remain red. This approach is referred to as the 'gold nanoparticle cross-linking method' because it uses the target molecule as a linker for bringing together gold particles. The approach was further exploited using different methods for bringing the gold particle into close contact *i.e.* head to head [19] or head to tail contact [20, 21]. However, the fact that a rather large aggregate of nanoparticles is required to produce a visually detectable color change, means that the Minimum Detection Limit (MDL) using these assays is relatively high. In order to improve on this, Storhoff *et al.* [22], utilized scattered, instead of absorbed, light for the detection of AuNP aggregates. This approach decreased the MDL for the MRSA *mecA* gene to 3.3 ng/μl of target DNA, with a further decrease to 66 pg/μl, if 4 instead of 2 AuNPs were combined at adjacent sites. Notably, the proposed methodology improved the detection of aggregates even in the presence of an excess of non-aggregated particles. In 2005 Li *et al.* [23] proposed an interesting alternative to this methodology by incorporating a high-fidelity Tth DNA ligase for detecting point mutations. This assay uses an allele-specific discriminating probe and a common probe, both immobilized on the surface of gold nanoparticles by strong sulphur–Au adsorption. Hybridization of the target strand with the probes results in the formation of an extended polymeric Au nanoparticle–polynucleotide aggregate, triggering a red to purple color change in the solution. A perfect match between the base at the 3′-end of the discriminating probe and the target allows the ligase to covalently join the two adjacent probes that flank the mutation site, while a mismatch does not. When the reaction mixture is heated to denature the duplex formed, the purple color of the perfect-match solution does not turn a red color, whilst a red color is observed when there is a mismatch. The result may be detected by colorimetry or spectrophotometry, and the method offers the advantage of single-base discrimination without the need for precise temperature control. Further, the thermally stable Tth ligase used enables the hybridization reaction to be performed at a relatively high temperature, increasing specificity. Du *et al.* [24], used a different approach by exploiting a highly sensitive light-scattering assay *via* the use of a common spectrofluorimeter equipped with a 150W high pressure Xenon lamp, which further decreased the MDL for a fragment of the human p53 gene (exon 8) to 0.1 pM.

The cross-linking properties of nanoparticles was recently applied to the construction of reporter and detection systems for DNA–protien interactions based on the regulated interaction between a DNA-binding protein (the lac repressor) and its cognate DNA binding site (the lac operator) [25]. Bai *et al.* [26] used cross-linked gold nanoparticles to make DNA target-induced aggregation visually detectable. Thirteen nanometer AuNP-DNA conjugates hybridized to a target sequence at 35°C and were then transferred to a solution containing CTAB (cetyltrimethyl ammonium bromide) and ascorbic acid. HAuCl4 was finally added to initiate the chemical deposition process, generating distinct colours in different solutions dependant on their target concentrations, and allowing visual detection of 50–200 pM of perfectly matched DNA.

The aggregation of gold nanoparticles through a target molecule can also be achieved using a protein in the role of the linker. In this case gold nanoparticles are not functionalized with oligonucleotides but with peptides or proteins. This method was applied by Thahn and Rosenzweig [27] who were able to detect as few as 1 µg/ml of *Staphylococcus aureus* protein A using a frame absorption spectrometer. A similar approach was utilized by Hirsch *et al.* [28] for the detection of rabbit IgG. The assay relied on the use of silica nanoparticles layered with a gold shell that was covered with anti-rabbit IgG antibodies. This combination allowed detection of 0.88 ng/ml of rabbit IgG in whole blood samples from experimentally infected animals.

b. Non cross-linking method: The manner in which nanoparticles react to a change of solution dielectric has been used as the basis for the development of alternative methodologies for the detection of AuNP-conjugates. In this case, particles that DO NOT hybridize to a specific target that actually aggregate and precipitate once a change in the solution's dielectric occurs (Fig. **2** and **3**). Using this approach, a change of color is observed in the ABSENCE of the target molecule *i.e.* when the test sample is negative. In this respect, Baptista *et al.* [29] used this method of selective aggregation to detect AuNP-RNA of the FSY1 gene of *Sacharomyces bayanus* (adding salt to increase the solution dielectric). One year later, Baptista *et al.* [30] applied the same method for the detection of *Mycobacterium tuberculosis* in 73 clinical specimens from patients with suspected pulmonary and extrapulmonary tuberculosis. The samples that were examined by the Ziehl-Neelsen stain were tested using the AuNP assay and compared with reference to the established INNO-LiPA-Rif-TB method. DNA was amplified by one round of PCR and used for hybridization to AuNPs functionalized with oligonucleotides complementary to the target molecule. Again aggregation was induced by an increase in the solution's salt concentration to 2 mM. The concordance of the results obtained between the two methods in relation to the positive samples was 100%, whereas the relevant percentage for the samples that produced a negative result by INNOLiPA- Rif-TB was almost 90%.

A different approach for the modification of the solution's dielectric was followed more recently by our team for the detection of mycobacteria at the genus level [31]. AuNPs 20 nm in size were functionalized with oligonucleotide probes against the 16s-23s ITS DNA region, which is highly conserved among the members of *Mycobacterium*. Nanoparticle probes were synthesized with a thiol group at their 5′-end and were used for hybridization with the target DNA at 65°C. The solution containing the functionalized conjugates exhibited a pink color and an absorption peak at ~525 nm. The addition of HCl in the absence of the target sequence caused an absorption peak shift towards a longer wavelength, generating a color change from pink to purple. Notably, in the case of positive samples no nanoparticle deposition was recorded even when the test tubes were incubated overnight at room temperature. The MDL of the assay was 18.75 ng of DNA diluted in a sample volume of 10 µl. In order to assess the ability of this method to detect target DNA in heavily contaminated samples containing mixed bacterial populations in excess, we applied the method to non-amplified DNA isolated from 12 positive and an 12 negative control fecal samples. The former (which produced a positive real time PCR (RT-PCR) result for the detection of *Mycobacterium avium* subsp. *Paratuberculosis*) were collected from goats with paratuberculosis. The concordance of the two methods in relation to positive and negative results was 87.5% and 100%, respectively. As expected, the results indicated that the AuNP assay was not influenced by PCR inhibitors, an advantage that together with a lower cost and simplicity (no dedicated equipment, or expert personnel, and time-to-diagnosis within approximately 20 minutes) suggests a suitability for use in point-of-care applications.

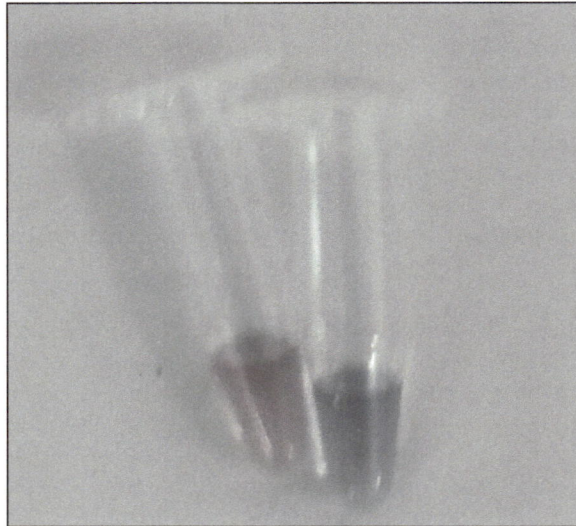

Fig (2). Results obtained using the non cross-linking method and functionalized nanoparticles to detect the DNA isolated from *Mycobacterium avium* subsp *paratuberculosis*) (red tube). In contrast, the negative control (water) remains purple/grey.

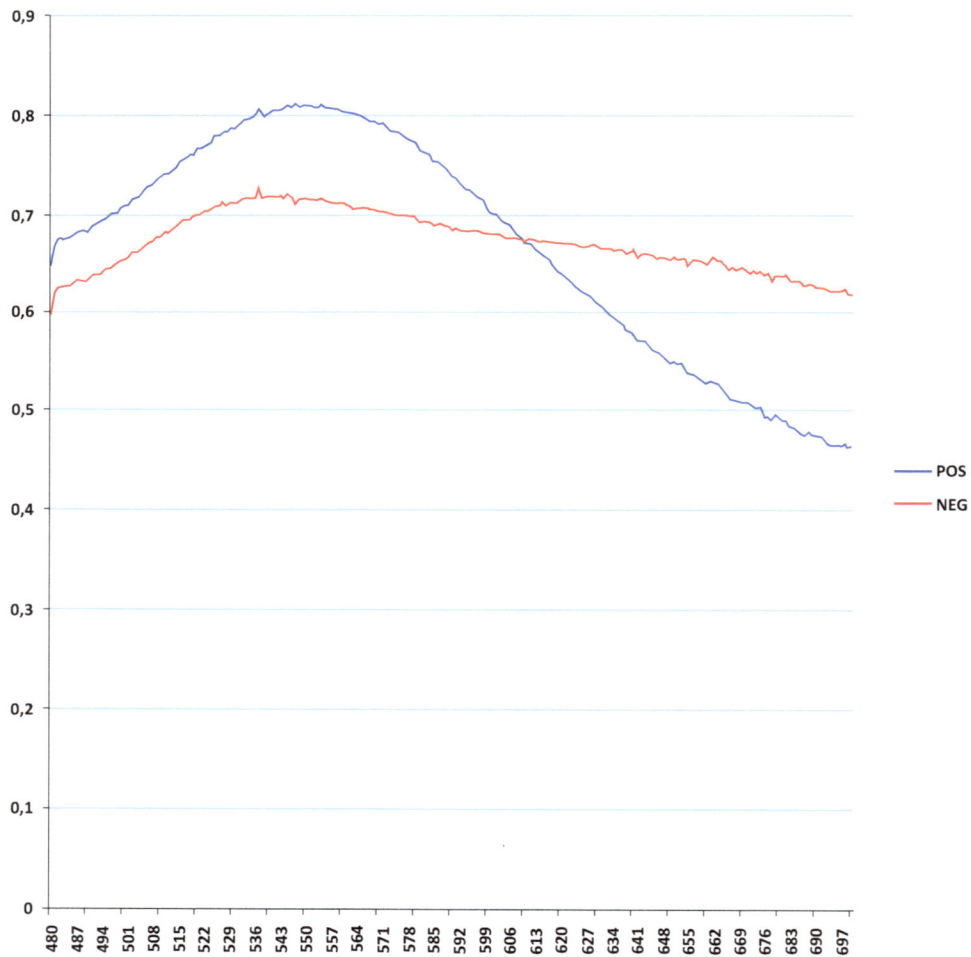

Fig (3). Graphical representation of the absorption spectra of positive and negative controls (Fig. **2**) using the non cross-linking method.

Another very interesting application of the non-cross-linking method is salt-induced nanoparticle aggregation, which was used for the detection of two point mutations on the human epidermal growth factor gene [32]. The procedure comprised 3 stages, of which the first comprised the denaturation of the target DNA, which was then hybridized to unmodified oligonucleotide probes. In the second stage, the hybridized mixture was incubated to interact with AuNPs for 10 minutes. Aggregation was induced at the final stage by the addition of NaCl, causing a color change in the wild type (as opposed to the mutant version, which did not generate hybridization). The addition of salt effectively diminishes the electrostatic repulsion between particles and induces easier aggregation of the gold nanoparticle suspension, particularly with respect to the perfectly matched dsDNA when compared to mismatched dsDNA. This method does not rely on modified oligonucleotides as probes, which simplifies the procedure and makes it more easily adaptable for other targets. Finally Conde *et al.* [33] recently applied the non-cross-linking method for the detection of non-amplified RNA of the BCR-ABL fusion product that is of importance in the diagnostic investigation of chronic myeloid leukaemia. They demonstrated the possibility of using AuNPs for the direct detection of BCR-ABL RNA in samples.

c. Bio-barcode assay: AuNPs are the cornerstone of the bio-barcode assay (BCA), which has been proposed as a potential alternative to PCR [34]. This method incorporates many of the advances made from previous DNA-AuNP studies into the multiplex and ultra-sensitive detection of proteins and nucleic acids [35]. Further, the method can be extended to detect any target capable of being sandwiched between a pair of probes, resulting in an extremely flexible and broad (in terms of its potential applications) technique [35].

The BCA involves isolation of target molecules by means of a sandwich format consisting of oligonucleotide-modified AuNPs and magnetic microparticles. The barcodes are single stranded molecules of DNA, shorter than 100 base pairs, that can be easily modified using a number of different chemical functional groups and fluorophores. The low MDL of BCA results from the release of a large number of barcode DNA strands, which occurs after the binding of each target molecule.

In 2003 Nam *et al.* [36] described this approach for the detection of proteins *via* the use of gold nanoparticles. In this case, AuNPs were not used as labels but as carriers of different DNA sequences (that act as barcodes), as well as an antibody that had been constructed to be complimentary to the target molecule. In more detail, magnetic beads carry monoclonal antibodies that bind to the specific protein of interest (*e.g.* prostate-specific antigen, PSA), whilst AuNPs carry polyclonal antibodies against the same specific protein and bar-code oligonucleotides that allow recognition of this polyclonal antibody. PSA is bound by both the magnetic beads and AuNPs to form a "sandwich". Magnetic separation of the beads that have hybridized to the PSA target, followed by release (dehybridization) and identification of the AuNP barcode, allows the determination of the presence of the target protein. Further, because the nanoparticle carries a large number of oligonucleotides per captured protein molecule, there is a substantial enhancement of the signal, allowing the detection of 30 attomoles of PSA. Alternatively, amplification of the oligonucleotide barcodes by PCR can improve the MDL of the assay to 3 attomolar. For comparison, the MDL of the clinically accepted "gold standard" assay used for the detection of PSA is approximately 3 picomole *i.e.* 6 orders of magnitude higher. In fact, this same group extended this approach in 2004 [37] to the detection of target DNA by simply substituting the antibodies present on both the magnetic beads and the AuNPs with specific oligonucleotides. Since 2004, this approach has been used in the diagnostic investigation of Alzheimer's Disease [38, 39], as well as the simultaneous detection of HBV, VV, HIV, EV [40]. Also, Zhang *et al.* [41] used 2 DNA probes designed to be specific for the insertion element (Iel) of *Salmonella enteritidis* and adapted the detection mechanism described above to the detection of the specific pathogen by incorporating signal amplifier Au-NPs that were functionalized with one or two capture probes and with FAM labelled oligonucleotides. These FAM labelled oligonucleotides could be detected by spectrophotometry, whilst the functionalized magnetic beads were used to concentrate the target molecule. In this case, the fluorescent signal of the released DNA barcodes showed an exponential relationship to the target DNA concentration, resulting in an MDL of 1 ng/ml target DNA.

d. Other uses of AuNPs in liquid phase: In 2001 Dubertret *et al.* [42] demonstrated that gold nanoparticles could be used as quenchers in molecular beacons with a quenching efficiency of 99.966 ± 0.026. The quenching of AuNPs could be theoretically optimized to a specific wavelength through the production of particles with defined shapes and dimensions. This meant that it is possible to optimize gold quenchers for virtually each dye that can be used in Real Time PCR assays. In 2005 Li *et al.* [43] used gold nanoparticles as PCR enhancers. According to this team, the use of 13 nm AuNPs improved the amplification yield of PCR by 10^4 - 10^6 fold, probably due to the excellent heat dispersion of gold colloids. Interestingly, Wan and Yeow [44] investigated the effect of 5, 10 and 20 nm AuNPs on PCR efficiency, concluding that AuNPs of larger size have stronger inhibitory effect on PCR than smaller particles (at the same particle concentration). This effect was attributed to the binding of AuNPs to Taq polymerase, effectively reducing the amount of free polymerase in the PCR solution, and resulting in a decrease in the reaction yield.

4.2. Solid Phase Detection

Nanoparticles can also be incorporated into solid phase detection systems, solid phase systems facilitating either the removal of unbound material, and/or signal amplification. Further, different approaches can be used in order to reveal target molecule / biosensor interactions. These approaches fall into the following 3 types of detection technologies: AuNP microarrays, Quartz Crystal Microbalances (QCM) and Dipsticks.

a. Microarrays: The power of microarray technology is the ability to detect hundreds to thousands of DNA or RNA sequences in a single assay. Microarrays are based on the immobilization on solid surfaces of capture probes (either oligonucleotides or antibodies) that are complementary to the targeted molecule. The standard approach for the demonstration of any binding event is *via* fluorescent dye labels. Though broadly used and well-established these dyes cannot however be considered ideal, mainly due to photo bleaching, a fluorescence that depends on the chemical environment, and the need for specific filters for excitation and detection [45]. These factors, as well as a need to decrease the cost of microarray testing, have provided an opportunity for nanoparticle researchers [46]. The use of AuNPs as labels for the detection of conjugated targets on microarrays could overcome the disadvantages of traditional dyes since they are stable and their signal is not dependent upon their environment [47]. Furthermore the fact that their detection is possible through scanometric, potentiometric, or Surface Enhanced Raman Spectroscopy (SERS), may improve the cost/benefit ratio of AuNP microarrays (Table **1**). In more detail, the scanometric assay involves AuNP labeled probes that can be detected by visual observation, or after silver deposition (in the presence of a reducing agent *e.g.* hydroquinone), even if the concentration of the target is low [48]. This approach was first reported by Taton *et al.* [49], who used sandwich hybridization with AuNP labeled probes for gene detection. Recently, improved optics were incorporated to decrease the MDL of this type of technology to the high attomolar to high femtomolar concentration range, with impressive grey-scale quantification capabilities [50].

A potentiometric readout is achieved by functionalizing microelectrode gaps with intervening target capture sequences for the detection of sandwiched targets using gold nanoparticle probes. Upon silver development (see above), the gap is able to pass a current whose amplitude is dependent upon the concentration of the bound target sequence [35]. These devices are proving very promising tools for the detection of extremely small quantities of analytes, and at the same time are easy and cheap to produce. Further, the instrumentation required is relatively simple and can be easily miniaturized to the circuit-board level, facilitating the development of disposable potentiometric devices [51].

SERS is based on the finding that the light scattering across sections of molecules adsorbed onto roughened noble metal surfaces, (typically Au and Ag and to a lesser extent copper (Cu)), are significantly enhanced upon laser excitation. Gold nanoparticles are functionalized with a target-specific molecule and also an extra Raman dye (different Raman "bar-code" dye colors may be utilized). Bar-code detection occurs upon silver enhancement and Raman spectroscopy. Raman scattering is dependent on two phenomena, a weakly enhancing short-range chemical enhancement mechanism (CE) and a stronger long-range electromagnetic Enhancement Mechanism (EM) [52].

b. Quartz Crystal Microbalances: QCMs offer an alternative detection strategy for monitoring mass changes dependant upon the binding of target molecules on quartz crystal microbalances [53]. In order to increase the signal and the analytical sensitivity of the method, a second probe labelled with AuNPs may be

Table 1: Applications of scanometric, potentiometric or surface enhanced Raman spectroscopy for the microarray detection of nanoparticles.

Type of assay	Ref.	Detection by	Target	Method Characteristics /specifications
Scanometric detection of DNA	50	AuNP labeled probes	Gene detection	Sandwich hybridization with a pair of probes specific for each target
	84	Streptavidin conjugated AuNPS		The method eliminates the need of oligonucleotide probes specific for each target. Results of the colorimetric detection using silver deposition comparable to fluorescence-detection by confocal scanner
	85	Two-probe sandwich hybridization/nanoparticle	HBV & HCV	Visual detection of silver-staining enhanced coloring of hybridized PCR products
	86	Probe sandwich hybridization/nanoparticle	Multiplex SNP[1] profiling	Visual detection of silver-staining enhanced coloring of non-amplified DNA. MDL[2] of 500 ng of genomic DNA.
	87	Probe sandwich hybridization/nanoparticle	Human total RNA	Target molecules are hybridized with oligo dT-modified AuNP silver enhanced probes. Detection by light scattering resulting to a 1000-fold increase of signal.
	88	Probe sandwich hybridization/nanoparticle	*Ureoplasma urealyticum* and *Chlamydia trachomatis*	Simultaneous detection of targets directly from clinical samples without PCR amplification.
	47	250-nm AuNP	DNA control samples	Highly positive charged nanoparticles to label negatively charged target. MDL 2pg of DNA.
Scanometric detection of proteins	89	Probe sandwich hybridization/nanoparticle with silver enhancement	Human IgG	MDL comparable to fluorescent method
	90	Immunosensor	cAbPSA-N7	Sandwich assay involving biotinylated PSA-specific mouse monoclonal antibodies and streptavidin-AuNP conjugates
	91	AuNP labelled peptides	*Treponema pallidum* antibody	MDL 1 ng/mL
	92	LSP[4]-based immunochip	tau protein	100-fold increase in assay sensitivity over the conventional fluorophore techniques and near 4-fold increase in specificity
Potentiometric	93	chip-based DNA detection	Actinomycetes	Detection does not require optical equipment, therefore the assay can be realized in an inexpensive manner.
	94	Immunosensor	Anti-sperm Ab in human serum	electron-transfer resistance of the electrode increases when anti-sperm Ab bind in the surface-immobilized sperm antigen
	95	AuNP-DNA/RNA conjugates including a RAMAN active molecule	SNPs	MDL of 1 fmol/l
SERS	96	AuNP-protein conjugates	HBV surface antigen	Immunogold nanolabelling and silver staining enhancement method with the SERS for quantitative detection with MDL of 0.5 mg/ml
	52	AuNP-DNA conjugates	West Nile Virus	Detection is based on the capture-mediated positioning of Au nanoparticles in close proximity to a Raman label bound to Ag coated films

hybridized to the QCM. The resulting mechanism allows simple, rapid and real-time measurement of DNA binding and hybridization at the sub-nanogram level [54]. QCM has been extensively investigated as a transducer in hybridization-based DNA biosensors for the detection of mutations [55], genetically modified organisms [56], and various pathogens [57-59]. Mo *et al.* [53] have functionalized gold-coated QCMs with oligonucleotides and then used these substrates to capture DNA targets and nanoparticle–oligonucleotide conjugates in a sandwich format. They were thus able to achieve a 50-fold improvement of MDL over conventional techniques. Pang *et al.* 2006 [60] applied a nanoparticle-amplified QCM for the capture of target DNA in solution for the detection of point mutations. Thiol-modified capture probes were immobilized on the gold electrode surface of QCM. Successive hybridization of the capture probe with the target probe and the nano-Au-labeled DNA detection probe, lead to the formation of double-stranded DNA (dsDNA) bridged by the target DNA. A DNA ligase reaction was then used to close the nick between the capture and the detection probe (ligation does not take place in the case of a single-base mismatch). After denaturation, the AuNP- labelled DNA probe only remained on the QCM sensor surface provided that there was a perfect match to the target. Chen *et al.* [61] utilized a similar approach for the detection and identification of *Escherichia coli* O157:H7. Target DNA was captured using a single-stranded DNA-probe, and the signal was amplified using a sequence specific probe conjugated to AuNPs. The application of the QCM system was tested in real food samples (apple juice, milk, and ground beef). The method detected PCR-amplified DNA fragments of the target pathogens at an MDL of 1.2×10^2 CFU/ml.

c. Dipstick: The strong interest in the development of simple and low-cost detection methods suitable for the routine clinical laboratory and/or point-of-care led to the development of dipstick dry reagent assays. These seem to be a very promising diagnostic tool due to their low cost, disposability and simplicity. Kalogianni *et al.* [62] reported the first dry-reagent DNA biosensor in a disposable dipstick format, for the visual detection and sequence confirmation of Genetically Modified Organisms (GMO) within minutes. Oligonucleotide-conjugated AuNPs were used as probes and constituted an integral part of the sensor. The user need only to apply the sample and immerse the sensor in the appropriate buffer. As a model, the biosensor was applied to the detection of genetically modified soybean in certified reference materials and samples. The biosensor consisted of a wicking (immersion) pad, a conjugation pad, a laminated membrane and an absorbent pad assembled on a plastic adhesive backing. The 4 parts were positioned in such a way that their ends overlapped in order to ensure continuous flow of the developing solution from the wicking pad up to the absorbent pad upon immersion. Oligo(dT)-conjugated gold nanoparticles were placed on the conjugate pad and were allowed to dry. The laminated membrane contained a zone of immobilized streptavidin (test zone) and a zone of immobilized oligo(dA) (control zone). The sensors were stored dry at ambient temperature. For GMO screening, a 10 µl aliquot of each biotinylated amplified product for 35S, NOS and lectin was mixed with 1µl of 0.9 M NaCl and 1 pmol of dATP-tailed specific probe. The mixture was heated at 95°C for 2 min and then hybridization was allowed to proceed for 5 min at 37°C. Both the denaturation and hybridization steps were performed in the thermal cycler. A 5µl aliquot of the above mixture was applied to the conjugate pad of the dipstick next to the gold nanoparticles. The wicking pad of the sensor was then immersed into 200 µL of developing solution. The visual detection of amplified sequences was completed within 10 min. Another variation of this approach was developed by Huang [63] for the detection of *Staphylococcus aureus* protein A. Anti-protein A IgG and goat anti-rabbit antibody were applied respectively to the test and the control lines on the nitrocellulose membrane that was dried at 35°C. An untreated absorption pad was used. The AuNP-conjugate with anti-protein A IgG antibody was applied on an untreated glass-fiber membrane and completely dried at 35°C. The nitrocellulose membrane, the absorption pad, the glassfiber membrane and the pretreated sample pad were attached to the strip. A sample was pipetted into a reaction holder to determine the result of the strip test. All of the 130 isolates of *S. aureus* that were tested produced the same result using the immunochromatographic test, the coagulase test, and the latex agglutination test, confirming test sensitivity of 100% with an MDL of 25 ng. Kalogianni *et al.* [64] introduced a similar rapid molecular test in a dry reagent disposable dipstick format, for the visual detection and sequence confirmation of 6 bacterial species commonly implicated in arthroplasty infections *i.e. Escherichia coli, Staphylococcus aureus, Staphylococcus epidermidis, Streptococcus pneumoniae, Enterococcus faecium,* and *Haemophilus influenza.* The test allowed detection of PCR products by hybridization within minutes without the need for specialized instrumentation. The authors used a similar approach and a single pair of universal primers to amplify highly conserved regions of the 23S rRNA gene. The resultant PCR mix was pipetted onto the sample area of a conjugate pad, and the strip was immersed in the developing buffer. The developing solution migrated upward by capillary action and rehydrated oligo(dT) conjugated AuNPs on the conjugate pad. The oligo(dT) strands hybridize with the dA tails of the probe, and the hybrids were captured by immobilized streptavidin in the test zone of the strip. A red line was formed due to the accumulation of the gold nanoparticles in this zone. The dipstick test demonstrated a 4 times greater detection result than agarose gel electrophoresis. Finally Konstantou *et al.* [65] reported another dipstick assay that enables simultaneous visual detection of genetic alleles within minutes using a single strip. Allele discrimination is based on a primer extension (PEXT) reaction. The PEXT reaction products are applied directly to the strip without prior purification. Oligonucleotide-conjugated AuNP-nanoparticles deposited in dry form on the strip were used as reporters. The assay was evaluated for the genotyping of two SNPs of the toll-like receptor 4 (TLR4) gene (Asp299Gly and Thr399Ile), one SNP of the cytochrome P450 gene CYP2C19 (CYP2C19*3) and one SNP of the TPMT (TPMT*2) gene.

5. DETECTION OF QDs

Conjugation of QDs to antibodies renders them ideal reporters for cellular imaging and immuno-staining of different cellular structures [66-71]. Their superior properties, with respect to normal fluorophores allow a 10-100 fold increase in sensitivity. On the other hand the application of QDs in diagnostic assays has only recently been exploited. QDs have been applied in immunoassay formats for the detection of biologically important molecules like Prostate Specific Antigen (PSA) [72] and Thyroid Stimulating Hormone (TSH) [73] or toxins. The wide absorption spectrum and the narrow emission of QDs renders them ideal for the simultaneous detection of different targets, each of which is labeled with a QD that emits light in a different wavelength. Goldman *et al.* [74] used a sandwich immunoassay for the detection of 4 different toxins (cholera toxin, ricin, shiga-like toxin 1, and staphylococcal enterotoxin B) in single wells of a microtiter plate allowing simultaneous quantification of all 4 toxins with an MDL of 3-300 ng/ml dependant on the target. With regard to pathogens, QDs have been applied to the detection of hepatitis B surface antigen (HBsAg) [75], adenovirus [76], *Bacillus anthracis* [77], *E. coli* O157 [78] and *Salmonella Typhimurium* [79]. Klostranec *et al.* [80] achieved picomolar sensitivity for the detection of antibodies against hepatitis HBV, HCV, and HIV with an assay that requires no more than 100 µl of sample and can be performed within less than 2 hours. Zhu *et al.* [81] exploited the characteristic optical properties of QDs for the simultaneous detection of *Crysptosporidium parvum* and *Giarda lamblia*.

Our team [82], has recently utilized a pair of biotinylated oligonucleotide probes as detectors of mycobacterial DNA through a sandwich hybridization reaction, with cadmium selenide QDs conjugated to streptavidin and species-specific probes that were used to produce a fluorescent signal. Further, magnetic beads conjugated to streptavidin and a genus-specific probe were used to isolate and concentrate DNA targets from the sample, dispensing with the need for PCR amplification. The MDL of the assay was determined as 12.5 ng of DNA (diluted in a sample volume of 20 µl). In order to obtain an indication of the method's performance on clinical samples, we applied the optimized assay to the detection of: i) *Mycobacterium tuberculosis* in DNA isolated from bronchoalveolar lavage of patients with tuberculosis, and ii) *Mycobacterium avium* subsp. *paratuberculosis* in faeces and paraffin embedded tissues. We compared the results to culture, Ziehl-Neelsen stain and Real Time PCR. The concordance of these methods compared to the QD system, and in respect to positive and negative samples, varied between 53.84% - 87.23% and 84.61% - 100%, respectively. The overall accuracy of the QD assay compared to Real Time PCR was 70% - 90% dependant on the type of clinical material used. More recently we utilized the same approach for the detection of mycobacterial surface antigens. In this case, streptavidin coated magnetic beads were functionalized with a biotinylated polyvalent genus-specific antibody that was complimentary to the target. A solution of mouse monoclonal antibodies against the mycobacterial antigens MTB-FDR 5B8.1, MTB-HBHA 1D4.1, MTB-FDR 4H9.1, MTB FDR 1A7.1 MTBHbHA BH4.1 MTB FDR 2B12.1 MTB HbHA 4A8.1, and Hsp65 was used to detect several different sites of the targeted mycobacterial cells. An anti-mouse biotinylated antibody was then added to the mixture and conjugation made detectable after the addition of cadmium selenide QDs, the idea being that the magnetic beads would capture any target bound monoclonal antibodies, leading to conjugation of subsequently added anti-mouse antibody, and then visualization *via* the QDs (Fig. **4**).

Fluorescence can be detected in mycobacterial positive reaction tubes, even using simple visual observation. The combination of the two assays (DNA and antigen) will facilitate the diagnostic investigation of mycobacterial infections by targeting both microbial DNA or antigen or both. The method can also be very easily adjusted to detect circulating antibody.

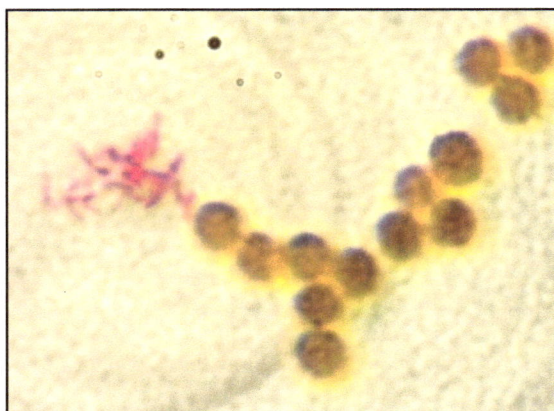

Fig (4). BCG strain captured by genus-specific antibody-coated Magnetic Beads (Ziehl-Neelsen stain 1000X).

Finally, one different but equally interesting approach for the detection of bacteria was made with the use of modified bacteriophages. Their host-specificity, combined with their rapid and prolific replication, bypasses the need for the molecular amplification of a target since their population increases very rapidly, making them easily detectable using QDs [83].

6. CONCLUSION

It can be conclusively stated that the current opportunities provided by nanotechnology provide an excellent foundation for the development of a broad spectrum of microbial detection devices and applications, including the diagnostic investigation of infectious diseases. Applications such as: i) species (or even strain) identification; ii) the detection of drug resistance genes; iii) the determination of pathogenic determinants; or even iv) the investigation of genetic polymorphisms associated with the chain of events that follow exposure to a pathogen, can be performed in a much simpler and cost effective way using nanotechnology. The possible applications of nanotechnology are numerous and will almost certainly create a revolution comparable to that observed after the introduction of molecular biology techniques, such as PCR, into the clinical research and diagnostic laboratory.

REFERENCES

[1]   World Health Organisation - WHO. http://www.who.int/mediacentre/factsheets/fs310/en/index2.html.

[2]   Michalet X, Pinaud FF, Bentolila LA, *et al.* Quantum Dots for live cells, *in vivo* imaging, and diagnostics. Science 2005; 307: 538-44.

[3]   Alivisatos AP. Birth of nanoscience building block. ACS nano 2008; 2: 1514-6.

[4]   Jain PK, Lee KS, El-sayed IH, El-sayed MA. Calculated adsorption and scattering of gold nanoparticles of different size, shape and composition: Applications in biological imaging and biomedicine. J Phys Chem B 2006; 110: 7238-48.

[5]   Pissuwan D, Cortie CH, Valenzuela SM, Cortie MB. Functionalised gold nanoparticles for controlling pathogenic bacteria. Trends Biotechnol 2010; 28: 207-13.

[6]   Niemeyer CM, Mirkin CA. Nanobiotechnology. Singapore: Markono print media Pte Ltd, 2004.

[7]   Buhro WE, Colvin VL. Semiconductor nanocrystals: Shape matters.Nat Mater 2003;2: 138-9.

[8]   Alivisatos AP. Semiconductor clusters, nanocrystals and quantum dots. Science 1996; 271: 933-7.

[9]   Dabbousi BO, Rodriguez-Viejo J, Mikulec FV, *et al.* (CdSe)ZnS Core−Shell Quantum Dots: Synthesis and characterization of a size series of highly luminescent nanocrystallites. J Phys Chem 1997; 101: 9463-75.

[10]   Parak WJ, Geron D, Zanchet D *et al.* Conjugation of DNA to silanized colloidal semiconductor nanocrystal quantum dots. Chem Mater 2002; 14: 2113-9.

[11]   Weissleder R. A clearer vision for *in vivo* imaging. Nat Biotechnol 2001; 19: 316-7.

[12]   Kaji N, Tokeshi M, Baba Y. Quantum dots for single bio molecule imaging. Anal Sci 2007; 23:21-4.

[13]   Green NM. Avidin. Adv Protein Chem 1975; 29: 85-133.

[14]   Sperling RA, Parak WJ. Surface modification, functionalization and bioconjugation of colloidal inorganic nanoparticles. Philos Transact A Math Phys Eng Sci 2010; 368: 1333-83.

[15]   Brust M, Walker M, Bethell D, Schiffrin DJ, Whyman R. Synthesis of thiol derivatised gold nanoparticles in a two phase liquid/liquid system. J Chem Soc Chem Commun 1994; 801-2.

[16]   Templeton AC, Hostetler MJ, Warmoth EK *et al.* Gateway reactions to diverse, polyfunctional monolayer protected gold clusters. J Am Chem Soc 1998; 120: 45-49.

[17]   Zharov VP, Woo Kim J, Curiel DT, Everts M. Self-assembling nanoclusters in living systems: application for integrated photothermal nanodiagnostics and nanotherapy. Nanomedicine 2005; 1: 326-45.

[18]   Mirkin CA, Letsinger RL, Mucic RC, Storhoff JJ. A DNA-based method for rationally assembling nanoparticles into macroscopic materials. Nat 1996; 382: 607-9.

[19]   Elghanian R, Storhoff JJ, Mucic RC, Letsinger RL, Mirkin CA. Selective colorimetric detection of polynucleotides based on the distance-dependent optical properties of gold nanoparticles. Science 1997; 277: 1078-81.

[20]   Storhoff JJ, Elghanian R, Mucic RC, Mirkin CA, Letsinger RL. One pot colorimetric differentiation of polynucleotides with single base imperfections using gold nanoparticle probes. J Am Chem Soc 1998; 120: 1959-64.

[21]   Reynolds RA, Mirkin CA, Letsinger RL. Homogeneous nanoparticle-based quantitative colorimetric detection of oligonucleotides. J Am Chem Soc 2000; 122: 3795–96.

[22]   Storhoff JJ, Lucas AD, Garimella V, Bao YP, Müller UR. Homogeneous detection of unamplified genomic DNA sequences based on colorimetric scatter of gold nanoparticle probes. Nat Biotechnol 2004; 22: 883-7.

[23]   Li J, Chu X, Liu Y, *et al.* A colorimetric method for point mutation detection using high-fidelity DNA ligase. Nuc Acid Res 2005; 33: e168.

[24]   Du BA, Li ZP, Liu CH. One-step homogeneous detection of DNA hybridization with gold nanoparticle probes by using a linear light-scattering technique. Angew Chem Int Ed Engl 2006;45:8022-5.

[25]   Fang J, Yu L, Gao P, Cai Y, Wei Y. Detection of protein-DNA interaction and regulation using gold nanoparticles. Anal Biochem 2010; 399: 262-7.

[26]   Bai X, Shao C, Han X, Li Y, Guan Y, Deng Z. Visual detection of sub-femtomole DNA by a gold nanoparticle seeded homogeneous reduction assay: toward a generalized sensitivity-enhancing strategy. Biosens Bioelectron 2010; 25: 1984-8.

[27]   Thanh NT, Rosenzweig Z. Development of an aggregation-based immunoassay for anti-protein A using gold nanoparticles. Anal Chem 2002; 74: 1624-8 .

[28]   Hirsch LR, Jackson JB, Lee A, Halas NJ, West JL. A whole blood immunoassay using gold nanoshells. Anal Chem 2003; 75: 2377-81.

[29]   Baptista P, Doria G, Henriques D, Pereira E, Frnaco R. Colorimetric detection of eukaryotic gene expression with DNA-derivatized gold nanoparticles. J Biotechnol 2005; 119: 111-7.

[30]   Baptista PV, Koziol-Montewka M, Paluch-Oles J, Doria G, Franco R. Gold-nanoparticle-probe-based assay for rapid and direct detection of *Mycobacterium tuberculosis* DNA in clinical samples. Clin Chem 2006; 52: 1433-4.

[31]   Liandris E, Gazouli M, Andreadou M, *et al.* Direct detection of unamplified DNA from pathogenic mycobacteria using DNA-derivatized gold nanoparticles. J Microbiol Methods 2009; 78: 260-4.

[32]   Lee H, Kang T, Yoon KA, Lee SY, Joo SW, Lee K. Colorimetric detection of mutations in epidermal growth factor receptor using gold nanoparticle aggregation. Biosens Bioelectron 2010; 25: 1669-74.

[33]   Conde J, de la Fuente JM, Baptista PV. RNA quantification using gold nanoprobes - application to cancer diagnostics. J Nanobiotechnol 2010; 24: 8.

[34]   Azzazy HM, Mansour MM. *In vitro* diagnostic prospects of nanoparticles. Clin Chim Acta 2009; 403: 1-8.

[35]   Thaxton CS, Georganopoulou DG, Mirkin CA. Gold nanoparticle probes for the detection of nucleic acid targets. Clin Chim Acta 2006; 363: 120-6.

[36]   Nam JM, Thaxton CS, Mirkin CA. Nanoparticle-based bio-bar codes for the ultrasensitive detection of proteins. Science 2003; 301: 1884-6.

[37]   Nam JM, Stoeva SI, Mirkin CA. Bio-bar-code-based DNA detection with PCR-like sensitivity. J Am Chem Soc 2004; 126: 5932-3.

[38]   Georganopoulou DG, Chang L, Nam JM, *et al.* Nanoparticle-based detection in cerebral spinal fluid of a soluble pathogenic biomarker for Alzheimer's disease. PNAS 2005; 102: 2273-6.

[39]   Keating C. Nanoscience enables ultrasensitive detection of Alzheimer's biomarker. PNAS 2005; 102: 2263–4.

[40]   Stoeva SI, Lee JS, Thaxton CS, Mirkin CA. Multiplexed DNA detection with biobarcoded nanoparticle probes. Angew Chem Int Ed Engl 2006; 45: 3303-6.

[41]   Zhang D, Carr DJ, Alocilja EC. Fluorescent bio-barcode DNA assay for the detection of *Salmonella enterica* serovar Enteritidis. Biosens Bioelectron 2009; 24: 1377-81.

[42]   Dubertret B, Calame M, Libchaber AJ. Single-mismatch detection using gold-quenched fluorescent oligonucleotides. Nat Biotechnol 2001; 19: 365-70.

[43]   Li M, Lin YC, Wu CC, Liu HS. Enhancing the efficiency of a PCR using gold nanoparticles. Nucleic Acids Res 2005; 33: e184.

[44]   Wan W, Yeow JT. The effects of gold nanoparticles with different sizes on polymerase chain reaction efficiency. Nanotechnology 2009; 20: 325702.

[45]   Iyer VR, Eisen MB, Ross DT, *et al.* The transcriptional program in the response of human fibroblasts to serum. Science 1999; 283: 83–87.

[46]   Sun Y, Fan WH, McCann MP, Golovlev V. Microarray gene expression analysis free of reverse transcription and dye labeling. Anal Biochem 2005; 345: 312-9.

[47]   Fritzsche W, Taton TA. Metal nanoaprticles as labels for heterogeneous chip-based DNA detection. Nanotechnology 2003; 14: 63-73.

[48]   Reichert J, Csaki A, Kohler JM, Fritzsche W. Chip-based optical detection of DNA hybridization by means of nanobead labelling. Anal Chem 2000; 72: 6025-9.

[49]   Taton TA, Mirkin CA, Letsinger RL. Scanometric DNA array detection with nanoparticle probes. Science 2000; 289:1757-60.

[50]   Storhoff JJ, Marla SS, Bao P, *et al.* Gold nanoparticle-based detection of genomic DNA targets on microarrays using a novel optical detection system. Biosens Bioelectron 2004; 19: 875-83.

[51]   Tang DP, Yuan R, Chai YQ, *et al.* Novel potentiometric immunosensor for hepatitis B surface antigen using a gold nanoparticle-based biomolecular immobilization method. Anal Biochem 2004; 333: 345-50.

[52]   Harpster MH, Zhangb H, Sankara-Warrier AK, *et al.* SERS detection of indirect viral DNA capture using colloidal gold and methylene blue as a Raman label. Biosens Bioelectron 2009; 25: 674-81.

[53]   Mo Z, Wang H, Liang Y, Liuab F, Xueb Y. Highly reproducible hybridization assay of zeptomole DNA based on adsorption of nanoparticle-bioconjugate. Analyst 2005; 130: 1589-94.

[54]   Liu T, Tang J, Han M Jiang L. Novel microgravimetric DNA sensor with high sensitivity. Biochem Biophys Res Commun 2003; 304: 98-108.

[55]   Su X, Robelek R, Wu Y, Wang G, Knoll W. Detection of point mutation and insertion mutations in DNA using a quartz crystal microbalance and MutS, a mismatch binding protein. Anal Chem 2004; 76: 489-94.

[56]   Mannelli I, Minunni M, Tombelli S, Mascini M. Quartz crystal microbalance (QCM) affinity biosensor for genetically modified organisms (GMOs) detection. Biosens Bioelectron 2003; 18: 129-40.

[57]   Mo X, Zhou Y, Lei H, Deng L. Microbalance-DNA probe method for the detection of specific bacteria in water. Enzyme Microb Technol 2002; 30: 583-89.

[58]   Hewa TP, Tannocka GA, Mainwaringa DE, Harrisona S, Fecondoa JV. The detection of influenza A and B viruses in clinical specimens using a quartz crystal microbalance. J Virol Meth 2009; 162: 14-21.

[59]   Wang H, Lei C, Li J, Wu Z, Shen G, Yu R. A piezoelectric immunoagglutination assay for *Toxoplasma gondii* antibodies using gold nanoparticles. Biosens Bioelectron 2004; 19: 701-9.

[60]   Pang L, Li J, Jiang J, Shen G, Yu R. DNA point mutation detection based on DNA ligase reaction and nano-Au amplification: A piezoelectric approach. Anal Biochem 2006; 358: 99-103.

[61]   Chen H, Wu V, Chuang Y, Lin C. Using oligonucleotide-functionalized Au nanoparticles to rapidly detect foodborne pathogens on a piezoelectric biosensor. J Microbiol Meth 2008; 73: 7-17.

[62]   Kalogianni D, Koraki T, Christopoulos T, Ioannou R. Nanoparticle-based DNA biosensor for visual detection of genetically modified organisms. Biosens Bioelectron 2006; 21: 1069-76.

[63]   Huang SH. Gold nanoparticle-based immunochromatographic test for identification of *Staphylococcus aureus* from clinical specimens. Clin Chim Acta 2006; 373: 139-43.

[64]   Kalogianni D, Goura S, Aletras A, *et al.* Dry reagent dipstick test combined with 23S rRNA PCR for molecular diagnosis of bacterial infection in arthroplasty. Anal Biochem 2007; 361: 169-75.

[65]   Konstantou J, Ioannou P, Christopoulos T. Dual-allele dipstick assay for genotyping single nucleotide polymorphisms by primer extension reaction. Eur J Hum Gen 2009; 17: 105-11.

[66] Bruchez M Jr, Moronne M, Gin P, Weiss S, Alivisatos AP. Semiconductor nanocrystals as fluorescent biological labels. Science 1998; 281: 2013-6.

[67] Wu X, Liu H, Liu J, *et al.* Immunofluorescent labeling of cancer marker Her2 and other cellular targets with semiconductor quantum dots. Nat Biotechnol 2003; 21: 41-6.

[68] Dubertret B, Skourides P, Norris DJ, Noireaux V, Brivanlou AH, Libchaber A. *In vivo* imaging of quantum dots encapsulated in phospholipid micelles. Science 2002; 298: 1759-62.

[69] Rosenthal SJ, Tomlinson I, Adkins EM, *et al.* Targeting cell surface receptors with ligand-conjugated nanocrystals. J Am Chem Soc 2002; 124: 4586-94.

[70] Sukhanova A, Devy J, Venteo L, *et al.* Biocompatible fluorescent nanocrystals for immunolabeling of membrane proteins and cells. Anal Biochem 2004; 324: 60-7.

[71] Akerman ME, Chan WC, Laakkonen P, Bhatia SN, Ruoslahti E. Nanocrystal targeting *in vivo.* PNAS 2002; 99: 12617-21.

[72] Härmä H, Soukka T, Lövgren T. Europium nanoparticles and time resolved fluorescence for ultra sensitive detection of prostate-specific antigen. Clin Chem 2001; 47: 561-68.

[73] Pelkkikangas AM, Jaakohuhta S, Lövgren T, Härmä H. Simple, rapid, and sensitive thyroid-stimulating hormone immunoassay using europium(III) nanoparticle label. Anal Chim Acta 2004; 517: 169-76.

[74] Goldman ER, Clapp AR, Anderson GP, *et al.* Multiplexed toxin analysis using four colors of quantum dot fluororeagents. Anal Chem 2004; 76:684-8.

[75] Valanne A, Huopalahti S, Vainionpää R, Lövgren T, Härmä H. Rapid and sensitive HBsAg immunoassay based on fluorescent nanoparticle labels and time-resolved detection. J Virol Methods 2005; 129: 83-90.

[76] Valanne A, Huopalahti S, Soukka T, Vainionpää R, Lövgren T, Härmä H. A sensitive adenovirus immunoassay as a model for using nanoparticle label technology in virus diagnostics. J Clin Virol 2005; 33: 217-23.

[77] Zahavy E, Heleg-Shabtai V, Zafrani Y, Marciano D, Yitzhaki S. Application of fluorescent nanocrystals (q-dots) for the detection of pathogenic bacteria by flow-cytometry. J Fluoresc 2010; 20: 389-99.

[78] Hahn MA, Keng PC, Krauss TD. Flow cytometric analysis to detect pathogens in bacterial cell mixtures using semiconductor quantum dots. Anal Chem 2008; 80 :864-72.

[79] Branen JR, Hass MJ, Douthit ER, Maki WC, Branen AL. Detection of *Escherichia coli* O157, *Salmonella enterica* serovar Typhimurium, and staphylococcal enterotoxin B in a single sample using enzymatic bio-nanotransduction. J Food Prot 2007; 70: 841-50.

[80] Klostranec JM, Xiang Q, Farcas GA, *et al.* Convergence of quantum dot barcodes with microfluidics and signal processing for multiplexed high-throughput infectious disease diagnostics. Nano Lett 2007; 7: 2812-8.

[81] Zhu L, Ang S, Liu WT. Quantum dots as a novel immunofluorescent detection system for *Cryptosporidium parvum* and *Giardia lamblia.* Appl Environ Microbiol 2004; 70: 597-8.

[82] Gazouli M, Liandris E, Andreadou M, *et al.* Specific detection of unamplified mycobacterial DNA using fluorescent semiconductor quantum dots and magnetic beads. J Clin Microbiol 2010; 48: 2830-5.

[83] Edgar R, McKinstry M, Hwang J, *et al.* High-sensitivity bacterial detection using biotin-tagged phage and quantum-dot nanocomplexes. PNAS 2006; 103: 4841-5.

[84] Alexandre I, Hamels S, Dufour S, *et al.* Colorimetric silver detection of DNA microarrays. Anal Biochem 2001; 295: 1-8.

[85] Wang YF, Pang DW, Zhang ZL, Zheng HZ, Cao JP, Shen JT. Visual gene diagnosis of HBV and HCV based on nanoparticle probe amplification and silver staining enhancement. J Med Virol 2003; 70: 205-11.

[86] Bao YP, Huber M, Wei TF, Marla SS, Storhoff JJ, Müller UR. SNP identification in unamplified human genomic DNA with gold nanoparticle probes. Nucleic Acids Res 2005; 33: e15.

[87] Huber M, Wei TF, Müller UR, Lefebvre PA, Marla SS, Bao YP. Gold nanoparticle probe-based gene expression analysis with unamplified total human RNA. Nucleic Acids Res 2004; 32: e137.

[88] Cao X, Wang YF, Zhang CF, Gao WJ. Visual DNA microarrays for simultaneous detection of *Ureaplasma urealyticum* and *Chlamydia trachomatis* coupled with multiplex asymmetrical PCR. Biosens Bioelectron 2006; 22: 393-8.

[89] Liang RQ, Tan CY, Ruan KC. Colorimetric detection of protein microarrays based on nanogold probe coupled with silver enhancement. J Immunol Methods 2004; 285: 157-63.

[90] Huang L, Reekmans G, Saerens D, *et al.* Prostate-specific antigen immunosensing based on mixed self-assembled monolayers, camel antibodies and colloidal gold enhanced sandwich assays. Biosens Bioelectron 2005; 21: 483-90.

[91]   Wang Y, Gao W, Wang H, Luo Y. Preparation of a visual protein chip for detection of IgG against *Treponema pallidum*. Mol Biotechnol 2005; 31: 121-8.

[92]   Vestergaard M, Kerman K, Kim DK, Ha MH, Tamiya E. Detection of Alzheimer's tau protein using localised surface plasmon resonance-based immunochip. Talanta 2008; 74: 1038-42.

[93]   Möller R, Schüler T, Günther S, Carlsohn MR, Munder T, Fritzsche W. Electrical DNA-chip-based identification of different species of the genus *Kitasatospora*. Appl Microbiol Biotechnol 2008; 77: 1181-8.

[94]   Shen G, Tan S, Nie H, Shen G, Yu R. Electrochemical and piezoelectric quartz crystal detection of antisperm antibody based on protected Au nanoparticles with a mixed monolayer for eliminating nonspecific binding. J Immunol Methods 2006; 313: 11-9.

[95]   Cao YWC, Jin RC, Mirkin CA. Nanoparticles with Raman spectroscopic fingerprints for DNA and RNA detection. Science 2002; 297: 1536-40.

[96]   Xu S, Ji X, Xu W, *et al.* Immunoassay using probe-labelling immunogold nanoparticles with silver staining enhancement *via* surface-enhanced Raman scattering. Analyst 2004; 129: 63-8.

CHAPTER 7

Loop-Mediated Isothermal Amplification (LAMP) in Medical Microbiological Research and Diagnosis

M. Parida[*], J. Shukla, S. Sharma and P.V. Lakshmana Rao

Division of Virology, Defence Research & Development Establishment, Gwalior – 474002, M.P, India

Abstract: "LAMP" or Loop-mediated Isothermal Amplification is a simple, rapid, specific and cost-effective nucleic acid amplification method that is characterized by the use of 6 different primers (3 different primer pairs) that are specifically designed to recognize 8 distinct regions on the target gene. LAMP amplification takes place at a constant temperature *via* a strand displacement reaction. Amplification and detection of genes can be completed in a single step, by incubating a mixture of samples, primers, a DNA polymerase (possessing DNA strand displacement activity) and accompanying substrates, at a constant temperature of 60 - 65°C. The high amplification efficiency of the LAMP process means that the presence of amplified products can be monitored by the naked eye either through visual turbidity or visual fluorescence. LAMP technology is emerging as a promising nucleic acid amplification tool that offers rapid, accurate, and cost-effective diagnosis of infectious diseases. The technology has already been developed into commercially available detection kits for a variety of pathogens including bacteria and viruses. Further, the combination of LAMP and novel microfluidic technologies may facilitate the realization of gene-based microbiological point-of-care testing systems, which may be available in both developed and developing countries in the near future.

Keywords: Loop-Mediated Isothermal Amplification (LAMP), Isothermal Amplification, Loop Primers, Gene Quantification.

1. INTRODUCTION

Recent developments in rapid molecular testing methods have greatly enhanced the ability of diagnostic and research laboratories to identify and characterize microbial pathogens, with nucleic acid amplification strategies and advances in amplicon detection having been key aspects in the progress of molecular microbiology-based detection. Indeed, sophisticated new combinations of amplification/detection technologies are resulting in an increasing number of applications with respect to laboratory testing for infectious diseases. The development of technologies possessing rapid and sensitive detection capabilities, and increased throughput, have become crucial in the global response to an increasing number of threats posed by emerging and re-emerging microorganisms, especially viruses.

Nucleic acid amplification technologies are the leading methods used to detect and analyze the small quantities of nucleic acids found in microorganisms. Of these, the Polymerase Chain Reaction (PCR) is the most widely used method for DNA amplification for the detection/identification of infectious diseases, genetic disorders and other research purposes. Unfortunately however, despite the high magnitude of amplification, these PCR based methods require either high precision instrumentation for efficient and accurate amplification of DNA, and/or elaborate methods for the detection of any successfully amplified products. In addition, these methods are often cumbersome to adapt for routine clinical use in peripheral health care settings and private clinics. Further, traditional PCR amplification technology possesses several intrinsic disadvantages, including: a requirement for thermal cycling; careful optimization to yield sufficient specificity and high amplification efficiency; separate methods to detect amplified products (*e.g.* gel electrophoresis); and a major reliance on diagnostic PCR assays that reported qualitative ('yes/no' format), rather than quantitative results. Finally, the time required to achieve a result using traditional PCR technology is relatively long. More recently however, so-called "real-time"-based assays have been

---

*****Address correspondence to M. Parida:** Division of Virology, Defence Research & Development Establishment, Gwalior – 474002, M.P, India; Email:paridamm@rediffmail.com

John P. Hays and W. B. van Leeuwen (Eds)

developed, that complement traditional PCR-based assay systems, and provide solutions to many of the problems associated with traditional PCR methodologies.

The development of real-time PCR (including the ability to accurately quantify nucleic acids) has brought PCR-based nucleic acid detection technology out of the pure research laboratory and into the diagnostic laboratory, with real-time PCR amplification technology combining traditional PCR-based amplification with fluorescently labeled, microorganism specific, probes. These fluorescent probes are able to detect amplified DNA during the amplification reaction. This fluorescent chemistry coupled with advances in optical detection now means that real-time PCR is more sensitive than conventional gel based PCR [1]. Over the past two years, several real-time PCR assays have been developed to address the need for reliable detection systems for the early detection, as well as quantification, of virus load in the acute phase of illness. In addition, real-time PCR automates the laborious process of amplification by quantifying reaction products for each sample in every cycle. Data analysis, including standard curve generation and copy number calculation, is performed automatically. Real-time PCR has enhanced wider acceptance of PCR due to its improved rapidity, sensitivity, reproducibility and the reduced risk of carry-over contamination. More recently, several investigators have reported the development of fully automated real-time PCR assays for the detection of viruses in acute-phase serum samples. Unfortunately however, all of these PCR-based nucleic acid amplification methodologies possess several intrinsic disadvantages, and require high precision instrumentation for amplification and/or detection of amplified products. Real-time PCR requires an instrumentation platform that consists of a thermal cycler, computer, optics for fluorescence excitation and emission collection, as well as data acquisition and analysis software. Only a few laboratories with good financial resources can afford to purchase such high precision instrumentation. Finally, "trust" issues associated with the replacement of "gold standard" microbiological detection methodologies by new technological screening systems, currently means that it is widely accepted that test results should be confirmed by more than one type of assay technology.

Novel developments in the *in vivo* synthesis of DNA have provided a basis for the development of technologies that allow the amplification of DNA under isothermal conditions, without the need for a thermocycling apparatus (a requirement of PCR-based amplification technology). The recent identification of various DNA polymerase accessory proteins has enabled the development of new *in vitro* isothermal DNA amplification methods, which may mimic the mechanisms found *in vivo*. In fact, there are currently several types of isothermal nucleic acid amplification methodologies described, including: i) transcription mediated amplification [2]; ii) nucleic acid sequence-based amplification [3]; iii) signal mediated amplification of RNA technology [4]; iv) strand displacement amplification [5]; v) rolling circle amplification [6]; vi) isothermal multiple displacement amplification [7]; vii) helicase-dependent amplification single primer isothermal amplification [8]; vii) circular helicase-dependent amplification [9]; and viii) loop-mediated isothermal amplification of DNA (as described in this chapter). Indeed, LAMP technology has now been developed into commercially available test kits, some of which have been adopted as officially recommended methods for the routine identification and surveillance of pathogens (in Japan) [10]. This new generation of simple, rapid and cost effective gene amplification technologies possess all of the characteristics required for: i) the routine detection of microbial pathogens; and ii) monitoring of the re-emergence and resurgence of large scale microbiological epidemics. In this chapter, the authors describe the potential application of Loop-Mediated Isothermal Amplification (LAMP), a technology that is gaining popularity among researchers and diagnosticians, due to its simple operation, rapid time-to-diagnosis, and easy detection. The chapter describes the usefulness of this novel gene amplification technology in microbiological diagnosis and medical microbiological research.

2. LOOP-MEDIATED ISOTHERMAL AMPLIFICATION TECHNOLOGY (LAMP)

The principal of LAMP is based on nucleic acid amplification *via* an autocyclic strand displacement reaction, which is performed at a constant temperature of approximately 63°C. The method employs a DNA polymerase and a set of 6 specially designed primers that recognize a total of 8 distinct sequences on the target DNA. The process itself comprises both non-cyclic and cyclic steps, which will be explained later in this chapter. Further, the amplification and detection of a specific gene can be completed in a single step, using a mixture of target sample, specifically designed primers, a DNA polymerase possessing strand displacement activity, and relevant substrates [1]. Importantly, the high amplification efficiency of the LAMP reaction yields a large quantity of by-product, pyrophosphate ion, leading to the formation of a white precipitate of magnesium pyrophosphate in the LAMP reaction mix. The production of this precipitate leads to a subsequent increase in the turbidity of the reaction mix, with the turbidity of the precipitate being correlated to the amount of DNA synthesized. This means that the real-time monitoring of LAMP reactions can be performed using real-time measurement of turbidity formation [11]. In fact, the whole LAMP protocol can be performed at a constant temperature by simply incubating the reagents in an incubator, water bath, heating block, or any other heat source that can provide a constant temperature of 60-65°C for 30 minutes. Being an isothermal-based amplification methodology, LAMP does not require a sophisticated thermal cycling apparatus, and as previously mentioned, the detection of specific amplification products can be determined without the use of sophisticated detection devices. This means that LAMP has the potential to be developed into a cost effective, point of care testing technology. Finally, with specific respect to medical microbiological diagnosis, LAMP technology has been used for the detection of a wide range of bacterial, viral, fungal and parasitic diseases of humans, animals and plants (see section 'Applications of LAMP in Medical Diagnostics below').

3. THE DESIGN OF LAMP PRIMERS

The design of highly sensitive and specific primer sets are crucial when developing a LAMP amplification protocol. To help in this process, the correct design of LAMP primers may be accomplished using the software program "Primer Explore", a LAMP primer design and support software program available at the Net laboratory, Japan: http://venus.netlaboratory.com. This program takes into account primer base composition, GC content, and the formation of secondary structure. The total primer set required for LAMP amplification utilizes a mix of 6 primers (3 primer pairs), which comprise 2 "outer", 2 "internal" and 2 "loop" primers that recognize 8 specific nucleic acid sequences present within the target sequence (Fig. 1). The 2 outer primers comprise a forward outer primer (F3) and a backward outer primer (B3), which play a role in strand displacement during the non-cyclic step only. The 2 internal primers FIP and BIP (forward and backward internal primers), possess both sense and antisense sequences in such a way that they have the ability to form "loops" (FIP contains sequences F1C and F2, whilst BIP contains sequences B1 and B2C). The 2 loop primers themselves comprise a Forward Loop Primer (FLP) and a Backward Loop Primer (BLP), which are designed to accelerate the amplification reaction by binding to additional sites that are not accessed by the internal primers. In fact, LAMP amplification can be achieved using the 2 outer (F3 & B3] and 2 internal (FIP & BIP) primers alone, though the use of the 2 loop primers (FLP & BLP) accelerate the amplification process, thereby shortening amplification time (to a detectable signal) by 1/3 to 1/2 [1].

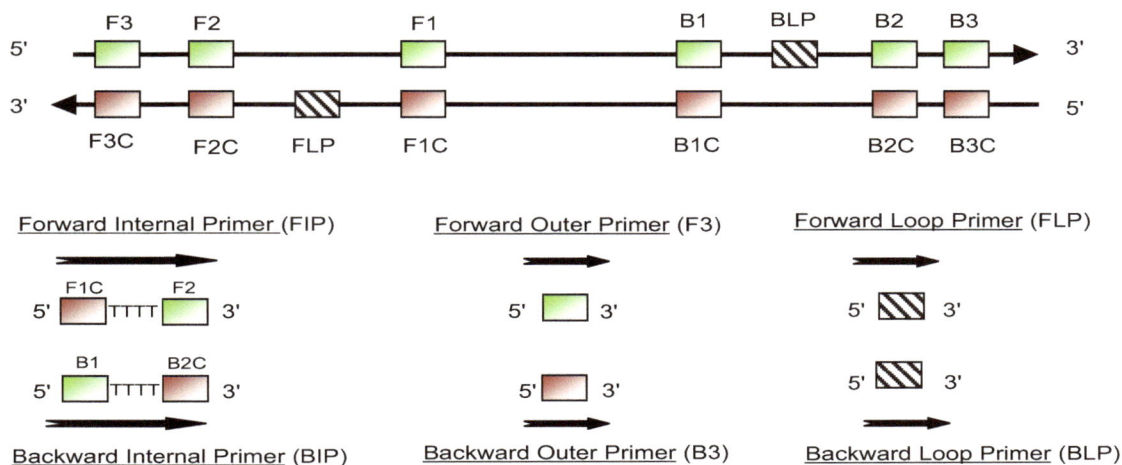

Fig. (1). Schematic representation of the primer combinations utilized in LAMP-based nucleic acid amplification assays showing the position of the 6 primers that span 8 distinct regions of the target gene.

The design of the above mentioned 6 primers (3 primer pairs) are based on the following 8 distinct regions of the target gene: the F3c, F2c and F1c & FLP regions at the 3'-end of the target nucleic acid, and the B1, B2, B3 & BLP regions at the 5'-end of the target nucleic acid. The Forward Internal Primer (FIP) consists of an F2 sense sequence region at its 3'-end, as well as an F1c sequence (complementary to the F1 sequence) at its 5'-end. The Forward Outer Primer consists of the F3 region, which is complementary to the F3c region. The Backward Inner Primer consists of the B2 region (at the 3'-end), which is complementary to the B2c region, and an identical sequence as the B1c region at its 5'-end. The Backward Outer Primer consists of the B3 region, which is complementary to the B3c region. F1P consists of a complementary sequence of F1 and a sense sequence of F2. BIP consists of a complementary sequence of B1 and a sense sequence of B2. FIP and BIP are long primers purified by High Performance Liquid Chromatography (HPLC). The FLP and BLP primers are composed of sequences that are complementary to the sequence between F1&F2 and B1&B2 regions respectively [12]. Fig. **1.** is a schematic representation of the design of LAMP primer sequences.

4. THE PRINCIPLE OF LAMP AMPLIFICATION

The chemistry of LAMP amplification is based on the principle of an autocyclic strand displacement reaction performed at a constant temperature. This method employs a DNA polymerase and a set of 6 specially designed primers that recognize a total of 8 distinct sequences on the target DNA. LAMP amplification *per se* may be divided into both Non-cyclic and Cyclic (Amplification) steps [13].

Non-Cyclic Step

The non-cyclic step is characterized by the formation of stem loop DNA conformations, with stem-loops at each end of the target DNA serving as the starting structure for LAMP amplification cycles. This step can be divided into 11 individual stages whereby: 1) at the reaction temperature of 65°C, double stranded DNA is found in a condition of dynamic equilibrium, meaning that 1 of the LAMP primers is able to anneal to the complimentary sequence of double stranded target DNA, thereby initiating DNA synthesis *via* the strand displacing DNA polymerase; 2) the DNA polymerase displaces and releases single stranded DNA [2,13], such that (unlike PCR-based amplification reactions), there is no need for heat denaturation of the double stranded DNA into a single strands; 3) the DNA polymerase synthesizes a DNA strand complementary to the template DNA starting from the 3'-end of the F2 region of the FIP; 4) the F3 primer anneals to the F3c region, outside of the FIP, on the target DNA and initiates strand displacement DNA synthesis thereby releasing the FIP-linked complementary strand; 5) a double strand is formed from the DNA strand synthesized from the F3 Primer and the template DNA strand; 6) the FIP-linked complementary strand is released as a single strand due to the displacement of the DNA strand synthesized from the F3 Primer (this released single strand forms a stem-loop structure at the 5'-end because of the complementary F1c and F1 regions); 7) this single strand DNA in turn serves as a template for BIP-initiated DNA synthesis and subsequent B3-primed strand displacement DNA synthesis; 8) the BIP anneals to the DNA strand produced in step 7) above; 9) synthesis of complementary DNA takes place starting from the 3'-end of the BIP (the DNA reverts from a loop structure to a linear structure in this process); 10) the B3 Primer anneals to the outside of the BIP and then, through the activity of the DNA polymerase and starting at the 3'-end, the DNA synthesized from the BIP is displaced and released as a single strand, until finally; 11) DNA synthesis occurs *via* the B3 Primer. In essence, the displaced BIP-linked complementary strand forms a structure with stem-loops at each end, which looks like a dumbbell structure. This dumbbell-like DNA structure is quickly converted into stem-loop DNA *via* self-primed DNA synthesis, and it is this structure that serves as the starting template for exponential amplification in the cyclic step of LAMP amplification.

Cyclic (Amplification) Step

The cyclic (amplification) step of LAMP cycling is characterized by 5 stages. Essentially, an inner primer hybridizes to the loop structure on the template generated during the non-cyclic step, thereby initiating strand displacement DNA synthesis and yielding both the original stem–loop DNA as well as a new stem–loop DNA with a stem twice as long as the original. Briefly, this process involves: 1) the annealing of FIP to the single stranded region in the stem-loop DNA of the non-cyclic step product, priming strand displacement DNA synthesis, and releasing the previously synthesized strand; 2) this released single strand then forms a stem-loop structure at its 3'-end because of the complementary B1c and B1 regions; 3) DNA synthesis starts from the 3'-end of the B1 region using DNA as a template, releasing the FIP-linked complementary strand; 4) this released single strand then forms a dumbbell-like structure as both ends possess complementary F1 - F1c and B1c - B1 regions, respectively, finally; 5) BIP anneals to the B2c region and primes strand displacement DNA synthesis, releasing the B1-primed DNA strand. As a result of this cyclic (amplification-step) process, various sized structures consisting of alternate inverted repeats of the target sequence on the same strand of DNA, are formed. In fact, this cycling reaction can continue, resulting in the accumulation of up to 10^9 copies of target in less than an hour. The final products are stem–loop DNAs with several inverted repeats of the target, and 'cauliflower-like' structures with multiple loops that have been formed by annealing between alternate inverted repeats of the target to the same strand (Fig. **2**).

It should be noted that LAMP amplification can also be accomplished using only the two outer (F3 & B3) and two internal primers (FIP & BIP), though the use of the two loop primers (FLP & BLP) results in an acceleration of the amplification reaction, thereby reducing the tine to amplification for a given amount of product copies (and hence reducing the time to acquire a positive signal). In fact, the time required for amplification of target DNA to a specific concentration with Loop Primers is one-third to one-half of that required without Loop Primers. The use of Loop Primers means that a detectable positive signal can be achieved within 30 minutes [1].

5. PROTOCOL FOR LAMP AMPLIFICATION

LAMP amplification reactions are usually performed in a total reaction volume of 25 µl that contains: i) 50 pmol each of the primers FIP and BIP; ii) 5 pmol each of the outer primers F3 and B3; iii) 25 pmol each of loop primers FLP and BLP; iv) a 2x reaction mixture comprising 20mM Tris-HCl pH8.8, 10mM $(NH_4)_2SO_4$, 8mM $MgSO_4$, 10mM KCl, 1.4mM dNTPs, 0.8M Betaine, 0.1% Tween20, 8 units Bst DNA polymerase (New England Biolabs) and 2 µl of DNA template. Positive and negative controls should be included in each run, and all precautions to prevent cross-contamination of reaction mixes should be observed. Studies on the optimum temperature required for efficient amplification using the LAMP protocol have indicated that a temperature of 63°C is required for the optimum activity of the Bst DNA polymerase [14].

The amplification of RNA templates using the LAMP methodology has been accomplished using a "Reverse Transcription-Loop-mediated Isothermal Amplification (RT-LAMP)" assay, which employs a reverse transcriptase for initial reverse transcription of RNA into cDNA in addition to the Bst DNA polymerase and other components (primers, DNA polymerase with strand displacement activity, substrates, *etc.*). After mixing and incubating at a constant temperature between 60-65°C, RNA amplification and detection can be performed in a single step [1,14,15].

6. MONITORING OF LAMP AMPLIFICATION

Turbidometric monitoring is the easiest way of monitoring gene amplification by LAMP amplification [11], and the real-time monitoring of LAMP amplification can be accomplished using, for example, a Loopamp Realtime turbidimeter (LA-200, Teramecs, Japan) that records the turbidity in the form of O.D. units at 400 nm every 6 seconds (Figs. **3**, **4A**). A turbidimeter is relatively inexpensive as compared to a real-time PCR machine. In fact, turbidity is a unique characteristic associated with LAMP amplification, a characteristic associated with the high amplification efficiency of LAMP reactions. In order to observe this turbidity (in the form of a white precipitate), a DNA yield of ≥ 4 µg is required so as to generate a pyrophosphate ion (P_2O_7) concentration in the reaction mix that is > 0.5 ppm. LAMP reactions typically produce DNA yields of ≥ 10 µg per 25 µl reaction volume compared to 0.2 µg for 25 µl PCR-based nucleic amplification reactions. During PCR-based amplification, the low amount of pyrophosphate ion formed becomes hydrolysed to phosphate (PO_4) due to the high DNA disassociation temperatures (>94°C) used. However, unlike real-time PCR-based amplification assays, where "positivity" is decided on the basis of Ct values (*i.e.* the number of cycles required to achieve a signal above a pre-determined threshold value), the criterion for LAMP-amplification "positivity" is based on "time-to-positivity" (Tp) values. This varies from organism to organism and is based on the primer set utilized and the nature of the selected template. The cut-off value for positivity for a particular gene using real time RT-LAMP assays can be determined by taking into account the time of positivity (Tp; in minutes) at which the turbidity increases above a fixed threshold value of 0.1, which is twice the average turbidity value of the negative controls of several replicates (47).

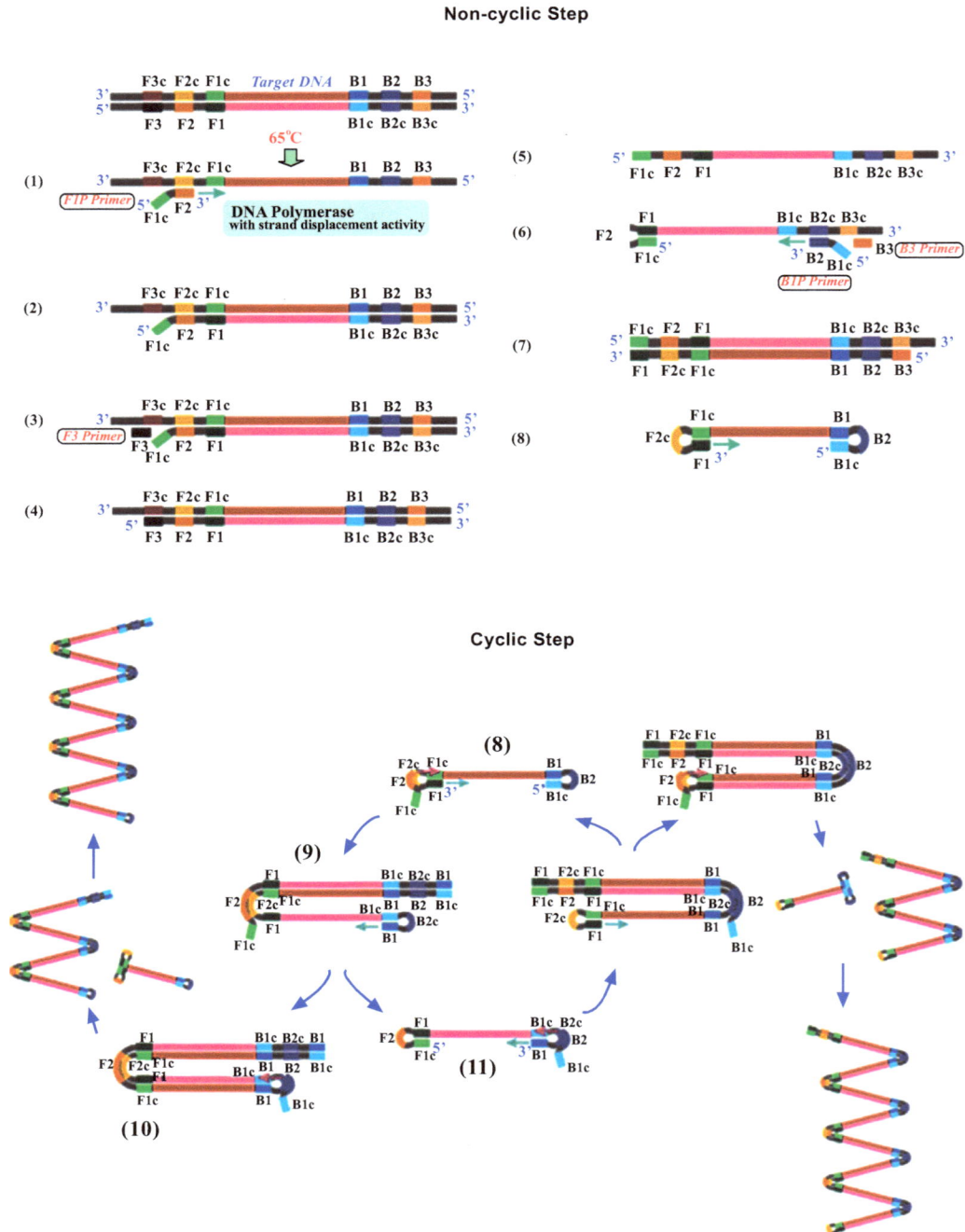

Fig. (2). Principles of LAMP amplification. Non-cyclic Step – during this step, stem loop DNA amplification products with dumbbell structures at both ends are generated, which then act as template for exponential amplification by internal and loop primers during the Cyclic Step of LAMP amplification. Printed with permission of the EIKEN CHEMICAL Co. Ltd who own copyright to these figures.

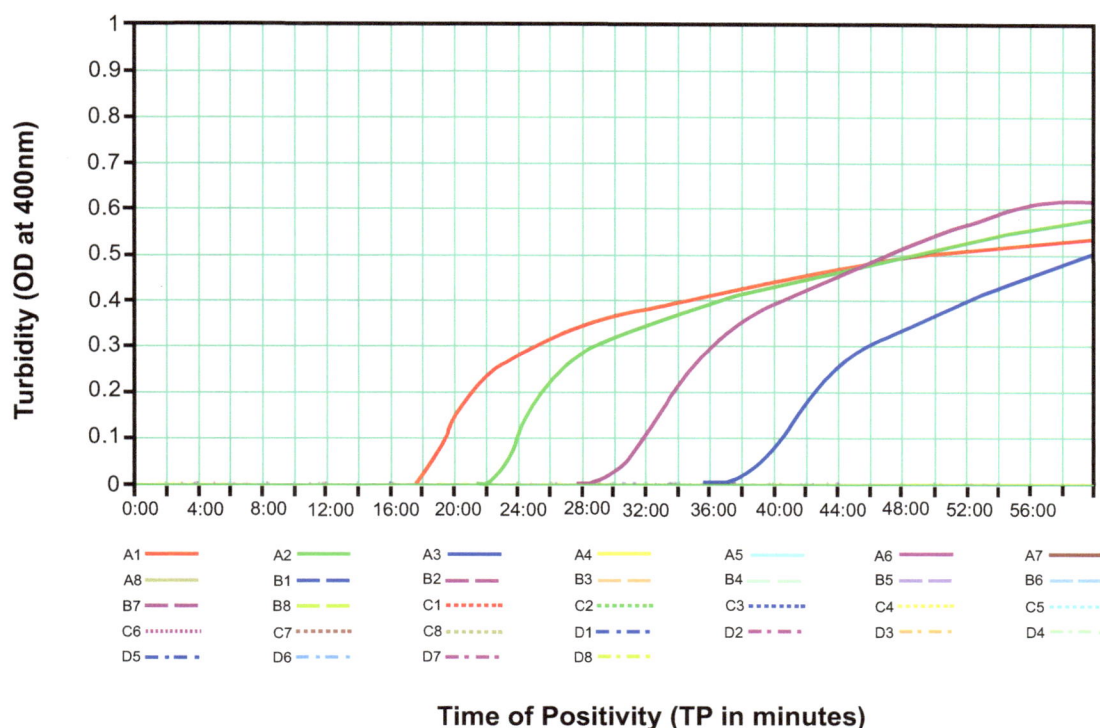

Time of Positivity (TP in minutes)

Fig. (3). Real-Time monitoring of LAMP amplification showing the amplification curve obtained when testing clinical samples for the presence of Chikungunya virus. The X-axis shows the time of positivity and the Y-axis the turbidity value in terms of O.D. at 400 nm. Numbers represent individual clinical samples. The reaction temperature was 63°C. O.D. values >0.1 are regarded as positive for the presence of Chikungunya virus (clinical samples A1, A2, A3 and A6).

Monitoring of LAMP amplification may also be performed using the naked eye, either in the form of visual turbidity or visual fluorescence. Following amplification, the tubes can be pulse centrifuged to deposit the precipitate in the bottom of the tube and inspected for the presence of a white pellet (Fig. **4C**) [16].

As well as turbidometric measurement, LAMP amplification products can also be analyzed using agarose gel electrophoresis. Following incubation at 63°C for 30 min, 10 µl aliquot of LAMP amplified products are electrophoresed on 3% NuSieve 3:1 agarose gel (BMA, Rockland, ME, USA) in Tris-borate buffer, followed by staining with ethidium bromide and visualization on an ultraviolet (UV) transilluminator at 302 nm (Fig. **4B**). LAMP amplification products may be better visualized in the presence of a fluorescent intercalating dye, for example ethidium bromide, SYBR Green I, Calcein *etc.*, *via* illumination using a UV lamp, whereby the fluorescence intensity increases as amplification products are generated. In practice, visual inspection is performed for a color change following addition of 1 µl of SYBR Green I to the tube. For LAMP-positive amplification, the original orange color of the dye will change to green that can be judged under natural light or under UV light (302nm) with the help of a hand held UV light [16]. If there are no amplification products, then the original orange color of the dye will be retained. Any change in color using this method is permanent meaning that the reaction can be stored for future reference (Fig. **4D**). On agarose gel analysis, the LAMP amplicons generated reveal a ladder-like pattern (in contrast to the single amplification product band observed using PCR-based amplification technologies). This is due to the 'cauliflower-like' structures and multiple loops formed by annealing between alternative inverted repeats present within the amplified target products and present within the same template product strand. The specificity of the LAMP amplified products can be established by digesting the products with a restriction enzyme that specifically cuts one end of the selected target products. Specificity may also be confirmed using nucleic acid sequencing of the amplified products.

A. Real Time Monitoring

B. Agarose Gel Analysis

C. Visual Turbidity

D. Visual Fluorescence

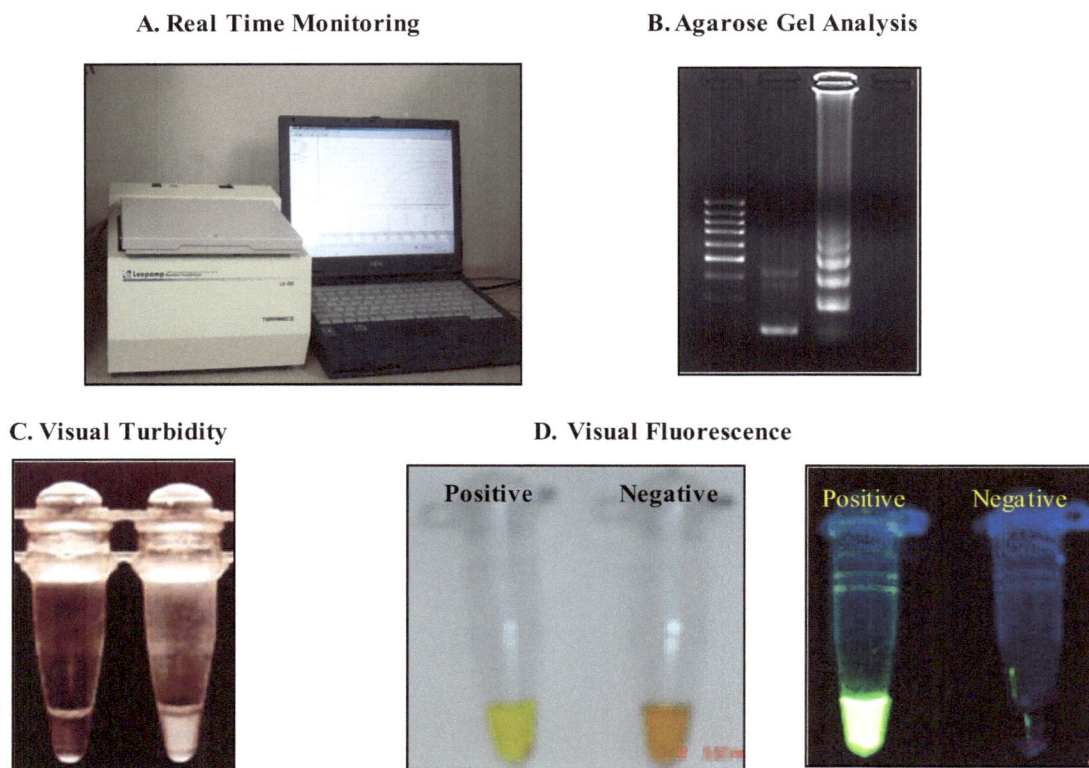

Fig. (4). Monitoring of LAMP Amplification. **A)** The turbidity of magnesium pyrophosphate, a by-product of the reaction, can be detected in real-time using a real-time turbidimeter. **B)** Agarose gel electrophoresis analysis reveals a typical "ladder-like" electrophoresis pattern for LAMP-generated amplification products comprising products of various sizes. **C)** Visual turbidity against a brown background. **D)** LAMP-amplification products after the addition of a fluorescent intercalating dye (under normal light conditions and illuminated by a UV lamp causing the fluorescent intensity to increase).

7. SENSITIVITY AND SPECIFICITY OF LAMP

As already discussed, the LAMP assay is based on the principle of an autocyclic strand displacement mechanism that amplifies the target nucleic acid with a high degree of specificity. This specificity is directly attributable to the 6 sets of primers used, which span 8 distinct sequences of the target gene being amplified. Only when all primer-target gene sequences are available will amplification proceed.

LAMP-based assays possess an increased sensitivity over corresponding PCR-based assays with an overall yield of 10 μg of DNA at the 25 μl reaction scale compared to 0.2 μg using conventional PCR. Further, from the authors' own experience, LAMP assays are 10 – 100 fold more sensitive than PCR-based amplification reactions for the detection of viruses, with a detection limit of 0.01 to 10 PFU of virus [14].

8. LAMP ASSAYS FOR THE QUANTIFICATION OF TARGET GENES

Capitalizing on its exquisite sensitivity, LAMP assays have been designed to quantify the amount of gene copies of potential microbiological pathogens within clinical samples of blood, thereby allowing physicians to monitor a patient's disease progression, pathogen load, and response to therapy. The ability to determine pathogen load before, during and after therapy has tremendous potential for improving the clinical management of infectious disease. In effect, the quantification of pathogen gene copy number and/or concentration may be accomplished *via* the generation of a standard curve by plotting a graph of known pathogen gene copy number (or concentration) against LAMP assay time to positivity. A linear relationship between pathogen gene copy number (or concentration) versus time of positivity is usually obtained using

LAMP-based amplification assays. Quantification of unknown gene copy number (or concentration) in the clinical samples can then be extrapolated from the standard curve on the basis of the unknown sample's time of positivity [17].

9. ADVANTAGES OF LAMP

The primary characteristic of LAMP is its ability to amplify nucleic acid under isothermal conditions (in the range of 65°C), which allows the use of simple and cost effective hardware (reaction and detection equipment) [18]. Both the amplification and detection of specific nucleic acid sequences can be completed in a single step by incubating a mixture of sample, primers, Bst DNA polymerase, and buffer components, at a constant temperature [2]. In addition the amplification efficiency of LAMP-based assays is very high, amplification proceeding extremely rapidly as there is no need for initial heat denaturation of the template DNA into single strands before each amplification cycle. The fact that LAMP does not require thermal cycling increases its potential application as a diagnostic tool, as well as in rapid molecular medicine and diagnosis [10].

One of the most important characteristics of LAMP is that large amounts of DNA are generated in a short period of time increasing the concentration of pyrophosphate ions. The resultant turbidity may be observed as a white precipitate enabling visual detection of positive LAMP reactions by the naked eye [19]. This also greatly reduces the time required for post-amplification analysis. Another important characteristic of LAMP isothermal amplification is its tolerance to PCR-based amplification inhibitory compounds, present in, for example, cell culture medium [20]. This generally means that LAMP-based assays are less affected by the various inhibitory components that affect PCR-based assays and may be found in many clinical samples. In effect this translates into the fact that LAMP assays generally do not require a DNA purification step. Finally, the amplification and detection of target genes by LAMP can be completed in a single step, saving time to diagnosis. For example, the time required for the confirmation of results using a standard reverse transcription-LAMP (RT-LAMP) assay is 30 min, compared to 3-4 hours for a standard RT-PCR assay (Table **1**).

Table 1: Comparative advantages and disadvantages of various diagnostic techniques.

		Isolation	Serology	Conventional PCR	Real-time PCR	LAMP
Advantage		• Gold standard • Confirmatory • Fulfills Koch's postulate	• Widely adapted as rapid screening test in routine diagnostic laboratory • Cost effective	• Alternate gold standard for isolation in absence of live agent • Early confirmatory diagnosis • Widely used molecular diagnostic format	• Simultaneous amplification and detection during exponential amplification • Real-time monitoring of amplification as it happens • Quantitative, thus useful for monitoring the microbial load • Lower carry over contamination due to closed tube operation • Increased sensitivity due to fluorescent	• Isothermal field based gene amplification without requiring thermal cycler • Amplification can be accomplished using a waterbath/ heating block • Real-time as well as quantitative • Higher amplification efficiency and sensitivity • Naked eye visual monitoring either through turbidity or color change by fluorescent

				chemistry • High throughput analysis due to software driven operation	intercalating dye (SYBR Green I)
Disadvantage	• Time consuming • Tedious • Requirement for a susceptible cell line (viruses) • Requirement of viable organism • Requirement for containment facility for processing high risk pathogens	• Not confirmatory, always considered as probable diagnosis • Paired sera analysis preferred • Time lag for appearance of antibodies • Not suitable for early diagnosis • Cross reaction among closely related species	• Qualitative (Yes or No format) • End-point detection in plateau phase • Post PCR handling leading to carry over contamination • Less sensitive, thereby missing border line cases with low gene copy numbers • Laboratory based • Time consuming (3-4 hrs) • Requirement of thermal cycler and gel documentation system	• Expensive detection equipment and consumable • Requirement for fluorescent probes • Restricted to laboratories with good financial support	• Complicated Design (requirement for 6 primer pairs) • Two long primers of HPLC grade purity required • Restricted availability of reagents and equipment within an international context

10. APPLICATIONS OF LAMP IN MEDICAL DIAGNOSTICS

LAMP is a gene amplification methodology that has found a variety of applications in a wide range of medical fields, including clinical diagnosis, SNP typing and the quantification of template DNA [21]. In particular, LAMP is considered to be effective as a gene amplification method for use in genetic point-of-care testing (g-POCT) devices [16]. Earlier detection of disease can mean earlier treatment and an earlier return to good health.

LAMP technology is particularly emerging as a simple, rapid and powerful gene amplification methodology useful in the early detection of microbial pathogens. In fact, though the first description of LAMP dates back to 1998 [1], the popularity of LAMP only really started after 2003, following the emergence of West Nile and SARS viruses. Since this period, LAMP assays have been increasingly adapted by researchers (mostly from Japan) for the clinical diagnosis of emerging diseases, including bacteria, viruses and parasitic diseases (Table **2**). As a consequence, LAMP assays are currently being put to practical use in the detection of many emerging viral pathogens, most notably with respect to the development of RT-LAMP assays for the rapid and real-time detection of RNA viruses (due to their recent increased importance with respect to potential epidemics of significant public health importance). These include; Dengue, Japanese Encephalitis (JE), Chikungunya, West Nile, SARS, Norwalk, H5N1 highly pathogenic avian influenza (HPAI) "Bird Flu", and the novel H1N1 swine flu of 2009 [14, 15, 22-27]. The usefulness of LAMP in the amplification of DNA viruses has also been reported for HBV (Hepatitis B

Table 2: Usefulness of LAMP in rapid detection of infectious and non-infectious diseases of human and animals.

Organism type		Etiology/ Disease	References
1. Virus	DNA	Parvovirus	31
(Human)		Human papillomavirus type 6, 11, 16, and 18.	32
		Varicella-zoster virus	33, 34
		Hepatitis B virus	35
		Cytomegalovirus	36
		Herpes simplex virus	37
		Human herpesvirus 6	38
		Human herpesvirus 7	39
		Human herpesvirus 8	40
		BK virus	41
	RNA	Novel swine flu virus (H1N1)	27
		West Nile virus	16
		Japanese encephalitis virus.	22, 23
		Norovirus	42, 43
		H5 avian influenza virus	26
		Chikungunya virus	24
		Dengue viruses (1,2,3 &4)	14
		Severe acute respiratory syndrome (SARS) coronavirus.	25
		HIV-1	44
2. Bacteria		*Staphylococcus Aureus*	45
		Shiga toxin producing *E. coli*	46, 47
		Brucella	48
		Anthrax	49
		Salmonella	18
		Mycobacterium avium, Mycobacterium complex	50, 51
		E.coli	52, 53
		Costridium	13, 54
		Vibrio Cholerae	55
3. Parasite		*African trypanosomes*	12, 29, 30
		Trypanosoma brucei rhodesiense	56
		Leishmania	57
		Malaria	58
		Babesia	59

virus), HPV (Human papillomavirus) types 6, 11, 16 & 18, HSV, and VZV. Further, LAMP assays have been found to be superior in terms of sensitivity, specificity, rapidity, and simplicity, compared to established PCR and real-time PCR methodologies [1,10]. With respect to bacteria, LAMP assays have been successfully used for the rapid detection of *Mycobacterium tuberculosis, Porphyromonas gingivalis.* the *Trypanosoma brucei* group (including *T. brucei brucei, T. brucei gambiense, T. brucei rhodesiense,* and *T. evansi*), and *T. congolense.* Experiments showed that the lower detection limits of a 60-min LAMP reaction without loop primers were 1 µg/tube for *P. gingivalis*, 10 fg/tube for *T. forsythia*, and 1 ng/tube for *T. denticola* with a 100 fold greater sensitivity than that of PCR-based assays [28]. *In vivo* studies in mice infected with human-infective *T. brucei gambiense* further highlighted the potential clinical importance of LAMP as a diagnostic tool for the identification of African trypanosomiasis [12, 29, 30]

11. CONCLUSION

LAMP is a novel, simple, rapid, cost effective, highly sensitive and specific field-based novel gene amplification technology that can be used in the routine microbiological diagnostic laboratory, as well as in peripheral health care centers, without requiring expensive high-end equipment such as PCR thermocycling machines, gel electrophoresis and documentation systems *etc.* Specific target amplification may be monitored either in the form of a turbidity measurement or *via* a change of color (after the addition of intercalating DNA dyes) using the naked eye. The better appreciation of, for example, apple green fluorescence generated by DNA dye intercalation, can be achieved using a simple hand held UV light source.

12. FUTURE PERSPECTIVES

LAMP is an innovative, new generation, gene amplification methodology that possesses the ability to amplify target nucleic acid sequences with a high degree of sensitivity and specificity. Under isothermal conditions LAMP has all the characteristics of current real-time nucleic acid amplification assays of high sensitivity, can be used for gene/pathogen quantitation studies, and requires simple operational procedures for easy adaptability. Further, the future integration of LAMP-based isothermal amplification technology with electrophoresis performed on microchips will lead to novel "LAMP on a Chip" technologies for quick and accurate identification of disease producing pathogens and genes at the patient's bedside and at the point-of-care. Ultimately, LAMP-based technology possesses the advantages of rapid amplification, simple operation and easy detection, with potential uses in microbiological clinical diagnosis and the surveillance of infectious diseases, particularly in developing countries where healthcare finances are lacking.

13. ACKNOWLEDGEMENTS

The authors would like to thank Dr R. Vijaya Raghavan, Director, Defence Research and Development Establishment (DRDE), Ministry of Defence, Govt. of India for his keen interest, constant inspiration and for providing the necessary facilities to perform this work.

REFERENCES

[1]   Parida M, Sannarangaiah S, Kumar Dash P, Rao PVL, Morita K. Loop mediated isothermal amplification (LAMP): a new generation of innovative gene amplification technique; perspectives in clinical diagnosis of infectious diseases.Rev Med Virol 2008; 18: 407–421.

[2]   Shenai S, Rodrigues C, Almeida A, Mehta A. Rapid diagnosis of tuberculosis using transcription mediated amplification. Indian Journal of Medical Microbiology 2001; 19(4): 184-189.

[3]   Compton J. Nucleic acid sequence based amplification. Nature 1991; 350(6313): 91-2.

[4]   Hall MJ, Wharam SD, Weston A, Cardy DL, Wilson WH. Use of signal mediated-amplification of RNA technology (SMART) to detect marine cyanophage DNA. Biotechniques 2002; 32(3); 604-6, 608-11.

[5]   Walker GT, Fraiser MS, Schram JL, Little MC, Nadeau JG, Malinowsky DP. Nucleic acids Res 1992; 20: 1691-96.

[6]   Demidov VV. Rolling circle amplification in DNA diagnostics: the power of simplicity. Expert. Rev. Mol. Diagn. 2002; 2(6): 89-95.

[7]   Luthra R, Medeiros LJ.Isothermal Multiple Displacement Amplification 2004; J Mol Diagn: 6(3).

[8]   Goldmayer J, Kong H, Tang W. Development of a novel One-Tube Isothermal reverse transcription thermophilic helicase-dependent amplification platform for Rapid RNA detection. J Mol Diagn 2007; 9(5): 639-44.

[9]   Xu Y, Kim H, Kays H, Rice J, Kong H. Simultaneous amplification and screening of whole plasmids using the T7 bacteriophage replisome. Nucleic Acid Res 2006; 34(13): e98.

[10] Yasuyoshi M, Notomi T. Loop mediated isothermal amplification (LAMP): a rapid, accurate, and cost effective diagnostic method for infectious diseases. J Infect Chemother 2009; 15: 62-69.

[11] Mori Y, Nagamine K, Tomita N, Notomi T. Detection of Loop mediated isothermal amplification reaction by turbidity derived from magnesium pyrophosphate formation. Biochem Biophy Res Com 2001; 289: 150 -154.

[12] Njiru Z K, Mikosza AS, Matovu E African trypanosomiasis: Sensitive and rapid detection of the sub-genus Trypanozoon by loop-mediated isothermal amplification (LAMP) of parasite DNA. Int J Parasitol 2008; 38: 589-99.

[13] Sakuma J, Kurosaki Y,Fujinami Y, Takizawa T, Yasuda J. Rapid and simple detection of *Clostridium botulinum* types A and B by loop mediated isothermal amplification. J Appl Microbiol 2009; 106(4): 1252-9.

[14] Parida M M, Guillermo P, Inoue S, Hasebe F, Morita K. Real-Time Reverse Transcription Loop mediated isothermal amplification for rapid detection of West Nile Virus. J Clinical Microbiology 2004; 42 (1): 257-263.

[15] Parida MM, Horioke K, Ishida H, Rapid detection and differentiation of dengue virus serotypes by a real-time reverse transcription-loop-mediated isothermal amplification assay. J Clin Microbiol 2005; 43: 2895-2903.

[16] Mori Y, Kitao M, Tomita N, Notomi T. Real-time turbidimetry of LAMP reaction for quantifying template DNA. Journal of Biochemical and Biophysical Methods 2004; 59: 145-157.

[17] Li X, Zhang S, Zhang H, Zhang L, Tao H, Yu J, Zheng W, Liu C, Lu D, Xiang R, Liu Y. A loop –mediated isothermal amplification method targets the *phoP* gene for the detection of Salmonella in food samples. Int J Food Microbiol 2009; 133(3); 252-8.

[18] Mackay IM, Arden KE, Nitsche A. Real-time PCR in virology. Nucleic Acid Res 2002; 30: 1292-1305.

[19] Nagamine K, Hase T, Notomi T. Accelerated reaction by loop mediated isothermal amplification using loop primers. Mol Cell Prob 2002; 16: 223-229.

[20] Mori Y, Hirano T, Notomi T. Sequence specific visual detection of LAMP reactions by addition of cationic polymers. BMC Biotechnology 2006; 6: 3.

[21] Iwasaki M, Yonekawa T, Otsuka K Validation of the loop-mediated isothermal amplification method for single nucleotide polymorphism genotyping with whole blood genome. Letters 2003; 2(3): 119-126(8).

[22] Parida M M, Santhosh SR, Dash PK Development and evaluation of reverse transcription Loop mediated isothermal amplification assay for rapid and Real-time detection of Japanese encephalitis virus. J Clin Microbiol 2007; 44 (11): 4172- 4178.

[23] Toriniwa H, Komiya T. Rapid detection and quantification of Japanese encephalitis virus by real-time reverse transcription loop-mediated isothermal amplification. Microbiol Immunol 2006; 50(5): 379-387.

[24] Parida MM, Santhosh SR, Dash PK Rapid and real-time detection of Chikungunya virus by reverse transcription loop mediated isothermal amplification assay. J Clin Microbiol 2007; 45 (2): 351-357.

[25] Hong T C, Mai QL, Cuong DV, Parida MM, Minekawa H, Notomi T, Hasebe F, Morita K. Development and evaluation of a novel loop mediated isothermal amplification (lamp) method for rapid detection of SARS coronavirus. J. Clinical Microbiology 2004; 42 (5): 1956-1961.

[26] Imai M, Ninomiya A, Minekawa H. Rapid diagnosis of H5N1 avian influenza virus infection by newly developed influenza H5 hemagglutinin gene-specific loop-mediated isothermal amplification method. Vaccine 2006 24(44-46): 6679-6682.

[27] Kubo T, Agoh M, Mai L Q Development of a reverse transcription loop mediated isothermal amplification assay for detection of pandemic (H1N1) 2009 virus as a novel molecular method for diagnosis of pandemic influenza in resource limited settings. J Clin Microbiol 2010; 48(3): 728-35.

[28] Yoshida A, Nagashima S, Ansai TLoop-mediated isothermal amplification method for rapid detection of the periodontopathic bacteria *Porphyromonas gingivalis*, *Tannerella forsythia*, and *Treponema denticola*. J Clin Microbiol 2005; 43(5): 2418-2424.

[29] Kuboki N, Inoue N, Sakurai T, Di Cello F, Grab DJ, Suzuki H, Sugimoto C, Igarashi I. Loop-mediated isothermal amplification for detection of African trypanosomes. J Clin Microbiol 2003; 41(12): 5517-5524.

[30] Thekisoe OM, Kuboki N, Nambota A Species-specific loop-mediated isothermal amplification (LAMP) for diagnosis of trypanosomosis. Acta Trop 2007; 102(3): 182-189.

[31] Chen HT, Zhang J, Yang SH,Ma LN, Ma YP,Liu XT, Cai XP,Zhang YG,Liu YS. Rapid detection of porcine parvovirus DNA by sensitive loop mediated isothermal amplification. J Virol Methods 2009; 158(1-2).

[32] Hagiwara M, Sasaki H, Matsuo K, Honda M, Kawase M, Nakagawa H. Loop-mediated isothermal amplification method for detection of human papillomavirus type 6, 11, 16, and 18. J Med Virol 2007; 79(5): 605-615.

[33] Kaneko H, Iida T, Aoki K, Ohno S, Suzutani T. Sensitive and rapid detection of herpes simplex virus and varicella-zoster virus DNA by loop-mediated isothermal amplification. J Clin Microbiol 2005; 43(7): 3290-3296.

[34] Okamoto S, Yoshikawa T, Ihira M, Suzuki K, Shimokata K, Nishiyama Y, Asano Y. Rapid detection of varicella-zoster virus infection by a loop-mediated isothermal amplification method. J Med Virol 2004; 74(4): 677-682.

[35] Cai T, Lou G, Yang J, Xu D, Meng Z. Development and evaluation of real time loop mediated isothermal amplification for hepatitis B virus DNA quantification: a new tool for HBV management. J Clin Virol 2008; 41(4)270-6.

[36] Suzuki R, Yoshikawa T, Ihira M, Enomoto Y, Inagaki S, Matsumoto K, Kato K, Kudo K, Kojima S, Asano Y. Development of the loop-mediated isothermal amplification method for rapid detection of cytomegalovirus DNA. J Virol Methods 2006; 132(1-2): 216-221.

[37] Enomoto Y, Yoshikawa T, Ihira M. Rapid diagnosis of herpes simplex virus infection by a loop-mediated isothermal amplification method. J.Clin.Microbiol 2005; 43(2): 951-955.

[38] Ihira M, Akimoto S, Miyake F, Fujita A, Sugata K, Suga S, Ohashi M, Nishimura N, Ozaki T, Asano Y, Yoshikawa T. Direct detection of human herpesvirus 6 DNA in serum by the loop-mediated isothermal amplification method. J Clin Virol 2007; 39(1): 22-26.

[39] Yoshikawa, T., M. Ihira, and S. Akimoto. 2004. Detection of human herpesvirus 7 DNA by loop-mediated isothermal amplification. J Clin Microbiol 42(3): 1348-1352.

[40] Kuhara T, Yoshikawa T, Ihira M Rapid detection of human herpesvirus 8 DNA using loop-mediated isothermal amplification. J Virol Methods 2007; 144(1-2): 79-85.

[41] Bista BR, Ishwad C, Wadowsky RM, Manna P, Randhawa PS, Gupta G, Adhikari M, Tyagi R, Gasper G, Vats A. Development of a loop-mediated isothermal amplification assay for rapid detection of BK virus. J. Clin. Microbiol 2007; 45(5): 1581-1587.

[42] Fukuda S, Takao S, Kuwayama M, Shimazu Y, Miyazaki K. Rapid detection of norovirus from fecal specimens by real-time reverse transcription-loop-mediated isothermal amplification assay. J Clin Microbiol 2006; 44(4): 1376-1381.

[43] Iturriza- Gomara M, Xerry J, Gallimore C I, Dockery C, Gray J. Evaluation of the loopamp (Loop mediated isothermal amplification) kit for detecting Norovirus RNA in faecal samples. JClin Virol 2008; 42: 389-93.

[44] Curtis K A, Rudolph D L, Owen S M. Rapid detection of HIV-1 by reverse transcription, loop mediated isothermal amplification (RT-LAMP). J Virol Methods 2008; 151: 264-70.

[45] Misawa Y, Yoshida A, Saito R Application of loop-mediated isothermal amplification technique to rapid and direct detection of methicillin-resistant *Staphylococcus aureus* (MRSA) in blood cultures. J Infect Chemother 2007; 13(3): 134-140.

[46] Hara-Kundo Y, Niizuma J, Goto I, Lizuka S, Kaji Y, Kamakura K, Suzuki S, Takatori K. Surveillance of Shiga toxin-producing Escherichia coli in beef with effective procedures, independent of serotype. Foodborne pathog Dis 2008; 5 (1): 97-103.

[47] Song T, Toma C, Nakasone N, Iwanaga M. Sensitive and rapid detection of *Shigella* and enteroinvasive *Escherichia coli* by a loop-mediated isothermal amplification method. FEMS Microbiol Lett 2005; 243(1): 259-263.

[48] Ohtsuki R, Kawamoto K, Kato Y, Shah MM, Ezaki T, Makino SI. Rapid detection of *Brucella* spp. by the loop-mediated isothermal amplification method. J Appl Microbiol.2008; J Appl Microbiol; 104(6): 1815-23.

[49] Hatano B, Maki T, Obara T, Fukumoto H, Hagisawa K, Matsushita Y, Okutani A, Bazartseren B, Inoue S, Sata T, Katano H. LAMP using a disposable pocket warmer for anthrax detection, a highly mobile and reliable method for anti-bioterrorism. Jpn J Infect Dis 2010; 63(1): 36-40.

[50] Enosawa M, Kageyama S, Sawai K, Watanabe K, Notomi T, Onoe S, Mori Y, Yokomizo Y. Use of loop-mediated isothermal amplification of the IS900 sequence for rapid detection of cultured *Mycobacterium avium* subsp. paratuberculosis. J. Clin. Microbiol 2003; 41(9): 4359-65.

[51] Iwamoto TT, Sonobe, Hayashi K. Loop-mediated isothermal amplification for direct detection of *Mycobacterium tuberculosis* complex, *M. avium*, and *M. intracellulare* in sputum samples. J Clin Microbiol 2003; 41(6): 2616-2622.

[52] Hara-Kudo Y, Nemoto J, Ohtsuka K, Segawa Y, Takatori K, Kojima T, Ikedo M. Sensitive and rapid detection of Vero toxin-producing *Escherichia coli* using loop-mediated isothermal amplification. J Med Microbiol 2007; 56(3): 398-406.

[53] Hara-Kudo Y, Konishi N, Ohtsuka K, Hiramatsu R, Tanaka H, Konuma H, Takatori K. Detection of verotoxigenic *Escherichia coli* O157 and O26 in food by plating methods and LAMP method: A collaborative study. Int J Food Microbiol 2008; 122: 156-61.

[54] Kato H, Yokoyama T, Kato H, Arakawa Y. Rapid and simple method for detecting the toxin B gene of *Clostridium difficile* in stool specimens by loop-mediated isothermal amplification.J Clin Microbiol 2005; 43(12): 6108-6112.

[55] Ymazaki W, Seto K, Taguchi M, Ishibashi M, Inoue K. Sensitive and rapid detection of cholera toxin producing *Vibrio cholerae* using a loop mediated isothermal amplification. BMC Microbiol 2008; 8: 94.

[56] Njiru Z K, Mikosza AS, Armstrong T, Enyaru JC, Ndung'u JM, Thompson AR. Loop-mediated isothermal amplification (LAMP) method for rapid detection of *Trypanosoma brucei rhodesiense*. PLoS Negl Trop Dis 2008; 2(1): e147.

[57] Adams ER, Schoone GJ, Ageed AF, Safi SE, Schallig HD. Development of a reverse transcriptase loop mediated isothermal amplification (LAMP) assay for the sensitive detection of *Leishmania* parasites in clinical samples. Am J Trop Med Hyg 2010; 82(4): 591-6.

[58] Rodger A J, Cooke GS, Ord R, Sutherland CJ, Pasvol G. Cluster of falciparum malaria cases in UK airport. Emerg Infect Dis 2008; 14: 1284-6.

[59] Iseki H, Alhassan A, Ohta N, Theisoe O M, Yokoyama N, Inoue N, Development of a multiplex loop mediated isothermal amplification (mLAMP) method for the simultaneous detection of bovine Babesia parasites. J Microbiol Methods 2007; 71(3): 281-7.

CHAPTER 8

Phagocytic Cell Surface Markers in Medical Microbiological Research and Diagnosis

J. Nuutila*

Department of Biochemistry, University of Turku, Vatselankatu 2, 20014 Turku, Finland

Abstract: The rapid and reliable diagnosis of bacterial infection is crucial for three reasons: 1) delays in the identification of bacteraemia during the first 6 hours after hospital admission are associated with higher mortality rates; 2) delays in pathogen identification are associated with an increased utilization of hospital resources (*e.g.* for ICU treatment); and 3) the treatment of viral illnesses and non-infective causes of inflammation with antibiotics (because of inaccurate diagnoses) contributes to the development of antibiotic resistance, toxicity, and allergic reactions, all leading to increased medical costs. Therefore, the development of rapid and reliable diagnostic tests is an essential prerequisite for more accurate diagnosis and the effective use of antibiotics within hospitals and general practitioners' surgeries. One of the most promising technologies likely to impact on rapid and reliable diagnostic testing involves the flow cytometric quantitative analysis of new specific and sensitive cell surface markers (receptors) of bacterial infection on phagocytes. As an example of the usefulness of this method, this chapter presents an outline of how flow cytometric quantitative receptor analysis can be utilised for the clinical differential diagnosis of hospitalized febrile patients suspected of having an illness of microbiological origin.

Keywords: Flow Cyometric Aalysis, Phagocytes, CRP/CD11b Ratio, DNAVS Point, Neutrophil FcγRI, C3, CIS Point Analysis.

1. INTRODUCTION

Physicians depend on effective antimicrobial therapy in order to successfully treat illnesses caused by microorganisms, especially infections caused by bacteria. However, the clinical symptoms of many infectious diseases (such as meningitis, encephalitis, pneumonia, otitis, and tonsillitis) can be quite similar, regardless of whether the etiological agent involved is bacterial, fungal or viral in origin. Further, there is a current lack of reliable and rapid diagnostic microbiological technologies that are able to distinguish between bacterial, fungal and viral infections, meaning that clinicians often empirically prescribe so-called "broad spectrum" antibiotics (just to be on the safe side), in order to eliminate the risk of a severe and possibly life-threatening bacterial infection. However, the antibiotic treatment of fungal and viral illnesses, or non-infective causes of inflammation, is ineffective, and contributes to the development of antibiotic resistance in commensal bacteria, as well as toxicity and allergic reactions in the host, ultimately leading to increased patient morbidity and increased medical costs [1, 2].

In fact, antibiotic resistance has been called one of the world's most pressing public health problems. For example, society pays for the costs of hospital-acquired methicillin-resistant *Staphylococcus aureus* (MRSA) in increased tax or insurance charges, which have been estimated to be between $17 billion and $30 billion per year in the USA, discounting the costs of litigation. In the UK, MRSA has been estimated to cause an annual loss of between £3 billion and £11 billion to the economy [3, 56]. The correct use of antibiotics would allow a decrease, or even reverse, in the spread of resistance, and increase the cost-effectiveness of healthcare. One major factor adding to the unnecessary use of antibiotics is a lack of rapid and accurate diagnostic tests. In 2001, the Commission of the European Communities released a community strategy targeting antimicrobial resistance (Brussels, 20th June 2001, COM(2001) 333 final,

---

Address correspondence to J. Nuutila: Department of Biochemistry, University of Turku, Vatselankatu 2, 20014 Turku, Finland; E-mail: jarnuu@utu.fi

VOLUME 1), that included ways to limit the excessive and uncontrolled use of antimicrobial agents. In this strategy, the development of rapid and reliable diagnostic tests was included as an essential prerequisite for the prudent prescription of antibiotics.

Several methods have so far been developed that help clinicians to decide whether an infection is bacterial, fungal or viral in origin, including: a) microbial culture, the most widely used and accepted method of diagnosing bacterial, and to a lesser extent fungal and viral, infections (though microbiological culture is often time-consuming and is often negative in patients who are receiving antibiotic therapy [4, 5]); b) serology, including tests to determine the presence of microbial antigens or specific anti-microbial antibody titres; c) standard blood-based laboratory evaluation parameters of bacterial infection, such as leukocyte and neutrophil counts, serum C-Reactive Protein (CRP) levels, and Erythrocyte Sedimentation Rate (ESR), which all possess a relatively poor sensitivity and specificity for microbial infections [6]; d) the use of inflammatory mediators, such as M-CSF, TNF-α, IL-1β, IL-6, and IL-8 to detect infection and identify bacteraemia (a common problem however, is their lack of specificity [7-12]); e) the expression of FcγRI (CD64) on human neutrophils, which has been proposed as an improved diagnostic test for the evaluation of infection and sepsis as the expression of FcγRI on neutrophils and monocytes is increased in both bacterial and viral infections [13] (N.B. its usefulness as a marker for differential diagnosis has been somewhat limited [14-17], except from our own research where neutrophil FcγRI was exploited to distinguish between DNA and RNA virus infections [18]); f) the serum level of procalcitonin (PCT) is a potential marker of bacterial infection in critically ill patients (though this analyte appears to be correlated more to the severity of the infection [19, 20], particularly sepsis [21], rather than being an unequivocal marker of bacterial infection); and g) the use of nucleic acid amplification technology, including real-time PCR, which has been increasingly applied to detect the presence of specific microbial genes within clinical material, including blood. However, though a highly specific test, many target-specific PCR probes may be needed in order to successfully identify the relevant pathogen involved in an infection, which increases the number of tests that have to be performed per individual sample leading to an increased total cost per diagnosis). However, the sensitivity of the PCR technique is also its weakness. For example, a virus genome may be released from an infected tissue weeks after the actual infection has ended, possibly resulting in a false positive diagnosis.

Clearly then, there is an ongoing need for new sensitive and specific markers of bacterial infection that will help the clinician decide on the usefulness of antimicrobial therapy in patients presenting with systemic disease. One candidate technology that may help in this process is the flow cytometric determination of specific phagocyte surface receptors.

Flow Cytometric Analysis. Flow cytometry is a universally accepted technology used for detecting and counting particular types of cells (0.2 to 150 micrometers) such as immune cells, as well as detecting and quantifying receptors expressed on cellular surfaces. The sample to be tested comprises a suspension of cells which streams through the flow cytometry apparatus towards a point (in a flow chamber) where a beam of light (usually a laser) illuminates the sample. The passage of cells through a light beam generates a scattered and/or fluorescent light signal (*via* excited fluorescent dyes bound to specific cells) that may be detected by a "forward scatter", or "side scatter", using a fluorescence light detector. Fluctuations in light emission at each detector may be translated into information regarding the physical and chemical characteristics of the cells that have passed through the detector. Flow cytometry is now routinely used in many clinical laboratories, especially in the study of leukaemias. Of particular importance, flow cytometry analysis is a rapid technique, the time window from procuring a sample (*e.g.* blood), to data handling, being less than one hour (Fig. **1**). For a more complete review of the workings of a flow cytometer, the reader is referred to [22].

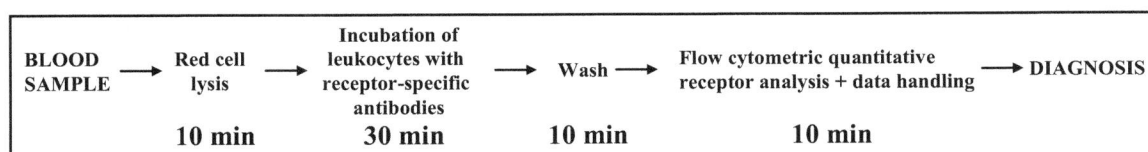

BLOOD SAMPLE	→	Red cell lysis	→	Incubation of leukocytes with receptor-specific antibodies	→	Wash	→	Flow cytometric quantitative receptor analysis + data handling	→	DIAGNOSIS
		10 min		**30 min**		**10 min**		**10 min**		

Fig. (1). Timeline for analysis of a blood sample using flow cytometry.

Nowadays, there are compact, fairly cheap (€30,000 euro), and easy to use flow cytometers available on the market, making the point of care diagnosis of bacterial infection possible even in health centres (as opposed to large hospitals).

In addition, the use of commercially available fluorescent calibration beads, now makes it possible to compare quantitative flow cytometry data between different laboratories, by allowing, for example, the reporting of receptor expression levels as absolute receptor numbers (expressed as the molecules of Equivalent Soluble Fluorochrome (MESF), or as Antigen Binding Capacity (ABC)) [7, 23, 24].

Phagocytes. Phagocytes are immune cells of the body that include: 1) monocytes - which circulate in the blood; 2) macrophages /dendritic cells - which are found in tissues throughout the body; and 3) neutrophils - which principally circulate in the blood but can move into tissues when required. Further, neutrophils also contain intracellular bodies or granules filled with potent bactericidal chemicals, hence they may also be called "granulocytes". Other granulocyte cells include eosinophils and basophils. For a more complete review of immune cells see [25].

The major breakthrough in phagocyte research happened over 100 years ago when Nobel prize winner Ilya Mechnikov theorized that certain white blood cells could engulf (phagocytose) and destroy harmful bodies such as bacteria. At that time, neutrophils were at the centre of intensive discussion about the nature of immunity and were considered by many as the most crucial cellular component of the immune system. Against this background, it is rather surprising that in recent immunological textbooks, for example, there are only a few pages dedicated to neutrophils, even though they are the most predominant cells in the blood stream and are the first cells to arrive at the site of infection! In this context, the author's own research group have, for the last 20 years, continued investigating phagocyte function and especially neutrophil function with respect to receptor expression, phagocytosis, and intracellular killing *via* the "respiratory burst". These studies have been performed in relation to infectious and inflammatory diseases, cancer, atopy and food allergy, as well as in healthy controls [16-18, 26-38]. Our results have been particularly relevant to investigating the processes of innate immunity and (more importantly with respect to this chapter) to clinical differential diagnostic applications.

Pro-Inflammatory Cytokines and Phagocytes in Infection. During infection, the well-orchestrated interplay between the soluble (humoral) and cellular components of the immune system is regulated by pro-inflammatory cytokines, as well as by low concentrations of other inflammatory mediators, which include LPS, fMLP, pathogen DNA/RNA fragments, and complement components C3a and C5a. Further, pro-inflammatory cytokines such as IL-6, IL-1β, TNF-α, INF-γ, and IL-8 are produced at the site of tissue injury / infection by a variety of cell types, mostly macrophages, monocytes, fibroblasts, and endothelial cells [39]. These cytokines are the main mediators that facilitate local inflammation and the response to infection, including eventual systemic responses.

Neutrophils are primed both locally and systemically by pro-inflammatory cytokines, as well as by low concentrations of inflammatory mediators such as LPS, fMLP, and complement component C5a [40, 41]. Priming occurs *via* the binding of inflammatory mediators to specific receptors present on the neutrophil cell surface (many of these mediators prevent neutrophil apoptosis [42]), with mediator binding contributing to amplification of the inflammatory response by prolonging the duration of phagocytoc events. Further, the general opinion is that primed neutrophils are not activated *per se*, but that their respiratory burst activity, and ability to effectively degranulate intracellular granules, is enhanced in response to subsequent stimuli, such as selectin- and CR3-dependent adhesion of chemo-attracted neutrophils to the vessel wall near the area of inflammation/infection [43]. Many receptors are only weakly expressed on the surface of resting (unprimed) neutrophils, being mainly stored in intracellular specific granules, gelatinase granules, and secretory vesicles [44]. It is the activation of primed neutrophils that leads to: i) the rapid and well-orchestrated degranulation of intracellular granules; and ii) the fusion of vesicles and granules with the plasma membrane, which leads to a quantitative up-regulation cell surface receptors.

The neutralization of microorganisms by phagocytes (neutrophils, monocytes, macrophages) can be separated into several stages including: a) chemotaxis; b) the weak (or strong) adhesion of chemo-attracted cells to blood vessel walls; c) endothelial migration of phagocytes into the inflamed tissue; where d) ingestion and intracellular killing of microorganisms eventually occurs. Distinct receptor types are involved in different stages of phagocyte recruitment from the circulation to the site of infection. For example, chemotaxis is a chemokine/cytokine receptor-dependent event, whilst weak adhesion of phagocytes to vessel walls is cellular lectin (selectin)-dependent, and strong adhesion/endothelial migration is Ig superfamily and integrin-dependent [43]. Finally, complement receptors and Fcγ-receptors are key molecules in the phagocytosis of complement- and IgG-opsonized microorganisms, respectively.

2. PHAGOCYTE COMPLEMENT RECEPTOR EXPRESSION IN INFECTIONS

Several important receptors for molecules of the complement system are expressed on the surface of phagocytes, and are therefore intimately involved in the humoral immune response to microbial pathogens. The most important receptors in this respect are Complement Receptor 1 (CR1) and Complement Receptor 3 (CR3).

The most common allelic form of human CR1, expressed in leukocytes and red blood cells, consists of 30 independently folding complementary Short Consensus Repeats (SCRs), each 56-70 amino acids long [45]. All but the two (transmembrane/intracellular) carboxyl-terminal SCRs can be organized into four Long Homologous Repeats (LHRs), termed A (outermost), B, C, and D (innermost), each 7 SCRs long. There are 2 functionally distinct active sites in CR1, site 1 and site 2, which are located in SCRs 1-3 of LHR A and in SCRs 8-10 of LHR B, respectively. Site 1 binds mainly C4b and site 2 binds both C3b and C4b [45]. In addition, data indicates that LHR D includes a binding site for C1q [46].

Another complement receptor, human CR3 (also known as CD11b/CD18, Mac-1, or $\alpha_M\beta_2$-integrin), is a member of the β_2 integrin subfamily and consists of a β-subunit of ≈750 amino acids, which is non-covalently linked to distinct but homologous α-subunits of ≈1100 amino acids. Ligand specificity (*i.e.* the specificity of receptor binding) for CR3 is broad and is largely conferred by the α-subunit (CD11b). The protein ligand binding portion of the α-subunit has been mapped to a specific region termed the I-domain [47]. The I-domain contains a distinct Metal Ion-Dependent Adhesion Site (MIDAS), which is important for protein ligand interaction [48]. The I-domain has been implicated in the binding of ICAM-1, fibrinogen [49], complement component C3bi [50], the yeast *Candida albicans* [51], and Neutrophil Inhibitory Factor (NIF) [52]. The α-subunit also recognizes mannose and β-glucan carbohydrate structures *via* a lectin-like binding domain which is located on the C-terminal of I-domain [53, 54]. The lectin domain binding ligands include zymosan, *Saccharomyces cereviseae*, and pure β-glucan.

Activation of the complement system and the involvement of peripheral blood phagocytes, mainly neutrophils, are the major effector pathways in bacterial infection. CR1 and CR3 are only weakly expressed on the surface of resting neutrophils, being mostly stored in intracellular granules (CR1 in secretory vesicles, and CR3 in specific, gelatinase granules, as well as in secretory vesicles) [44]. During infection, exposure to pro-inflammatory cytokines and chemo-attractants primes neutrophils for the rapid degranulation of their intracellular receptor containing granules. The fusion of these granules with the plasma membrane leads to a quantitative up-regulation of CR1 and CR3 on the cell surface. Primed monocytes behave like neutrophils, showing a significant increase in the expression of complement receptors after exposure to relevant stimuli [29].

As with neutrophils, up-regulation of complement receptors on monocytes is dependent on both intra- and extra-cellular calcium levels and modulated by rapid degranulation of secretory vesicle-like granules (SVLGs).

Up-regulated complement receptors CR1 and CR3, together with Fc-receptors, provide an essential link between the humoral and cellular immune response by functioning as key molecules in; a) the up-regulation of phagocytosis, b) the clearance of immune complexes, and c) in triggering the release of inflammatory mediators [55-57].

Phagocyte complement receptors also have functions not connected to the phagocytosis of complement-opsonized pathogens. For example, CR3 plays a crucial role in the migration of neutrophils from the bloodstream to the site of inflammation [43, 58], and CR1 can operate as a membrane-bound or soluble complement regulator, inhibiting both classical and alternative complement pathways (thereby protecting host cells against autologous complement lysis [59, 60]).

CR1 and CR3 in Distinguishing Between Bacterial and Viral Infections (the Clinical Infection Score Point*).* From our own experiments, the expression of neutrophil CR1 and CR3 is 3-fold and 2-fold higher, respectively, in classical bacterial than in viral infection [27] (Fig. **2a** and **2b**). In this context, the determination of the expression of complement receptors on neutrophils could be of value as a rapid tool in the aetiological diagnosis of bacterial versus viral infections. Using statistical Receiver Operating Characteristic (ROC) curve analysis, neutrophil CR1 expression showed a 92% sensitivity and 85% specificity with respect to distinguishing between bacterial and viral infections. This finding means that neutrophil CR1 expression analysis results in the most effective differential capacity as compared to other similar immunological measurements, *e.g.* neutrophil CR3 analysis, neutrophil count, C-Reactive Protein (CRP), and Erythrocyte Sedimentation Rate (ESR). Further, we showed in the same work that a computational variable, the Total Neutrophil Complement Receptor (TNCR) index (which incorporates neutrophil count and the number of CR1 and CR3 expressed on the surface of neutrophils), has a somewhat higher specificity (89%) than neutrophil CR1 alone when used for distinguishing between bacterial and viral infections. Though the behaviour of CRP and ESR are somewhat similar to the expression of neutrophil CR1 (in that they are significantly higher in bacterial than in viral infections), one advantage of using flow cytometric receptor analysis over CRP and ESR methods is the rapidity of diagnosis. In fact, the time window from procuring a blood sample to data handling is less than one hour for flow cytometry, a few hours quicker than CRP and ESR methods.

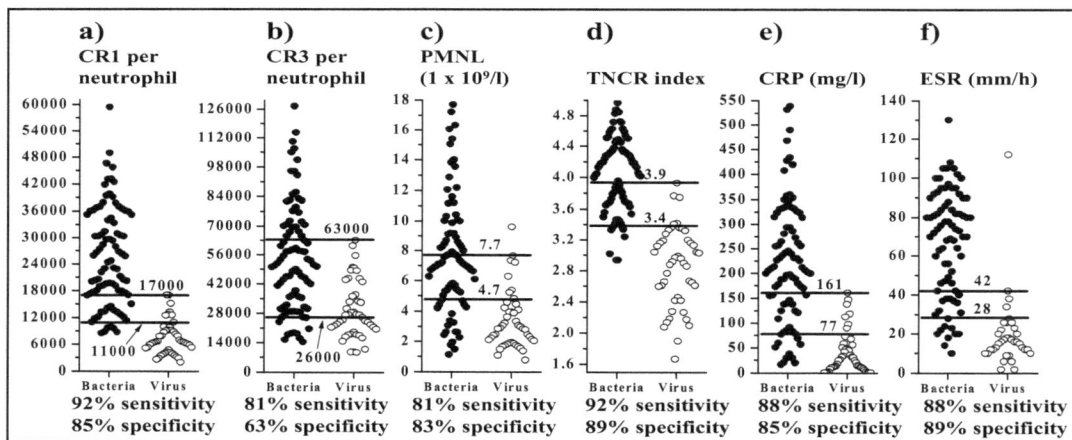

Fig. (2). Raw data of 6 immunological and serological markers (variables) of bacterial infection. The lower horizontal line and associated numerical value indicates the optimal receiver operating characteristic (ROC) curve cut-off point value of a variable in differentiating between bacterial (n=89) and viral (n=46) infection. The upper horizontal line and associated numerical value indicates the additional second cut-off value of a variable. Total neutrophil complement receptor (TNCR) index can be obtained by multiplying neutrophil count, number of CR1 on neutrophils, and number of CR3 on neutrophils and by taking the base-10 logarithm of this factorial thereafter [27].

Although a high expression of neutrophil CR1 correlates with the likelihood of bacterial infection, it is unlikely that any parameter (variable) of inflammation alone will be sufficiently robust to reliably allow the differentiation of bacterial and viral infections. In fact, it is more probable that diagnostic accuracy may be improved by incorporating several different variables. This idea is supported by a previous study where the Clinical Pulmonary Infection Score Point (CPIS), consisting of 6 clinical and laboratory variables (fever, leukocytosis, tracheal aspirates, oxygenation, radiographic infiltrates, and semi-quantitative cultures of tracheal aspirates with Gram stain), displayed a sensitivity of 93% and specificity of 96% for diagnosing ventilator-associated pneumonia [61].

From our own recent studies, the diagnostic accuracy of distinguishing between bacterial and viral infections was improved by generating a novel Clinical Infection Score (CIS) point consisting of 4 variables (Fig. **3**), including CRP levels, ESR, neutrophil count, and the amount of CR1 on neutrophils [27]. CIS points varied between 0 and 8, and differentiated between microbiologically confirmed bacterial and viral infections with a sensitivity of 97% and specificity of 97% when using a cut-off point of >2. The median CIS point value did not significantly differ between microbiologically confirmed and clinically diagnosed bacterial infections or between microbiologically confirmed systemic and local bacterial infections. We also found that CIS point-based differentiation between bacterial and viral infection is not affected by antibacterial treatment or underlying diseases. From our own experience, the CIS point method seems to be more powerful and faster than blood culture in differentiating between bacterial and viral pneumonia.

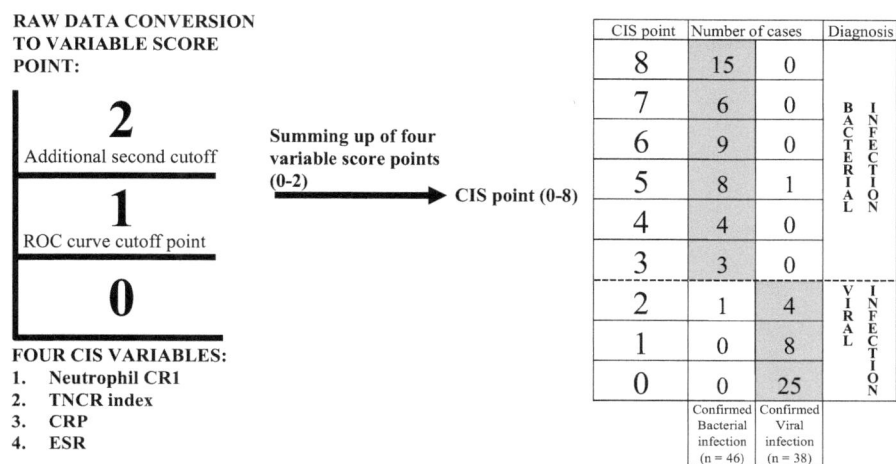

RAW DATA CONVERSION TO VARIABLE SCORE POINT:

2

Additional second cutoff

1

ROC curve cutoff point

0

FOUR CIS VARIABLES:
1. **Neutrophil CR1**
2. **TNCR index**
3. **CRP**
4. **ESR**

Summing up of four variable score points (0-2) → **CIS point (0-8)**

CIS point	Number of cases		Diagnosis
8	15	0	B A C T E R I A L I N F E C T I O N
7	6	0	
6	9	0	
5	8	1	
4	4	0	
3	3	0	
2	1	4	V I R A L I N F E C T I O N
1	0	8	
0	0	25	
	Confirmed Bacterial infection (n = 46)	Confirmed Viral infection (n = 38)	

Fig. (3). Calculation of the clinical infection score (CIS) points. On the left, is shown how an ROC curve and additional second cut-off values (Fig. **2**) are exploited in order to convert the variable raw data to the variable score points. The CIS point (which can vary between 0 and 8), can be obtained by combining the 4 variable score points. On the right, CIS point-based differentiation between microbiologically confirmed bacterial (n = 46) and viral (n = 38) infections [27] is shown.

C3 and CRP in Detecting Gram-Positive Sepsis (the CRP/CD11b ratio). Since severe sepsis with acute organ dysfunction can be fatal within hours, it is customary to start empirical broad-spectrum antimicrobial therapy in all patients hospitalised with a suspicion of systemic inflammatory response syndrome [62]. However, the inappropriate use of broad-spectrum antimicrobials has contributed to the emergence of drug resistant strains of bacteria, leading to increased patient morbidity and medical costs [1, 2]. Further, drug resistance among gram-positive bacteria, the leading cause of sepsis [63], is now endemic throughout the world and remains a serious therapeutic problem despite the availability of new antimicrobials. In order to avoid the inappropriate use of antibiotics, rapid and accurate identification of the causative agent of an infection is required, so that broad-spectrum antibiotic treatment may be replaced with targeted and appropriate narrow-spectrum antibiotic therapy, for example targeted therapy against either Gram-positive or Gram-negative bacteria. Since microbial culture (the "gold standard" method for identifying the causative agent of bacterial sepsis) is time consuming, and patients with sepsis require immediate antimicrobial therapy, there is an urgent need for new rapid method(s) for determining the type of infecting pathogen.

In a previous study, the authors found that increased serum CRP levels, coupled to a decreased amount of CR3 on neutrophils, correlates with the likelihood of Gram-positive bacterial infection, especially Gram-positive sepsis [28] (Fig. **4a** and **4b**). From this finding, we derived a "CRP/CD11b RATIO" by dividing the serum CRP value by amount of CR3 (equivalent to CD11b) on neutrophils, with the average CRP/CD11b RATIO being significantly higher in Gram-positive bacterial infections versus i) Gram-negative bacterial infections, ii) clinical bacterial infections (diagnosis made by the attending physician on grounds of symptoms and signs of the patient combined with the clinical course of the disease), and iii) viral infections. In detail, 13 (76%) patients we tested that presented with Gram-positive sepsis (n = 17) possessed CRP/CD11b RATIO ≥ a cutoff value of 5.7 μgl^{-1}neutrophil CR3^{-1} (Fig. **4c**). Of these 13 patients, 9 (70%) were diagnosed with *Streptococcus pneumoniae*, 2 with *Staphylococcus aureus*, 1 with *Enterococcus faecalis,* and 1 with both *Streptococcus intermedius* and *Streptococcus oralis* infection. The corresponding percentages of patients presenting with a CRP/CD11b RATIO ≥ a cut-off value of 5.7 μgl^{-1} neutrophil CR3^{-1} were 20% in local Gram-positive infection (n = 5), 14% in Gram-negative infection (n = 22), 30% in clinically diagnosed pneumonia (n = 24), and 15% in other clinically diagnosed infections (n = 20). Further, ROC curve analyses confirmed that the CRP/CD11b RATIO differentiated between Gram-positive sepsis (n = 17) and a combined group of patients (including the above mentioned groups of patients with local Gram-positive infection, Gram-negative infection, clinically diagnosed pneumonia, and other clinically diagnosed infections, where n = 71), with 76% sensitivity and 80% specificity. In comparison to the individual variables, serum CRP level and amount of CD11b on neutrophils, the CRP/CD11b RATIO test shows an increased ability to detect Gram-positive sepsis.

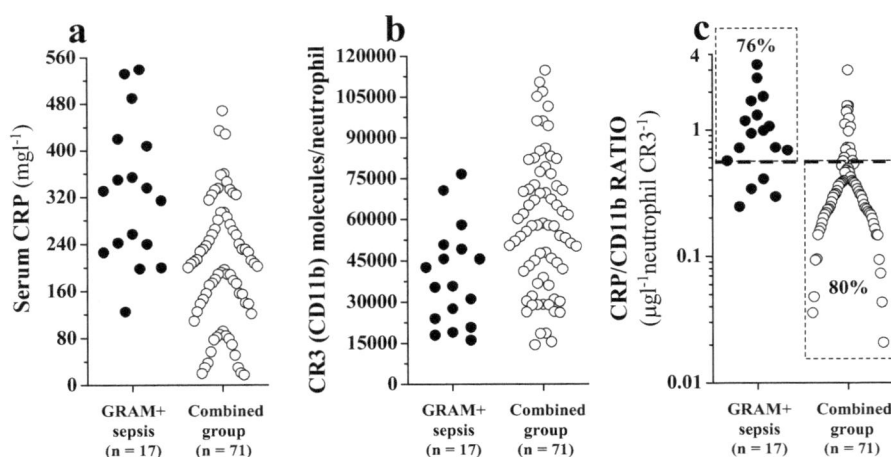

Fig. (4). The CRP/CD11b RATIO (c) is derived by dividing the serum CRP value (see **4a**) by the amount of CR3 (CD11b) on neutrophils (see **4b**). The horizontal dashed line indicates the optimal ROC curve cut-off value of 5.7 μgl^{-1}neutrophil CR3^{-1} when detecting gram-positive sepsis. The combined group consists of patients with local Gram-positive infection (n = 5), Gram-negative infection (n = 22), clinically diagnosed pneumonia (n = 24), or other clinically diagnosed infection (n = 20). [28].

The CRP/CD11b RATIO appears therefore to be able to differentiate between Gram-positive sepsis and other infectious diseases with statistical significance, though it is not an unequivocal marker of Gram-positive sepsis. Perhaps it could be used, together with a specific marker of bacterial infection, to distinguish between Gram-positive sepsis, local Gram-positive infections, Gram-negative infections, clinical bacterial infections, and viral infections. The CRP/CD11b RATIO may be particularly well suited for quickly detecting potential Gram-positive sepsis among intensive care unit patients with severe community-acquired or ventilator-associated nosocomial pneumonia. Previous data indicates that appropriate antibiotic therapy, when initiated very early in patients with ventilator-associated pneumonia, can reduce the patient mortality rate when compared to inappropriate antimicrobial therapy or when no therapy is given at all [64].

Combining the Clinical Infection Score Point and the CRP/CD11b RATIO. Using the clinical infection score point and CRP/CD11b RATIO together could be the first step in diagnosing a febrile patient suspected of having a Gram-positive, Gram-negative or viral infection. The CIS point could be used as a marker of bacterial infection, with the CRP/CD11b RATIO being used as a confirmatory test to indicate whether the patient has a Gram-positive sepsis or not. Patients positive for the CIS point test, but negative for the CRP/CD11b RATIO test would most probably have local Gram-positive infection, Gram-negative infection, or a clinical bacterial infection, whilst patients negative for the CIS point test would probably have a viral infection.

3. PHAGOCYTE FCΓRI RECEPTOR EXPRESSION IN INFECTIONS

Human cells of the myeloid lineage contain 3 classes of receptors for the Fc portion of IgG, designated FcγRI (CD64), FcγRII (CD32), and FcγRIII (CD16), which act in concert with complement receptors to provide an essential link between humoral and cellular immune systems by functioning as key molecules in phagocytosis, clearance of immune complexes, antigen presentation, and the release of inflammatory mediators [55-57,]. In contrast to FcγRII and FcγRIII, which bind monomeric IgG with low affinity ($\sim 10^6$ M^{-1}) and consequently interact preferentially with multimeric immune complexes [55], FcγRI binds monomeric human IgG1 and IgG3 with high affinity (10^9 M^{-1}), leading to saturation *in vivo* [25]. Further, apart from the Fc domains of IgG1 and IgG3, FcγRI also binds CRP, but with low affinity [66, 67].

Human FcγRI consists of α- and γ-chains. The α-chain alone is capable of mediating endocytosis [68] and calcium signaling [69], and forms a complex with the ITAM-containing homodimeric γ-chain that is indispensable for both surface membrane expression [70] and phagocytic function [68] of human FcγRI *in vivo*. Interactions between the human FcγRI α- and γ-chains are mediated solely by 21 amino acids in the transmembrane domain of the α-chain [71].

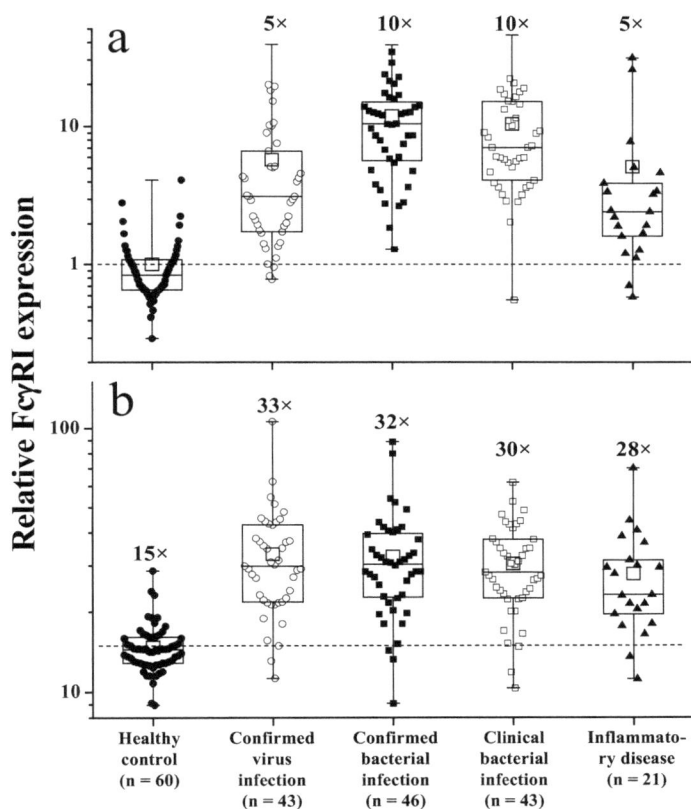

Fig. (5). Comparison of the relative number of FcγRI on neutrophils **(a)** and monocytes **(b)** in healthy adult controls and in different groups of patients with infection/inflammatory disease. The relative number of FcγRI on neutrophils of healthy controls has been normalised to 1 (corresponding to approximately 1400 receptors per cell). Box chart statistics: mean value (open square), median (the horizontal central line within the box), 75th and 25th percentiles (the upper and lower horizontal lines enclosing the box), and minimum/maximum values of the raw data, are also shown. The dotted horizontal lines represent the average relative values in healthy adult controls [17, 38].

In resting neutrophils, FcγRI is expressed at very low levels. However, upregulation of FcγRI on the surface of neutrophils is induced by inflammatory cytokines, such as interferon-gamma (INF-γ) [72] and Granulocyte Colony-Stimulating Factor (G-CSF) [73], which are produced during infections. Therefore, FcγRI expression on human neutrophils may be used as an improved diagnostic test for the evaluation of infections, particularly sepsis [13]. In contrast to neutrophils, human FcγRI is constitutively expressed in resting monocytes [74].

Phagocyte FcγRI as a Marker of Febrile Infection. In a previous study, we found that the average number of FcγRI on the surfaces of both neutrophils and monocytes is significantly increased in patients with febrile viral and bacterial infections, compared to healthy controls [17] (Fig. **5**). However, in most inflammatory patients (as well as in 0-6 month old healthy babies and kidney cancer patients), FcγRI expression on neutrophils seems to be at a relatively low level [75].

On average, the amount of FcγRI on neutrophils was found to be 5-10 times higher in febrile infections than in healthy controls, and almost twice as high in bacterial than viral infections. This was most probably due to exposure of the leukocytes to increased levels of several inflammatory mediators, including endo/exotoxins and inflammatory cytokines. These include TNF-α, Il-1, Il-6, G-CSF, and IFN-γ in bacterial infections, and predominantly, INF-γ in viral infections [73, 76, 77].

While human FcγRI is constitutively expressed on antigen-presenting cells expressing MHC class II molecules (APC; monocytes, macrophages, and dendritic cells), surprisingly limited data is available regarding FcγRI expression on monocytes in bacterial and viral infections. In fact, membrane-bound FcγRI is essential in mediating enhanced antigen presentation through internalization of antigen complexed with IgG *in vitro* [65], and FcγRI antigen targeting on APCs dramatically enhances T cell activation. Since antigen presentation is essential for stimulating effective immune responses regardless of the etiology of infection (bacterial or viral), it is plausible that the number of FcγRI on monocytes of bacterially and virally infected patients is higher than that of monocytes from healthy controls.

ROC curve analysis confirms the hypothesis that there exists distinct FcγRI expression on monocyte and neutrophil surfaces between febrile infected patients and healthy controls, with high sensitivities and specificities (Fig. **6a-c**). In particular, neutrophil FcγRI appears a highly sensitive marker of bacterial infection. On the other hand, FcγRI expression on both neutrophils and monocytes displays relatively poor sensitivity (73% and 52%) and specificity (65% and 52%) in distinguishing between bacterial and viral infections (Fig. **6d**), and does not differ significantly between systemic (sepsis), local, and clinically diagnosed bacterial infections. In conclusion, the amount of FcγRI on monocytes and neutrophils is a useful marker of infection, but (from our results) appears unable to effectively differentiate between bacterial and viral infections, or between systemic and local bacterial infections.

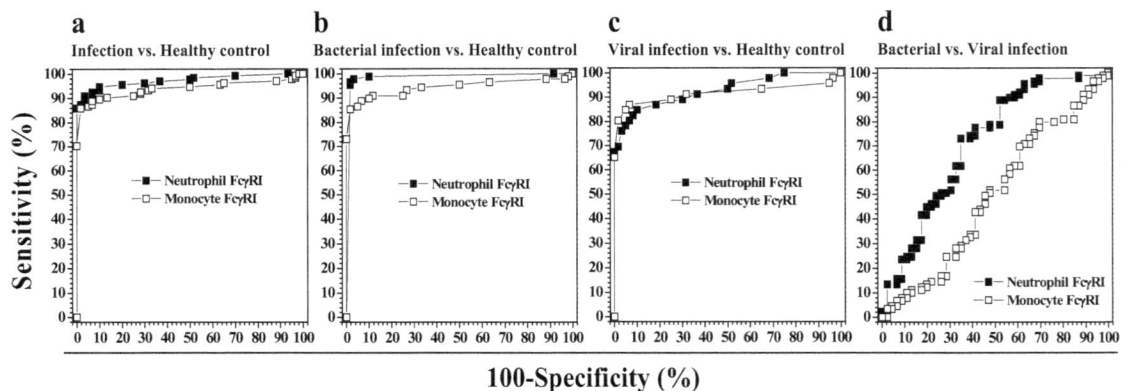

Fig. (6). Receiver operating characteristic (ROC) curves comparing neutrophil and monocyte FcγRI for separating: **a)** febrile infections (n = 135) from healthy controls (n = 60); **b)** bacterial infections (n = 89) from healthy controls (n = 60); **c)** viral infections (n = 46) from healthy controls (n = 60); and d) bacterial infections (n = 89) from viral infections (n = 46).

Inspired by the CIS point method (see above), we developed a novel marker of febrile infection, the "CD64 score point", which reliably distinguishes between febrile infections and healthy controls with 94%

sensitivity and 98% specificity [17] (Fig. **7**). The simultaneous quantitative analysis of FcγRI expression on both neutrophils and monocytes is the foundation of the CD64 score point method. In comparison to neutrophil FcγRI expression analysis alone, the reliability of the CD64 score point in detecting a true negative test result is enhanced over a wider range of febrile infection prevalence.

The CD64 score point method may be a highly sensitive and specific screening method for detecting an infection in patients with postoperative fever. Postoperative fever is one of the most common problems seen by both surgeons and medical consultants. Dependent on the surgical procedure, the prevalence of infection among patients with postoperative fever can vary between 0 and 20% shortly after operation [78-80]. However, the situation can be quite different for patients who develop a fever on or after the fifth day following surgery, as approximately 90% of these patients have been found to have an identifiable infection [78]. Therefore, in order to commence correct treatment, as rapidly as possible, timely knowledge of whether the postoperative fever is a consequence of infection would be beneficial for the clinician (for example by using the CD 64 score point method).

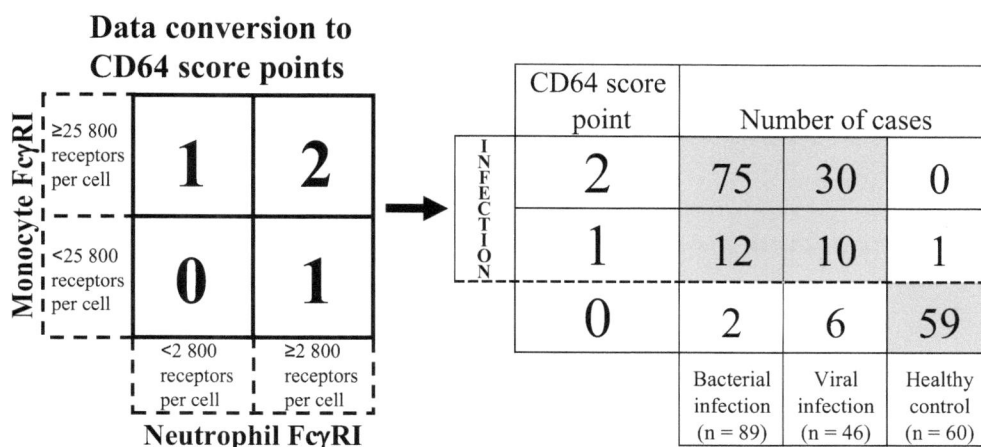

Fig. (7). Calculation and use of CD64 score points in differentiating between febrile infections and healthy controls. The figure on the left shows how to convert primary receptor expression data to CD64 score points. Vertical and horizontal lines represent the optimal cut-off point of 2800 receptors/cell and 25800 receptors/cell for neutrophil and monocyte FcγRI, respectively, in differentiating between febrile infections (n = 89) and healthy controls (n = 46). The figure on the right shows how the CD64 score points can be used to distinguish between febrile infections and healthy controls [17].

Neutrophil; FcγRI in Distinguishing Between RNA and DNA Virus Infections. Over the past few decades, several methods have been developed to help clinicians decide whether an infection is bacterial or viral in origin. However, little attention has been paid to the development of a fast and reliable method(s) for differentiating between DNA and RNA virus infections. In addition, reliable and specific antiviral agents are only available for a few viral agents, including nucleoside analogues for herpesviruses [81], neuraminidase inhibitors for influenza viruses [82], and antiretrovirals for HIV [83]. Nucleoside analogues and the phosphonic acid derivative foscarnet should be used to treat herpesvirus infections only, whilst neuraminidase inhibitors are ideally prescribed in cases of pneumonia caused by influenza viruses. Therefore, in order to commence effective antiviral therapy as rapidly as possible, timely knowledge of whether the infection is caused by a double stranded DNA (dsDNA) or a single stranded RNA (ssRNA) virus would be highly beneficial for the clinician.

The author's own data has indicated that the average amount of FcγRI on neutrophils (as well as the total and differential counts of lymphocytes), in febrile dsDNA virus infections, increased significantly compared to febrile ssRNA virus infections, suggesting that these parameters are suitable for distinguishing between DNA and RNA virus infections [18] (Fig. **8a-d**). However, none of these variables could reliably differentiate between DNA and RNA virus infections alone. In this context, we created a DNA virus score

(DNAVS) point, which incorporates the above mentioned variables (Fig. **8e** and **8f**). We calculated that at a cut-off point equal to or greater than 1.5, the DNAVS point differentiates between dsDNA and ssRNA virus infections with 95% sensitivity and 100% specificity. In comparison to the best individual variable (neutrophil FcγRI), the reliability of the DNAVS point in distinguishing between dsDNA and ssRNA virus infections is much superior, over a wider range of dsDNA virus prevalence. .

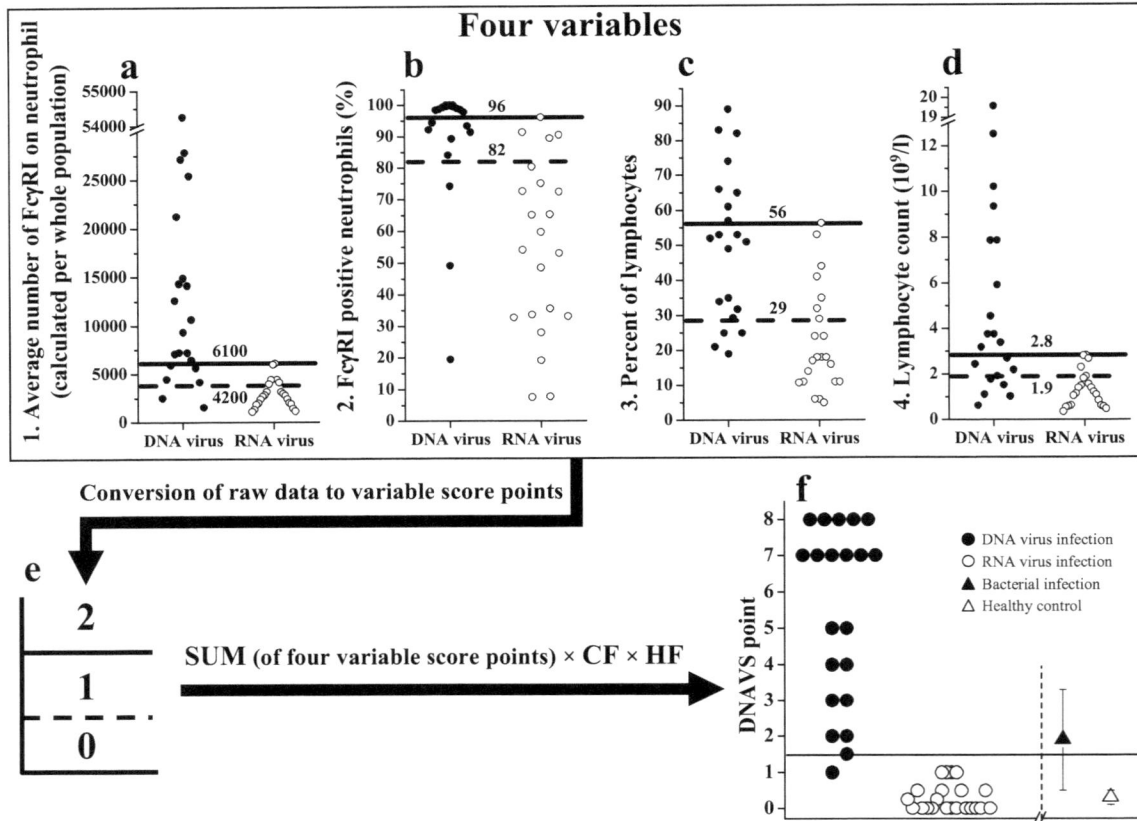

Fig. (8). Calculation of the DNA Virus Score (DNAVS) point. The raw data of the 4 DNAVS point variables (**a-d**) have to be first converted to variable score points by making use of an ROC curve cut-off values (the lower horizontal dashed line), as well as additional second cut-off values (here shown by an upper solid horizontal line that indicates the maximum value detected in patients with RNA virus infection). After data conversion (**e**), the SUM (*i.e.* the sum of the 4 variable score points) which can vary between 0 and 8, can be calculated. The actual DNAVS point can then be determined by multiplying the SUM value by the CD64 factor (CF) value, and the haematopoietic factor (HF) value (DNAVS point = SUM CF HF). A CF value of 0.25 should be used when the variable score point of both receptor variables (the amount of FcγRI on neutrophils) as shown in **a**), and the percentage of FcγRI positive neutrophils (as shown in **b**), is 0. If the variable score points of both haematopoietic variables (*i.e.* the percentage of lymphocytes) as shown in **c**,) and lymphocyte count (as shown in **d**) is 0, then an HF of 0.5 is used. In all other cases, CF and HF are 1. The DNAVS point-based differentiation between dsDNA (n = 21) / ssRNA (n = 22) virus infections is shown in **f** [18].

The use of neutrophil FcγR1 and CIS point analysis in distinguishing between bacterial infections, viral infections and inflammatory disease. As previously mentioned, the quantitative analysis of FcγRI expression alone on neutrophils cannot be used for distinguishing between bacterial, viral or inflammatory disease. However, this problem can be solved by creating a FcγRI/CIS point bivariate dot-plot graph, where the x-axis represents the amount of FcγRI expressed on neutrophils, and the y-axis represents the CIS point value [38]. By setting vertical and horizontal lines to represent the optimal cut-off point values of 3500 receptors/cell for neutrophil FcγRI and 2.5 for CIS point value, respectively, the bivariate dot-plot graph can be divided into four quadrants: an Upper Left Quadrant (ULQ); an Upper Right Quadrant (URQ); a Lower Left Quadrant (LLQ); and a Lower Right Quadrant (LRQ) (Fig. **9**). Using the FcγRI/CIS point - bivariate dot-plot graphing methodology, allowed the following conclusions to be drawn: 1) if the

FcγRI/CIS point - bivariate dot-plot value from a febrile patient lies within the URQ, then there is a very high probability that the patient is suffering from a bacterial infection, and a low probability of inflammatory disease (viral infection being virtually ruled out); 2) if the FcγRI/CIS point - bivariate dot-plot value from a febrile patient lies within the LRQ, then there is a very high probability that the patient is suffering from a viral infection and a low probability of a bacterial infection (inflammatory disease being virtually ruled out); 3) if the FcγRI/CIS point - bivariate dot-plot value from a febrile patient lies within the LLQ, then there is a very high probability that the patient is suffering from a viral infection and a low probability of inflammatory disease (bacterial disease being virtually ruled out); and 4) if the FcγRI/CIS point - bivariate dot-plot value from a febrile patient lies within the ULQ, then there is a high probability of inflammatory disease and a moderate probability of bacterial infection (with a low probability of viral infection). Additionally, using the DNAVS point calculation, patients with dsDNA and ssRNA virus infections will most probably be found in RLQ and LLQ, respectively. Further, it appears that the ULQ is an inflammatory disease-specific quadrant.

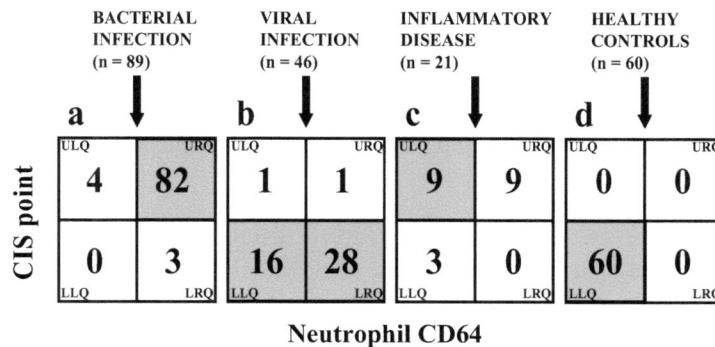

Fig. (9). FcγRI/CIS point - bivariate dot-plot graphs in bacterial (**a**) and viral (**b**) infections, as well as inflammatory diseases (**c**) and healthy adult controls (**d**). The quadrants which are typical of each patient group have been marked in grey. The vertical line in figures **a-d** indicates the optimal cut-off value of 3500 FcγRI receptors per neutrophil. The horizontal line in **a-d** indicates the optimal cut-off value of 2.5 using the CIS point method (see also Fig. 3).

It is also possible to replace the CIS point value in the bivariate dot-plot graph with data obtained from the quantitative analysis of CR1 on neutrophils [38]. Despite being slightly less powerful in distinguishing between bacterial, viral, and inflammatory disease, the advantage of the (flow cytometric) FcγRI/CR1 bivariate dot-plot method over the FcγRI/CIS point bivariate dot-plot method is cost-effectiveness, as time consuming CRP and ESR measurements are not required to calculate the CIS point value.

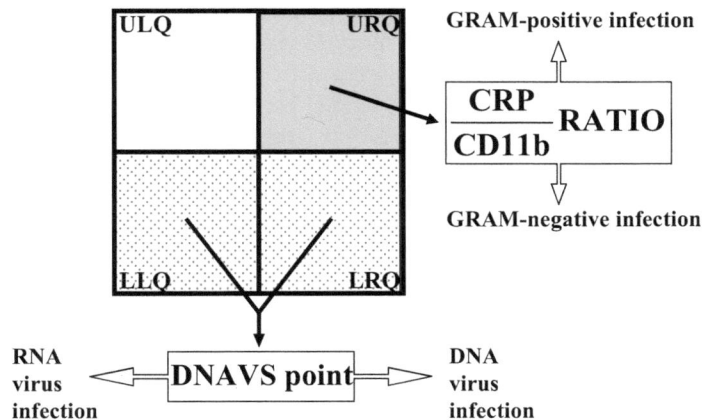

Fig. (10). Bacterially infected patients (in the URQ) can be subdivided into those with Gram-positive and Gram-negative bacterial infection by calculating their CRP/CD11b RATIO. Similarly, using the DNAVS point, virally infected patients (in the LLQ and LRQ) can be subdivided into those infected by either a dsDNA or ssRNA virus [18, 28, 38].

Calculation of the CRP/CD11b RATIO in bacterially infected patients present in the URQ allows further subdivision into Gram-positive and Gram-negative bacterial infection (Fig. **10**).

Similarly, using the DNAVS point, viral infected patients in LLQ and LRQ can be subdivided into patients with either DNA or RNA virus infection.

4. SUMMARY AND FUTURE OUTLOOK

In this chapter, the author has attempted to show the value of using flow cytometric quantitative receptor analysis in the differential diagnosis of hospitalized febrile patients suspected of having an infection. As indicated, receptor analyses may improve the differential diagnosis of hospitalised febrile patients, especially when several receptor variables are measured simultaneously and used to generate a combined diagnosis, for example using CIS point values combined with the CRP/CD11b RATIO. Although the CIS point method has very high sensitivity and specificity in differentiating between bacterial and viral infections, the greatest weakness of this approach is that it incorporates the results of four separate measurements (ESR, CRP, neutrophil count, and quantitative receptor analysis), making it a quite complex and time-consuming method. However, the CIS point method is applicable using a variety of measurements, and it may be possible to substitute new variables into the CIS point calculation in order to increase its "usability" value by, for example, replacing ESR and CRP measurements.

The author's own data has shown that the variation of the receptor amounts in healthy controls is narrow and independent of age or sex. Even though it is quite likely that the geographical location has no big effect on phagocyte receptor expressions, we cannot be absolutely sure of this. Further, all of the experiments discussed above have been performed on northern latitude of 60°27'00"N (city of Turku, Finland). Therefore, in the future, one should examine whether the cut-off points related to CD64 score point, CIS point, DNAVS point, and CRP/CD11b RATIO are relevant worldwide.

Sample storage is still one critical factor affecting the receptor values obtained, especially when heparin is used as an anticoagulant (as is the situation in all of the previously mentioned studies). In infectious patients, the levels of CR1 and CR3 have been found to be relatively constant within 3 hours after blood sampling [27]. On the other hand, the levels of these receptors in healthy controls started to increase after 1 hour of sampling. Therefore, the recommendation is that when the reference values of the controls are established, the blood samples should be analysed within 1 hour. The time window of handling of patient samples is not so crucial. Of course, fixing the specimen (if indeed successful), would remove the problems associated with sample storage.

In an ongoing research project, we are currently studying the expression patterns of 15 potential phagocyte cell surface markers (receptors) of infection. The ultimate goal is to discover whether some of these novel cell surface markers could be substitutes for the current CIS point variables, ESR and CRP, which would help produce a novel and rapid flow cytometric bacterial infection tool that would be able to distinguish between bacterial and viral infections in approximately 1 hour. We are currently in the process of patenting a suitable method (patent pending).

The following conclusions can be drawn from our research results so far:

1. The clinical usefulness of individually measured variables increases upon combination (*e.g.* the CD64 score point, CIS point, DNAVS point, and CRP/CD11b RATIO). [17, 18, 27, 28, 30, 38].

2. Although the high number of FcγRI on neutrophils is a sensitive marker of bacterial infection, these receptors are also highly expressed in DNA virus infections. As a result, neutrophil FcγRI cannot be used to distinguish between bacterial (either Gram-positive or Gram negative) and viral infections. [17, 18].

3. FcγRI on neutrophils cannot be used to reliably detect RNA virus infections, inflammatory diseases, and cancer [38, 75].

4. The best clinical benefit using the quantitative analysis of neutrophil FcγRI is obtained when the results are combined with a reliable marker of bacterial infection, such as the CIS point method [38].

5. The DNAVS point is an efficient method for differentiating between DNA and RNA virus infections [18].

6. The CRP/CD11b RATIO is an efficient method for differentiating between Gram-positive and Gram-negative bacterial infections [28].

REFERENCES

[1] Livermore DM. Minimising antibiotic resistance. Lancet Infect Dis 2005; 5: 450-459.

[2] French GL. Clinical impact and relevance of antibiotic resistance. Adv Drug Deliv Rev 2005; 57: 1514-1527.

[3] Gould IM. Costs of hospital-acquired methicillin-resistant *Staphylococcus aureus* (MRSA) and its control. Int J Antimicrob Agents 2006; 28: 379-384.

[4] Lutfiyya MN, Henley E, Chang LF, Reyburn SW. Diagnosis and treatment of community-acquired pneumonia. Am Fam Physician 2006; 73: 442-450.

[5] Mandell LA, Bartlett JG, Dowell SF, File TM, Jr., Musher DM, Whitney C. Update of practice guidelines for the management of community-acquired pneumonia in immunocompetent adults. Clin Infect Dis 2003; 37: 1405-1433.

[6] Korppi M, Heiskanen-Kosma T, Leinonen M. White blood cells, C-reactive protein and erythrocyte sedimentation rate in pneumococcal pneumonia in children. Eur Respir J 1997; 10: 1125-1129.

[7] Ng PC, Li K, Wong RP, Chui KM, Wong E, Fok TF. Neutrophil CD64 expression: a sensitive diagnostic marker for late-onset nosocomial infection in very low birthweight infants. Pediatr Res 2002; 51: 296-303.

[8] Wang SS, Lee FY, Chan CC, *et al.* Sequential changes in plasma cytokine and endotoxin levels in cirrhotic patients with bacterial infection. Clin Sci (Lond) 2000; 98: 419-425.

[9] Fischer JE, Benn A, Harbarth S, Nadal D, Fanconi S. Diagnostic accuracy of G-CSF, IL-8, and IL-1ra in critically ill children with suspected infection. Intensive Care Med 2002; 28: 1324-1331.

[10] Kitanovski L, Jazbec J, Hojker S, Gubina M, Derganc M. Diagnostic accuracy of procalcitonin and interleukin-6 values for predicting bacteremia and clinical sepsis in febrile neutropenic children with cancer. Eur J Clin Microbiol Infect Dis 2006; 25: 413-415.

[11] Mukai AO, Krebs VL, Bertoli CJ, Okay TS. TNF-alpha and IL-6 in the diagnosis of bacterial and aseptic meningitis in children. Pediatr Neurol 2006; 34: 25-29.

[12] El Solh A, Pineda L, Bouquin P, Mankowski C. Determinants of short and long term functional recovery after hospitalization for community-acquired pneumonia in the elderly: role of inflammatory markers. BMC Geriatr 2006; 6: 12.

[13] Davis BH, Olsen SH, Ahmad E, Bigelow NC. Neutrophil CD64 is an improved indicator of infection or sepsis in emergency department patients. Arch Pathol Lab Med 2006; 130: 654-661.

[14] Fjaertoft G, Pauksen K, Hakansson L, Xu S, Venge P. Cell surface expression of FcgammaRI (CD64) on neutrophils and monocytes in patients with influenza A, with and without complications. Scand J Infect Dis 2005; 37: 882-889.

[15] Leino L, Sorvajarvi K, Katajisto J, *et al.* Febrile infection changes the expression of IgG Fc receptors and complement receptors in human neutrophils *in vivo*. Clin Exp Immunol 1997; 107: 37-43.

[16] Hohenthal U, Nuutila J, Lilius EM, Laitinen I, Nikoskelainen J, Kotilainen P. Measurement of complement receptor 1 on neutrophils in bacterial and viral pneumonia. BMC Infect Dis 2006; 6: 11.

[17] Nuutila J, Hohenthal U, Laitinen I, *et al.* Simultaneous quantitative analysis of FcgammaRI (CD64) expression on neutrophils and monocytes: A new, improved way to detect infections. J Immunol Methods 2007; 328: 189-200.

[18] Nuutila J, Hohenthal U, Laitinen I, *et al.* A novel method for distinguishing between dsDNA and ssRNA virus infections. J Clin Virol 2008; 43: 49-55.

[19] Dubos F, Moulin F, Gajdos V, *et al.* Serum procalcitonin and other biologic markers to distinguish between bacterial and aseptic meningitis. J Pediatr 2006; 149: 72-76.

[20] Pecile P, Miorin E, Romanello C, *et al.* Procalcitonin: a marker of severity of acute pyelonephritis among children. Pediatrics 2004; 114: e249-254.

[21] van Rossum AM, Wulkan RW, Oudesluys-Murphy AM. Procalcitonin as an early marker of infection in neonates and children. Lancet Infect Dis 2004; 4: 620-630.

[22] Shapiro HM, Practical flow cytometry, 3rd ed. New York: Wiley-Liss, 1995.

[23] Allen E, Bakke AC, Purtzer MZ, Deodhar A. Neutrophil CD64 expression: distinguishing acute inflammatory autoimmune disease from systemic infections. Ann Rheum Dis 2002; 61: 522-525.

[24] Gratama JW, D'Hautcourt J L, Mandy F, *et al.* Flow cytometric quantitation of immunofluorescence intensity: problems and perspectives. European Working Group on Clinical Cell Analysis. Cytometry 1998; 33: 166-178.

[25] Gallin JI, Snyderman R, Inflammation: basic principles and clinical correlates, 3rd ed. Philadelphia, PA: Lippincott Williams & Wilkins, 1999.

[26] Jalava-Karvinen P, Hohenthal U, Laitinen I, *et al.* Simultaneous quantitative analysis of FcgammaRI (CD64) and CR1 (CD35) on neutrophils in distinguishing between bacterial infections, viral infections, and inflammatory diseases. Clin Immunol 2009.

[27] Nuutila J, Hohenthal U, Laitinen I, *et al.* Quantitative analysis of complement receptors, CR1 (CD35) and CR3 (CD11b), on neutrophils improves distinction between bacterial and viral infections in febrile patients: Comparison with standard clinical laboratory data. J Immunol Methods 2006; 315: 191-201.

[28] Nuutila J, Jalava-Karvinen P, Hohenthal U, *et al.* CRP/CD11b ratio: a novel parameter for detecting gram-positive sepsis. Hum Immunol 2009; 70: 237-243.

[29] Nuutila J, Jalava-Karvinen P, Hohenthal U, *et al.* Comparison of degranulation of easily mobilizable intracellular granules by human phagocytes in healthy subjects and patients with infectious diseases. Hum Immunol 2009.

[30] Nuutila J, Lilius EM. Distinction between bacterial and viral infections. Curr Opin Infect Dis 2007; 20: 304-310.

[31] Lilius EM, Nuutila JT. Particle-induced myeloperoxidase release in serially diluted whole blood quantifies the number and the phagocytic activity of blood neutrophils and opsonization capacity of plasma. Luminescence 2006; 21: 148-158.

[32] Salminen E, Kankuri M, Nuutila J, Lilius EM, Pellimiemi TT. Modulation of IgG and complement receptor expression of phagocytes in kidney cancer patients during treatment with interferon-alpha. Anticancer Res 2001; 21: 2049-2055.

[33] Gronlund MM, Nuutila J, Pelto L, *et al.* Mode of delivery directs the phagocyte functions of infants for the first 6 months of life. Clin Exp Immunol 1999; 116: 521-526.

[34] Isolauri E, Pelto L, Nuutila J, Majamaa H, Lilius EM, Salminen S. Altered expression of IgG and complement receptors indicates a significant role of phagocytes in atopic dermatitis. J Allergy Clin Immunol 1997; 99: 707-713.

[35] Pelto L, Isolauri E, Lilius EM, Nuutila J, Salminen S. Probiotic bacteria down-regulate the milk-induced inflammatory response in milk-hypersensitive subjects but have an immunostimulatory effect in healthy subjects. Clin Exp Allergy 1998; 28: 1474-1479.

[36] Pelto L, Salminen S, Lilius EM, Nuutila J, Isolauri E. Milk hypersensitivity--key to poorly defined gastrointestinal symptoms in adults. Allergy 1998; 53: 307-310.

[37] Nuutila J, Lilius EM. Flow cytometric quantitative determination of ingestion by phagocytes needs the distinguishing of overlapping populations of binding and ingesting cells. Cytometry A 2005; 65: 93-102.

[38] Jalava-Karvinen P, Hohenthal U, Laitinen I, *et al.* Simultaneous quantitative analysis of Fc gamma RI (CD64) and CR1 (CD35) on neutrophils in distinguishing between bacterial infections, viral infections, and inflammatory diseases. Clin Immunol 2009; 133: 314-323.

[39] Gabay C, Kushner I. Acute-phase proteins and other systemic responses to inflammation. N Engl J Med 1999; 340: 448-454.

[40] Svanborg C, Godaly G, Hedlund M. Cytokine responses during mucosal infections: role in disease pathogenesis and host defence. Curr Opin Microbiol 1999; 2: 99-105.

[41] Hallett MB, Lloyds D. Neutrophil priming: the cellular signals that say 'amber' but not 'green'. Immunol Today 1995; 16: 264-268.

[42] Colotta F, Re F, Polentarutti N, Sozzani S, Mantovani A. Modulation of granulocyte survival and programmed cell death by cytokines and bacterial products. Blood 1992; 80: 2012-2020.

[43] Etzioni A. Adhesion molecules--their role in health and disease. Pediatr Res 1996; 39: 191-198.

[44] Elghetany MT. Surface antigen changes during normal neutrophilic development: a critical review. Blood Cells Mol Dis 2002; 28: 260-274.

[45] Krych M, Hauhart R, Atkinson JP. Structure-function analysis of the active sites of complement receptor type 1. J Biol Chem 1998; 273: 8623-8629.

[46] Tas SW, Klickstein LB, Barbashov SF, Nicholson-Weller A. C1q and C4b bind simultaneously to CR1 and additively support erythrocyte adhesion. J Immunol 1999; 163: 5056-5063.

[47] Oxvig C, Springer TA. Experimental support for a beta-propeller domain in integrin alpha- subunits and a calcium binding site on its lower surface. Proc Natl Acad Sci U S A 1998; 95: 4870-4875.

[48] Lee JO, Rieu P, Arnaout MA, Liddington R. Crystal structure of the A domain from the alpha subunit of integrin CR3 (CD11b/CD18). Cell 1995; 80: 631-638.

[49] Zhou L, Lee DH, Plescia J, Lau CY, Altieri DC. Differential ligand binding specificities of recombinant CD11b/CD18 integrin I-domain. J Biol Chem 1994; 269: 17075-17079.

[50] Ueda T, Rieu P, Brayer J, Arnaout MA. Identification of the complement iC3b binding site in the beta 2 integrin CR3 (CD11b/CD18). Proc Natl Acad Sci U S A 1994; 91: 10680-10684.

[51] Forsyth CB, Plow EF, Zhang L. Interaction of the fungal pathogen *Candida albicans* with integrin CD11b/CD18: recognition by the I domain is modulated by the lectin-like domain and the CD18 subunit. J Immunol 1998; 161: 6198-6205.

[52] Zhang L, Plow EF. Identification and reconstruction of the binding site within alphaMbeta2 for a specific and high affinity ligand, NIF. J Biol Chem 1997; 272: 17558-17564.

[53] Thornton BP, Vetvicka V, Pitman M, Goldman RC, Ross GD. Analysis of the sugar specificity and molecular location of the beta- glucan-binding lectin site of complement receptor type 3 (CD11b/CD18). J Immunol 1996; 156: 1235-1246.

[54] Xia Y, Vetvicka V, Yan J, Hanikyrova M, Mayadas T, Ross GD. The beta-glucan-binding lectin site of mouse CR3 (CD11b/CD18) and its function in generating a primed state of the receptor that mediates cytotoxic activation in response to iC3b-opsonized target cells. J Immunol 1999; 162: 2281-2290.

[55] van de Winkel JG, Capel PJ. Human IgG Fc receptor heterogeneity: molecular aspects and clinical implications. Immunol Today 1993; 14: 215-221.

[56] Zhou MJ, Brown EJ. CR3 (Mac-1, alpha M beta 2, CD11b/CD18) and Fc gamma RIII cooperate in generation of a neutrophil respiratory burst: requirement for Fc gamma RIII and tyrosine phosphorylation. J Cell Biol 1994; 125: 1407-1416.

[57] Worth RG, Mayo-Bond L, van de Winkel JG, Todd RF, 3rd, Petty HR. CR3 (alphaM beta2; CD11b/CD18) restores IgG-dependent phagocytosis in transfectants expressing a phagocytosis-defective Fc gammaRIIA (CD32) tail-minus mutant. J Immunol 1996; 157: 5660-5665.

[58] Heit B, Colarusso P, Kubes P. Fundamentally different roles for LFA-1, Mac-1 and alpha4-integrin in neutrophil chemotaxis. J Cell Sci 2005; 118: 5205-5220.

[59] Kim DD, Song WC. Membrane complement regulatory proteins. Clin Immunol 2006; 118: 127-136.

[60] Mqadmi A, Abdullah Y, Yazdanbakhsh K. Characterization of complement receptor 1 domains for prevention of complement-mediated red cell destruction. Transfusion 2005; 45: 234-244.

[61] Pugin J, Auckenthaler R, Mili N, Janssens JP, Lew PD, Suter PM. Diagnosis of ventilator-associated pneumonia by bacteriologic analysis of bronchoscopic and nonbronchoscopic "blind" bronchoalveolar lavage fluid. Am Rev Respir Dis 1991; 143: 1121-1129.

[62] Bochud PY, Bonten M, Marchetti O, Calandra T. Antimicrobial therapy for patients with severe sepsis and septic shock: an evidence-based review. Crit Care Med 2004; 32: S495-512.

[63] Martin GS, Mannino DM, Eaton S, Moss M. The epidemiology of sepsis in the United States from 1979 through 2000. N Engl J Med 2003; 348: 1546-1554.

[64] Luna CM, Vujacich P, Niederman MS, *et al.* Impact of BAL data on the therapy and outcome of ventilator-associated pneumonia. Chest 1997; 111: 676-685.

[65] Gosselin EJ, Wardwell K, Gosselin DR, Alter N, Fisher JL, Guyre PM. Enhanced antigen presentation using human Fc gamma receptor (monocyte/macrophage)-specific immunogens. J Immunol 1992; 149: 3477-3481.

[66] Bharadwaj D, Stein MP, Volzer M, Mold C, Du Clos TW. The major receptor for C-reactive protein on leukocytes is fcgamma receptor II. J Exp Med 1999; 190: 585-590.

[67] Marnell LL, Mold C, Volzer MA, Burlingame RW, Du Clos TW. C-reactive protein binds to Fc gamma RI in transfected COS cells. J Immunol 1995; 155: 2185-2193.

[68] Davis W, Harrison PT, Hutchinson MJ, Allen JM. Two distinct regions of FC gamma RI initiate separate signalling pathways involved in endocytosis and phagocytosis. Embo J 1995; 14: 432-441.

[69] Indik Z, Chien P, Levinson AI, Schreiber AD. Calcium signalling by the high affinity macrophage Fc gamma receptor requires the cytosolic domain. Immunobiology 1992; 185: 183-192.

[70] van Vugt MJ, Heijnen AF, Capel PJ, *et al.* FcR gamma-chain is essential for both surface expression and function of human Fc gamma RI (CD64) *in vivo.* Blood 1996; 87: 3593-3599.

[71] Harrison PT, Bjorkhaug L, Hutchinson MJ, Allen JM. The interaction between human Fc gamma RI and the gamma-chain is mediated solely *via* the 21 amino acid transmembrane domain of Fc gamma RI. Mol Membr Biol 1995; 12: 309-312.

[72] Quayle JA, Watson F, Bucknall RC, Edwards SW. Neutrophils from the synovial fluid of patients with rheumatoid arthritis express the high affinity immunoglobulin G receptor, Fc gamma RI (CD64): role of immune complexes and cytokines in induction of receptor expression. Immunology 1997; 91: 266-273.

[73] Gericke GH, Ericson SG, Pan L, Mills LE, Guyre PM, Ely P. Mature polymorphonuclear leukocytes express high-affinity receptors for IgG (Fc gamma RI) after stimulation with granulocyte colony-stimulating factor (G-CSF). J Leukoc Biol 1995; 57: 455-461.

[74] van de Winkel JG, Anderson CL. Biology of human immunoglobulin G Fc receptors. J Leukoc Biol 1991; 49: 511-524.

[75] Nuutila J. The novel applications of the quantitative analysis of neutrophil cell surface FcgammaRI (CD64) to the diagnosis of infectious and inflammatory diseases. Curr Opin Infect Dis 2010; 23: 268-274.

[76] Gessl A, Willheim M, Spittler A, Agis H, Krugluger W, Boltz-Nitulescu G. Influence of tumour necrosis factor-alpha on the expression of Fc IgG and IgA receptors, and other markers by cultured human blood monocytes and U937 cells. Scand J Immunol 1994; 39: 151-156.

[77] Wagner C, Deppisch R, Denefleh B, Hug F, Andrassy K, Hansch GM. Expression patterns of the lipopolysaccharide receptor CD14, and the FCgamma receptors CD16 and CD64 on polymorphonuclear neutrophils: data from patients with severe bacterial infections and lipopolysaccharide-exposed cells. Shock 2003; 19: 5-12.

[78] Garibaldi RA, Brodine S, Matsumiya S, Coleman M. Evidence for the non-infectious etiology of early postoperative fever. Infect Control 1985; 6: 273-277.

[79] Fanning J, Neuhoff RA, Brewer JE, Castaneda T, Marcotte MP, Jacobson RL. Frequency and yield of postoperative fever evaluation. Infect Dis Obstet Gynecol 1998; 6: 252-255.

[80] Shaw JA, Chung R. Febrile response after knee and hip arthroplasty. Clin Orthop Relat Res 1999: 181-189.

[81] Hewlett G, Hallenberger S, Rubsamen-Waigmann H. Antivirals against DNA viruses (hepatitis B and the herpes viruses). Curr Opin Pharmacol 2004; 4: 453-464.

[82] Jefferson T, Demicheli V, Rivetti D, Jones M, Di Pietrantonj C, Rivetti A. Antivirals for influenza in healthy adults: systematic review. Lancet 2006; 367: 303-313.

[83] Wainberg MA. The emergence of HIV and new antiretrovirals: are we winning? Drug Resist Update 2004; 7: 163-167.

CHAPTER 9

Bead-Based Flow-Cytometry in Medical Microbiological Research and Diagnosis

N.J. Verkaik*, C.P. de Vogel, W. J.B. van W. and A. van Belkum

Department of Medical Microbiology & Infectious Diseases, Erasmus Medical Center, Rotterdam, The Netherlands.

Abstract: Bead-based flow cytometry (xMAP® and xTAG® Technology, Luminex Corporation) is a recently developed technology that allows for simultaneous quantification of multiple antibodies, antigens or oligonucleotides in a single sample. The newest generation of analyzers allow multiplexing of up to 500 unique tests within a single sample, which renders this technique much less time-consuming than conventional testing methodsologies. Numerous applications have already been developed for this technology in both medical microbiological research and diagnosis, with the number of reported applications still growing rapidly. Bead-based flow-cytometry has already firmly established itself as a supplemental and/or alternative technology to the more traditional routine diagnostic and research microbiology test platforms.

Keywords: Flow Cytometry, Luminex, XMap, Bead-based, Median Intensity Fluorescence, Immunity.

1. INTRODUCTION

Two topics are specially important when treating infectious diseases. First, it is essential to know which micro-organism is causing the infection, and second, it is important to know the patient's immune status in relation to the causative agent. With respect to microorganism detection, the causative agent may be identified using both traditional and modern direct detection techniques, such as bacterial culture and PCR-related genetic amplification techniques. With respect to patient immunity, the patient's immune status may be determined by measuring his/her humoral (antibody mediated) immunity using a variety of technologies, most of which were established as laboratory tools during the 1980's. These technologies include a variety of immunodiffusion tests, membrane-based Western blot assays and Enzyme Linked Immunosorbent Assays (ELISAs) [1]. Of these, it is the latter ELISA technology that is still most often associated with microbiological research and diagnosis, with individual ELISA test kits having been developed in a wide range of both antibody and antigen-specific test formats. Many of these test kits were developed by large-scale manufacturers and have now become successfully introduced into the microbiological market. However, though currently very successful, ELISA technology itself actually possesses some major disadvantages. These include: a) the requirement for a relatively large amount of test material (serum or other body fluid); b) a time-consuming protocol; and c) limitations with respect to the simultaneous testing of several different antigens or antibodies within a single test reaction (*i.e.* multiplex applications). In recent years however, these technological limitations have been largely overcome by the introduction of a new innovative bead-based immunofluorescence technology, the so-called xMAP® and xTAG® Technology (Luminex Corporation, Austin, Texas, USA). In general, xMAP® technology allows the detection of poly(peptides), (poly)saccharides, oligo-nucleotides, antigens and antibodies, whilst xTAG® technology allows the detection of nucleic acids (including viral genomes). Both technologies utilize a novel approach to overcome the disadvantages associated with ELISA-based test formats, as they both require small volumes of sera (or other body fluids), provide time savings with respect to microbiological diagnosis, and allow multiple antibodies and antigens to be tested simultaneously in the same sample (multiplexing testing is easy to perform).

*Address correspondence to N.J. Verkaik: Erasmus Medical Centre Rotterdam, Department of Medical Microbiology & Infectious Diseases's -Gravendijkwal 230, 3015 CE Rotterdam, The Netherlands. Email: n.j.verkaik@erasmusmc.nl

John P. Hays and W. B. van Leeuwen (Eds)

2. THE PRINCIPLE OF LUMINEX TECHNOLOGY

Luminex technology facilitates the use of low sample volumes and multiplex formats *via* specially designed, color-coded beads or "microspheres". These beads are 5.6 microns in diameter and internally color coded using 2 different fluorophores. By mixing the 2 fluorophores at different intensities, and then filling different batches of beads with the different fluorophore mixes, it is possible to create a set of approximately 100 (100-plex) distinguishable beads, each possessing its own spectral signature. Each of these 100 bead types can then be coated with specific biological materials and combined for multiplex testing applications. The coated beads (currently, antigens are the main biological coating material used) are then mixed with the test analyte *e.g.* a patient serum sample, so that interactions can take place between the antigen-bead and analyte components (the antigen coated bead is used to specifically capture antibodies present within the sample). After washing, a specific reporter molecule (*e.g.* a secondary anti-IgG antibody, labelled with a fluorescent dye) is added to the beads in order to detect the presence or absence of bound analyte components (in this case bound antibody) on the bead surface (Fig. **1A**). After re-washing, the beads are analysed using a flow cytometer equipped with two lasers. The first (red) laser excites the internal dyes present within the beads, and the second (green) laser excites the fluorescent dye on the reporter molecule (Fig. **1B**). High-speed digital-signal processors then identify each individually colored bead and determine whether the reporter molecule is attached to the surface of the bead, based on the presence/absence of a fluorescent reporter signal. The results are then reported in "Median Fluorescence Intensity" (MFI) values. Currently, the Luminex® flow cytometer can read 100 different color-coded beads, meaning that theoretically at least 100 different tests can be performed simultaneously on each sample. Further, using a 96-well microtiter plate for the analyses, means that theoretically 100 assays can be performed on 96 samples, producing 9,600 assay results within a very short period of time [2-4].

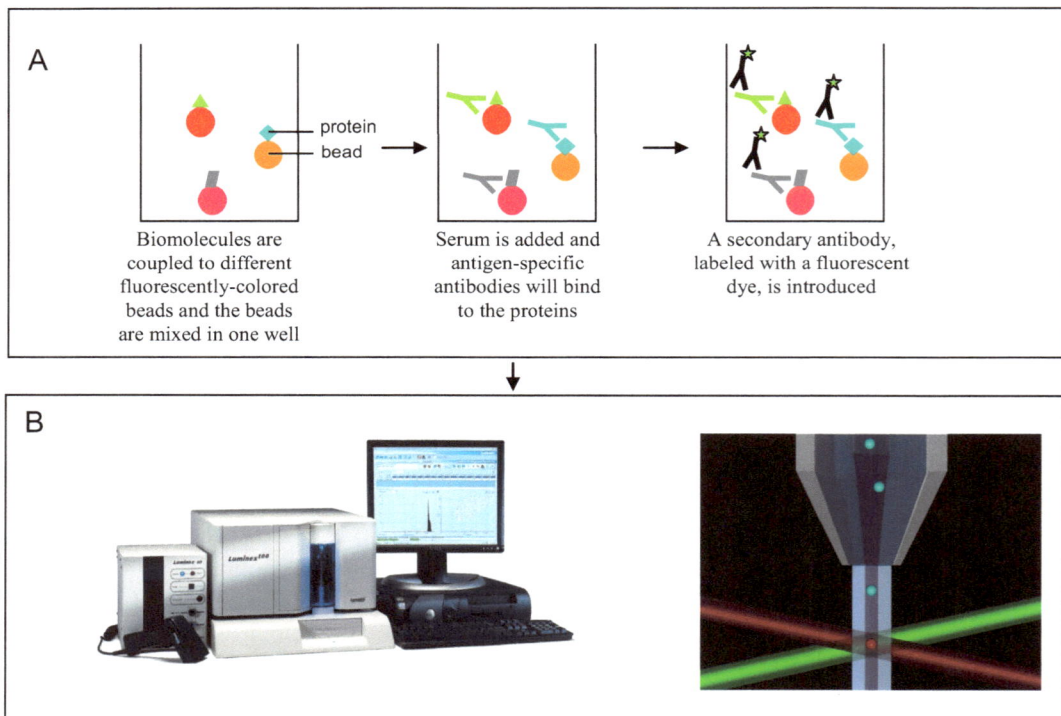

Fig. (1). Principle of the commercially available Luminex® bead-based flow cytometry system for simultaneous multiplex assay testing. **[A]** Flow of operations required for detecting specific antibodies in patient serum using antigen coupled beads. Black arrows indicate washing steps. **[B]** Assays are read using a compact analyzer, *e.g.* the Luminex® 100/200 system. The analyzer samples the well of a 96-well plate, beads passing rapidly through two lasers comprising a red laser for bead identification, and a green laser for the determination of fluorescence intensity (signal strength being determined by the presence/absence of bound fluorescently labelled secondary antibody attached to the bead). **[B]** is adapted from http://www.luminexcorp.com/products/index.html with permission.

3. MEDICAL MICROBIOLOGICAL APPLICATIONS

The majority of current applications for xMAP® and xTAG® bead-based flow cytometry technologies involve human-based research and diagnostics, including protein expression profiling (markers of human disease, cytokine measurement, metabolic markers), the diagnosis of genetic disease (cytochrome p450 and cystic fibrosis), and immunodiagnostics (autoimmune and HLA testing). In contrast, the application of bead-based flow cytometry techniques in medical microbiology research and diagnosis has been demonstrated for relatively fewer applications, though the number of articles published in this field is increasing exponentially. Further, many of these published applications are being directly adapted from the research to the diagnostic microbiology field.

Bead-based flow cytometry technology may be utilised to detect both microbial antigens and microbial-directed antibodies. For example, Luminex® technology may be used for the rapid identification of antigens or oligonucleotide sequences from fungi, parasites and bacteria, including *Aspergillus* species [5], *Cryptococcus neoformans* and *Cryptococcus gatti* [6], *Salmonella* species [7], *Cryptosporidium hominis* and *Cryptosporidium parvum* [8], vaginal microbiota [9], *Vibrio* species [10], *Plasmodium* species [11], *Candida albicans, Candida krusei, Candida parapsilosis, Candida glabrata, and Candida tropicalis* [12]. Further, with respect to the detection of antibodies, the technique may be useful in measuring the presence or absence of antibodies directed against a wide variety of microorganisms including human papillomavirus [13], West Nile virus [14], *Mycobacterium tuberculosis* [15], Epstein-Barr virus gp78 antigen [16], avian influenza virus [17], HIV, Hepatitis A and B [18], *Streptococcus mutans* glucosyltransferase (Gtf) / glucan binding protein B (GbpB) [19], tetanus, diphtheria, *Haemophilus influenzae* B [20], *Neisseria meningitidis* serogroup A, C, Y and W-135 [21] and pneumococcal polysaccharides [22, 23]. Further, new bead-based antibody detection protocols are continually being developed, often involving multiplex applications for the detection of many different microbial antibodies within a single diagnostic experiment (Table **1**). Finally, the use of secondary (detection) antibodies directed against different isotypes of antibody (including anti-IgG, anti-IgM, anti-IgA, anti-IgD and anti-IgE), as well as the use of secondary antibodies against immunoglobulin subtypes (anti-IgA1, antiIgG2, anti-IgG4 etc), allows investigations to be performed relating to the development of, for example, the immune response against acute infections, mucosal immunity and the development of antibody subtypes with age.

4. BEAD-BASED FLOW CYTOMETRY IN MEDICAL MICROBIOLOGICAL RESEARCH

In our own laboratory (Department of Medical Microbiology and Infectious Diseases, Erasmus MC, Rotterdam, The Netherlands), bead-based flow-cytometry technology has been extensively utilized to measure antibodies directed against several major pathogens, including *Staphylococcus aureus, Haemophilus influenzae* and *Moraxella catarrhalis*. With respect to *S. aureus*, we have developed a multiplex assay to simultaneously measure the antibody response to 40 different antigens of *S. aureus*, including the comparison of anti-staphylococcal antibody levels in healthy persistent carriers versus non-carriers of *S. aureus*. Although the antibody profiles were quite unique to each individual, we were able to identify characteristic differences in humoral response between these 2 groups [24]. In another investigation, we used the technology to study the anti-*S. aureus* humoral immune response in a longitudinal collection of sera from young children. Again, we were able to show that antibody profiles varied extensively between individuals, with IgA and IgM levels clearly increasing over the first 2 years after birth and maternal IgG antibodies decreasing steeply during the first six months of life. Additionally, maternal antibody levels did not appear to provide protection against *S. aureus* colonization, indicating that that several staphylococcal virulence factors are produced during the first confrontation between child and *S. aureus* [25]. Finally, we compared differences in anti-toxin antibodies generated by individuals suffering from distinct staphylococcal infections (bacteraemia, soft tissue-, respiratory tract-, and joint infections) and in patient controls [26]. Significantly elevated levels of antibodies against many *S. aureus* toxins were observed in infected patients as opposed to patient controls (Fig. **2**), suggesting that the production of these toxins are at least involved in the pathogenesis of *S. aureus* infections [26]. The basic methodology utilised in our own research is generally applicable to all medical microbiological research that utilises bead-based cytometry, and is briefly described below (pages 158 – 160) in Boxes 1 and 2. The first step involves the development of a multiplex immunoassay *via* the coupling of biomolecules *e.g.* specific microbial antigens, to microspheres (described in Box 1). Next, the multiplex assay (containing multiple antigens each attached to a specific colour-coded microsphere) is validated by comparing the MFI values (median fluorescent intensity signal) obtained using the new multiplex assay and a standard serum pool (for example human pooled serum), to the results obtained using individual singleplex assays and the same standard serum pool. The MFI values obtained for each antigen in the multiplex assay should be approximately 100% of the MFI values obtained using each antigen in its own singleplex assay. After coupling and validation, the precision of the assay should be determined, including both intra- and inter-assay variation. Intra-assay variation should be ideally determined by testing (at least) 10 serum samples, each sample assayed in three or four wells within a plate.

Table 1: Some of the infectious disease antibodies that can be detected in a multiplex format using Luminex® xMAP® technology.

Bacteria-Related	Virus-Related	
Bordetella pertussis	Adenovirus	HPV
Campylobacter jejuni	Cytomegalovirus	HSV-1 gD
Chlamydia pneumoniae	Ectromelia virus	HSV-1/2
Chlamydia trachomatis	Encephalitozoon cuniculi	HSV-2 gG
Cholera Toxin	Epstein-Barr EA	HTLV-1/2
Cholera Toxin b	Epstein-Barr NA	Influenza A
Clostridium piliforme	Epstein-Barr VCA	Influenza A H3N2
Diphtheria Toxin	HBV Core	Influenza B
Helicobacter pylori	HBV Envelope	Minute virus
Leishmania donovani	HBV Surface (Ad)	Mumps
Mycoplasma pneumoniae	HBV Surface (Ay)	Parainfluenza 1
Mycobacterium tuberculosis	HCV Core	Parainfluenza 2
Mycoplasma pulmonis	HCV NS3	Parainfluenza 3
Trypanosoma cruzi	HCV NS4	Parvovirus
Treponema pallidum 15kd	HCV NS5	Polio Virus
Treponema pallidum p47	Hepatitis A	Polyoma virus
Tetanus Toxin	Hepatitis D	Reovirus-3
Toxoplasma spp.	HEV orf2 3KD	RSV
	HEV orf2 6KD	Rubella
	HEV orf3 3KD	Rubeola
	HIV-1 gp120	Sendai virus
	HIV-1 gp41	Varicella zoster
	HIV-1 p24	

Adapted from http://www.luminexcorp.com/applications/infectious_disease.html with permission.

In contrast, inter-assay variation should be ideally determined by testing 10 serum samples on different days. To determine the inter-laboratory reproducibility, tests need to be performed at different sites (*in house* and in independent laboratories) using the same instruments. For this purpose, the use of a standardized serum sample (or ideally a panel of standardized serum samples) is recommended. As specificity controls, beads to which no antigenic protein has been coupled should be used in every experiment, in order to determine whether non-specific antibody binding is taking place. Further, in the case of non-specific binding, the non-specific binding MFI values should be subtracted from the antigen-specific results in order to account for the background "noise" of the system. Of course, if this noise approaches the signal generated by a weak positive sample, then the assay itself may have to be re-designed. In this respect, the availability of serum panels containing weak, intermediate and strong antibody responses will be invaluable. In addition, Phosphate Buffered Saline (PBS) should be incubated with antigen-coupled beads as controls in each experiment. This will control the effectiveness of the washing steps in removing secondary-labelled antibodies prior to fluorescence measurement.

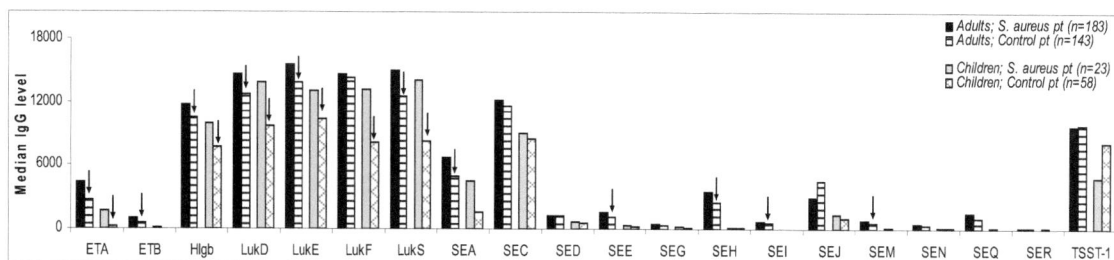

Fig. (2). Toxin-specific IgG levels in *S. aureus*-infected patients and control patients. IgG levels are reflected by Median Fluorescence Intensity (MFI) values. Results are shown for adults and children separately. Statistically significant differences are indicated by black arrows (Mann Whitney *U* test; *P*<0.05). ET, exfoliative toxin; HlgB, γ hemolysin B; Luk, leukocidin; SE, staphylococcal enterotoxin; TSST-1, toxic shock syndrome toxin-1. Anti-staphylococcal IgG levels are higher in adults than children and IgG levels are higher in *S. aureus*-infected patients than in hospital-admitted controls. This suggests that the anti-staphylococcal humoral immune state of an individual develops over the years and probably depends on the history of confrontations with *S. aureus*. Figure adapted in part from the article "Immunogenicity of toxins during *Staphylococcus aureus* infection", Clinical Infectious Diseases 2010; 50: 61-68, © 2009 by the Infectious Diseases Society of America [26].

MFI Values or Antibody Concentration? If it is important to determine the actual concentration of antibodies within samples (instead of MFI values), a calibration curve should be made in which the unknown sample is compared to a set of standardized samples containing known (low, intermediate and high) concentrations of relevant antibodies. Calibration should be performed for every antigen in the multiplex assay, and also whenever a new set of coupled beads is used. This is because of the differences in coupling efficiency that occur between individual coupling reactions, and the fact that some antigens may couple better than other antigens to their respectively colored beads (due to for example differences in antigen molecular weights).

5. BEAD-BASED FLOW CYTOMETRY

In Medical Microbiological Diagnostics

Two major applications for bead-based flow cytometry in medical microbiological diagnostic laboratories have been currently described, these include: 1) the determination of the immune response to pneumococal vaccination; and 2) the detection of viral respiratory infections.

Pneumococcal Immunity – *Streptococcus pneumonia* is one of the major causes of pneumonia and meningitis. In developing countries, the mortality attributed to pneumonia is significant. Between 2002 and 2003, pneumonia accounted for 19% of the 10.6 million yearly deaths among children younger than 5 years of age [27]. Further, vaccination can substantially reduce the risk of infection, especially in young children. A bead-based pneumococcal multiplex assay has been developed that simultaneously measures the IgG response to 14 different pneumococcal serotypes per serum sample, and provides data on the success or failure of pneumococcal vaccination strategies. This multiplex technique was evaluated by independent researchers who found that a pneumococcal immunity panel was useful in identifying low-responders to unconjugated pneumococcal vaccine [28].

The Detection of Respiratory Infections – Respiratory infections are among the most common infectious diseases of humans worldwide and cause significant morbidity. Clinical diagnosis is difficult, because a wide variety of respiratory viruses cause diseases that present with overlapping clinical symptoms. In this context, a bead-based respiratory virus panel (RVP) has been developed (see http://www.luminexcorp.com/rvp/overview.html) that allows the detection of 12 (FDA cleared) or 19 (CE marked) different respiratory virus families and subtypes, including (Para)Influenza, Respiratory Syncytial Virus, Metapneumovirus, Rhinovirus and Adenovirus. The process of testing this RVP panel involves xTAG® technology (see http://www.xtagrvp.com). Basically, a nasopharyngeal swab is taken, nucleic acids are isolated, and the nucleic acids amplified using a multiplex Polymerase Chain Reaction (PCR). The amplified genetic material is then combined with a mixture of short sequence primer DNA (a 'TAG') that is specific for each viral target. If genetic material derived from a particular virus is present, then the specific primer will bind to the viral genetic material and be lengthened *via* a process called "target specific primer extension". During this process, a label is also attached to the specifically extended primer. The labelled genetic material is then added to a mixture of color-coded beads, where each colour is specific for a particular virus type or subtype (*via* the presence of a complementary anti-TAG sequence). The multiplexed sample and beads are then mixed and the results read using a flow-cytometer to detect the colour of the bead (virus type or subtype), as well as the presence or absence of an associated label (presence or absence of specific viral genetic material) [2, 3]. Of course, one of the major advantages of this type of technology is the fact that the whole process can be multiplexed, saving both time and money compared to many traditional and modern virus detection techniques. A report from the Provincial Laboratory for Public Health Microbiology, Alberta, Canada, stated that the RVP assay sensitivity for viral targets was good (though the assay had a lower sensitivity than their in house nucleic acid amplification tests for the detection of adenovirus) [29]. Further, Krunic *et al.* concluded that RVP testing was comparable in analytical sensitivity to RT-PCR nucleic acid amplification methods [30]. For further information on this topic, the reader is referred to a range of articles published in the Journal of Clinical Virology, Volume 40, Supplement 1, Pages S1-S60 (October 2007), "Respiratory Viral Diagnostics – The Pathogens, the Challenges and the Solutions - Introducing the xTAG™ Respiratory Viral Panel".

6. CURRENT ADVANCES AND FUTURE PERSPECTIVES

Recently, a new bead-based cytometric analyzer was introduced to the market, the FLEXMAP 3D™ (Luminex Corporation, Austin, Texas, USA). In this system, each bead is color-coded with three instead of two internal dyes (red, infra red and orange red). Monitoring the relative intensity of the 3 signals allows the system to (theoretically) discriminate between up to 500 different multiplexed bead sets (instead of the previous 100 multiplex range). The 500 bead sets are combined with an instrument that enables multiplexing of up to 500 analytes in a single reaction well, allowing users to run up to 64,000 tests in 45 min (see http://www.luminexcorp.com/pdfs/177_FLEXMAP_TP_TS.pdf). Of course, increasing the multiplex capacity of assays will require extensive optimization and validation prior to universal acceptance in routine clinical diagnostic microbiology laboratories. However, it is this multiplexing capacity, coupled to the associated savings in costs and time-to-diagnosis, that makes it likely that bead-based cytometry technology will soon fulfil its potential and become an integral part of the medical microbiology diagnostic laboratory of the future.

With respect to medical microbiology research, the further development of protocols allowing the coupling of lipids, lipooligosaccharides (LOS), peptidoglycan, polysaccharides etc to microsphere beads, will increase the number of applications for which bead-based cytometric assays may be used. Just one example of such an application is the differentiation of bacterial LOS types in health and disease, as well as the determination of differences in the LOS antibody response to microbial infections.

Finally, an important development in bead-based flow cytometry microbiological research will be the collection and use of standard defined serum panels containing known quantities (low, intermediate and high) of antibodies against the specific antigens to be tested. These panels are necessary for creating calibration curves that are useful in converting MFI values into actual immunoglobulin levels. The creation and acceptance of such panels will hasten the switch from bead-based research to bead-based diagnostic microbiological applications.

REFERENCES

[1]   Tempelmans Plat-Sinnige MJ, Verkaik NJ, van Wamel WJ, de Groot N, Acton DS, van Belkum A. Induction of *Staphylococcus aureus*-specific IgA and agglutination potency in milk of cows by mucosal immunization. Vaccine 2009; 27(30): 4001-9.

[2]   http://www.luminexcorp.com

[3]   Beads of Life®. Luminex Corporation ©2009.

[4]   Verkaik N, Brouwer E, Hooijkaas H, van Belkum A, van Wamel W. Comparison of carboxylated and Penta-His microspheres for semi-quantitative measurement of antibody responses to His-tagged proteins. J Immunol Methods 2008; 335(1-2): 121-5.

[5]   Etienne KA, Kano R, Balajee SA. Development and validation of a microsphere-based Luminex assay for rapid identification of clinically relevant aspergilli. J Clin Microbiol 2009; 47(4): 1096-100.

[6]   Bovers M, Diaz MR, Hagen F, *et al.* Identification of genotypically diverse *Cryptococcus neoformans* and *Cryptococcus gattii* isolates by Luminex xMAP Technology. J Clin Microbiol 2007; 45(6): 1874-83.

[7]   Dunbar SA, Jacobson JW. Quantitative, multiplexed detection of *Salmonella* and other pathogens by Luminex xMAP suspension array. Methods in Molecular Biology. Clifton, NJ 2007; 394: 1-19.

[8]   Bandyopadhyay K, Kellar KL, Moura I, *et al.* Rapid microsphere assay for identification of *Cryptosporidium hominis* and *Cryptosporidium parvum* in stool and environmental samples. J Clin Microbiol 2007; 45(9): 2835-40.

[9]   Dumonceaux TJ, Schellenberg J, Goleski V, *et al.* Multiplex detection of bacteria associated with normal microbiota and with bacterial vaginosis in vaginal swabs by use of oligonucleotide-coupled fluorescent microspheres. J Clin Microbiol 2009; 47(12): 4067-77.

[10] Tracz DM, Backhouse PG, Olson AB, *et al.* Rapid detection of *Vibrio* species using liquid microsphere arrays and real-time PCR targeting the *ftsZ* locus. J Med Microbiol 2007; 56: 56-65.

[11] McNamara DT, Kasehagen LJ, Grimberg BT, Cole-Tobian J, Collins WE, Zimmerman PA. Diagnosing infection levels of four human malaria parasite species by a polymerase chain reaction/ligase detection reaction fluorescent microsphere-based assay. The American journal of tropical medicine and hygiene 2006; 74(3): 413-21.

[12] Page BT, Kurtzman CP. Rapid identification of *Candida* species and other clinically important yeast species by flow cytometry. J Clin Microbiol 2005; 43(9): 4507-14.

[13] Michael KM, Waterboer T, Sehr P, *et al.* Seroprevalence of 34 human papillomavirus types in the German general population. PLoS pathogens 2008; 4(6): e1000091.

[14] Wong SJ, Demarest VL, Boyle RH, *et al.* Detection of human anti-flavivirus antibodies with a west nile virus recombinant antigen microsphere immunoassay. J Clin Microbiol 2004; 42(1): 65-72.

[15] Khan IH, Ravindran R, Yee J, *et al.* Profiling antibodies to *Mycobacterium tuberculosis* by multiplex microbead suspension arrays for serodiagnosis of tuberculosis.Clin Vaccine Immunol 2008; 15(3): 433-8.

[16] Gu AD, Mo HY, Xie YB, *et al.* Evaluation of a multianalyte profiling assay and an enzyme-linked immunosorbent assay for serological examination of Epstein-Barr virus-specific antibody responses in diagnosis of nasopharyngeal carcinoma. Clin Vaccine Immunol 2008; 15(11): 1684-8.

[17] Watson DS, Reddy SM, Brahmakshatriya V, Lupiani B. A multiplexed immunoassay for detection of antibodies against avian influenza virus. J Immunol Methods 2009; 340(2): 123-31.

[18] Lukacs Z, Dietrich A, Ganschow R, Kohlschutter A, Kruithof R. Simultaneous determination of HIV antibodies, hepatitis C antibodies, and hepatitis B antigens in dried blood spots--a feasibility study using a multi-analyte immunoassay. Clin Chem Lab Med 2005; 43(2): 141-5.

[19] Nogueira RD, King WF, Gunda G, *et al.* Mutans streptococcal infection induces salivary antibody to virulence proteins and associated functional domains. Infect Immun 2008; 76(8): 3606-13.

[20] Pickering JW, Martins TB, Schroder MC, Hill HR. Comparison of a multiplex flow cytometric assay with enzyme-linked immunosorbent assay for quantitation of antibodies to tetanus, diphtheria, and *Haemophilus influenzae* Type B. Clin Diagn Lab Immunol 2002; 9(4): 872-6.

[21] Lal G, Balmer P, Joseph H, Dawson M, Borrow R. Development and evaluation of a tetraplex flow cytometric assay for quantitation of serum antibodies to *Neisseria meningitidis* serogroups A, C, Y, and W-135. Clin Diagn Lab Immunol 2004; 11(2): 272-9.

[22] Pickering JW, Martins TB, Greer RW, *et al.* A multiplexed fluorescent microsphere immunoassay for antibodies to pneumococcal capsular polysaccharides. Am J Clin Pathol 2002; 117(4): 589-96.

[23] Lal G, Balmer P, Stanford E, Martin S, Warrington R, Borrow R. Development and validation of a nonaplex assay for the simultaneous quantitation of antibodies to nine *Streptococcus pneumoniae* serotypes. J Immunol Methods 2005; 296(1-2): 135-47.

[24] Verkaik NJ, de Vogel CP, Boelens HA, *et al.* Anti-staphylococcal humoral immune response in persistent nasal carriers and noncarriers of *Staphylococcus aureus*. J Infect Dis 2009; 199(5): 625-32.

[25]   Verkaik NJ, Lebon A, de Vogel CP, *et al.* Induction of antibodies by *Staphylococcus aureus* nasal colonization in young children. Clin Microbiol Infect 2009; 16: 1312-1317.

[26]   Verkaik NJ, Dauwalder O, Antri K, *et al.* Immunogenicity of toxins during *Staphylococcus aureus* infection. Clin Infect Dis 2010; 50(1): 61-8.

[27]   Bryce J, Boschi-Pinto C, Shibuya K, Black RE. WHO estimates of the causes of death in children. Lancet 2005; 365(9465): 1147-52.

[28]   Borgers H, Moens L, Picard C, *et al.* Laboratory diagnosis of specific antibody deficiency to pneumococcal capsular polysaccharide antigens by multiplexed bead assay. Clinical immunology, Orlando, Fla 2009.

[29]   Pabbaraju K, Tokaryk KL, Wong S, Fox JD. Comparison of the Luminex xTAG respiratory viral panel with in-house nucleic acid amplification tests for diagnosis of respiratory virus infections. J Clin Microbiol 2008; 46(9): 3056-62.

[30]   Krunic N, Yager TD, Himsworth D, Merante F, Yaghoubian S, Janeczko R. xTAG RVP assay: analytical and clinical performance. J Clin Virol 2007; 40 Suppl 1: S39-46.

Box 1: Protocol for the coupling of proteins to microsphere beads

1. Resuspend the stock of uncoupled microspheres by vortexing briefly.
2. Transfer 5.0×10^6 of the stock microspheres to a microcentrifuge tube.
3. Pellet the stock microspheres by microcentrifugation (>12,000g, 1-2 minutes).
4. Remove the supernatant and resuspend the pelleted microspheres in 100 μL distilled H_2O by vortexing and sonication (20 seconds).
5. Pellet the microspheres by microcentrifugation.
6. Remove the supernatant and resuspend the washed microspheres in 80 μL 100 mM NaH_2PO_4, pH 6.2 by vortexing and sonication.
7. Add 10 μL of 50 mg/mL Sulfo-NHS (diluted in distilled H_2O) to the microspheres and mix gently by vortexing (this stabilizes the 1-ethyl-3-(3-dimethylaminopropyl)-mediated coupling of COOH with NH_2 groups).
8. Add 10 μL of 50 mg/mL 1-ethyl-3-(3-dimethylaminopropyl (EDC) (diluted in distilled H_2O) to the microspheres and mix gently by vortexing.
9. Incubate for 20 minutes at room temperature with gentle mixing.
10. Pellet the activated microspheres by microcentrifugation.
11. Remove the supernatant and resuspend the microspheres in 250 μL of 50 mM MES, pH 5.0 by vortexing and sonication.
12. Pellet the microspheres by microcentrifugation.
13. Repeat steps 11 and 12.
14. Remove the supernatant and resuspend the activated and washed microspheres in 100 μL of 50 mM MES, pH 5.0 by vortexing and sonication.
15. Add 125, 25, 5 or 1 μg protein to the resuspended microspheres (titration is required in order to determine the optimal amount of protein required for each specific coupling reaction).
16. Bring the total volume to 500 μL with 50 mM MES, pH 5.0.
17. Mix the coupling reaction by vortexing.
18. Incubate for 2 hours with mixing (by rotation) at room temperature.
19. Pellet the coupled microspheres by microcentrifugation.
20. Remove the supernatant and resuspend the pelleted microspheres in 500 μL of PBS, 0.1% BSA, 0.02% Tween-20, 0.05% azide (PBS-TBN), pH 7.4 by vortexing and sonication.
21. Incubate for 30 minutes with mixing (by rotation) at room temperature.
22. Pellet the coupled microspheres by microcentrifugation.
23. Remove the supernatant and resuspend the microspheres in 1 mL of PBS-TBN by vortexing and sonication.
24. Pellet the microspheres by microcentrifugation.
25. Repeat steps 23. and 24.
26. Remove the supernatant and resuspend the coupled and washed microspheres in 250-1000 μL of PBS-TBN.
27. Count the microsphere suspension using for example a hemacytometer.
28. Store coupled microspheres refrigerated at 2-8°C in the dark until use.

Key. Sulfo-NHS - *N*-hydroxysulfosuccinimide; EDC - 1-ethyl-3-(3-dimethylaminopropyl); MES - 2-(*N*-morpholino)-ethanesulfonic acid; PBS-TBN - PBS, 0.1% BSA, 0.02% Tween-20, 0.05% azide.

Adapted with permission from http://www.luminexcorp.com/support/protocols/index.html.

Box 2: Protocol for bead-based antibody capture immunoassay

1. Select the appropriate antigen-coupled microsphere sets.
2. Resuspend the microspheres by vortexing and sonication for approximately 20 seconds.
3. Prepare a Working Microsphere Mixture in PBS-1% bovine serum albumin (BSA). (Note: 50 µL of Working Microsphere Mixture is required for each reaction.)
4. Pre-wet a 96-well 1.2 µm filter plate (Millipore, Multiscreen BV, Catalogue number MABVN 1250) with 100 µL/well of PBS-1% BSA and aspirate using a vacuum manifold.
5. Aliquot 50 µL of the Working Microsphere Mixture into the appropriate wells of the filter plate.
6. Add 50 µL of PBS-1% BSA to each background well.
7. Add 50 µL of standard or test sample (*e.g.* serum) to the appropriate wells.
8. Mix the reactions gently by pipetting up and down several times with a multi-channel pipette.
9. Cover the filter plate and incubate for 30-60 minutes at room temperature on a plate shaker.
10. Aspirate the supernatant using a vacuum manifold.
11. Wash each well twice with 100 µL of PBS-1% BSA and aspirate using a vacuum manifold.
12. Resuspend the microspheres in 50 µL of PBS-1% BSA by gently pipetting up and down 5 times with a multi-channel pipette.
13. Dilute phycoerythrin-labeled anti-species IgG secondary detection antibody (NB other secondary detection antibody isotypes and subclasses may be used) to 5 µg/mL in PBS-1% BSA. Note: 50 µL of diluted detection antibody is required for each reaction.
14. Add 50 µL of the diluted secondary detection antibody into the appropriate wells of the filter plate.
15. Mix the reactions gently by pipetting up and down several times using a multi-channel pipette.
16. Cover the filter plate and incubate for 35 minutes at room temperature on a plate shaker.
17. Aspirate the supernatant using a vacuum manifold.
18. Wash each well twice with 100 µL of PBS-1% BSA and aspirate using a vacuum manifold.
19. Resuspend the microspheres in 100 µL of PBS-1% BSA by gently pipetting up and down 5 times with a multi-channel pipette.
20. Analyze 100 µL of bead solution using a suitable flow-cytometer according to the manufacturer's instructions.

Adapted with permission from http://www.luminexcorp.com/support/protocols/index.html

Index

A

Agarose degrading bacteria 5
Axima@Saramis® 62

B

Biosensors
      Antibody probe 27-35
      Electrical perturbance biosensor 32-33
      Interferometric sensor 36-38
      Magnetoelastic sensor 32
      Piezoelectric sensor 30

C

Capillary electrophoresis-mass spectroscopy (CE-MS) 81
Clinical Infection Score point 138-139
Conducting polymers (CPs) 92
Culture Chips 9

D

Devices
      Amperometric 33
      Impedance 33
      Potentiometric 34
      Surface Plasmon Resonance (SPR) 34

E

Electronic nose 90
      Conducting polymers (CP) 92
      Electrochemical sensor 93
      Metal oxide sensor (MOS) 92-93
      Quartz microbalance (QMB) 92
      Surface acoustic wave sensor (SAW) 30-31, 93
Enzyme Immuno Assay (EIA) 20
Enzyme-linked Immunosorbent Assay (ELISA) 20-21, 151

F

Flow cytometry 21, 135
      Bead-based 21-24, 151
Flux analysis 84
Fourier transform-ion cyclotron resonance-mass spectrometry (MALDI FT-ICR-MS) 81

G

Gas chromoatography-mass spectrometry (GC-MS) 80
Gold Standard 3, 19-20, 26, 38-40, 79, 94, 109, 127, 139,
Gram positive sepsis
      C3/CD11b ratio 139

H

Human Microbiome Project 74